Mobile Communications and Public Health

Mobile Communications and Public Health

Edited by
Marko Markov

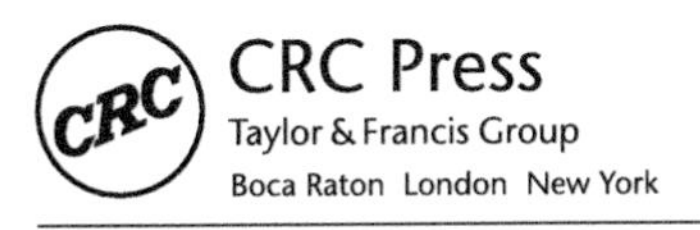

CRC Press is an imprint of the
Taylor & Francis Group, an **informa** business

CRC Press
Taylor & Francis Group
6000 Broken Sound Parkway NW, Suite 300
Boca Raton, FL 33487-2742

First issued in paperback 2023

ISBN 13: 978-1-032-65308-2 (pbk)
ISBN 13: 978-1-138-56842-6 (hbk)
ISBN 13: 978-0-203-70510-0 (ebk)

DOI: 10.1201/b22486

Visit the Taylor & Francis Web site at
http://www.taylorandfrancis.com

and the CRC Press Web site at
http://www.crcpress.com

Contents

Preface: To the Reader

At the end of the second decade of the twenty-first century, we evidence a dramatic increase of all means of mobile communications, which includes space signals, smartphones, and smart meters. Recent data indicate that the number of mobile devices surpasses 7.5 billion users. The integration between the mobile devices and smart home environments and the emerging advances in mobile phone technology including recent 4G and 5G modalities open the discussions on the potential hazard for the biosphere and mankind.

Unfortunately, the scientific, medical, and public health communities, after more than a quarter of century of discussions, still do not have a common opinion on the issue of if, and to what extent, the EMF from mobile communications represent a hazard for public health. The entire world population is exposed to various RF EMF signals. The problem here is that the population has no knowledge of the exposure or of the parameters of the received EMF. It would be correct to say that the international system for control and regulation had failed.

Obviously, it is impossible to evaluate the daily, monthly, and yearly rate of use, or the total value of the absorbed energy. This is even more important because mobile devices and cell phones may be seen in the hands of children as young as 1–3 years in age. It is already recognized that children have a unique vulnerability to external adverse factors of the environment.

As wireless broadband technology has evolved from generation to generation, the manufacturers were able to upgrade and adapt to necessary changes in the products. Today, the situation is different—the problem is not to upgrade—any new generation is basically new technology, and 5G is an especially deep step in the millimeter range of the electromagnetic spectrum. In addition to the new frequency range, the distribution of the signal requires a large number of antenna elements which need to be integrated into advanced device packaging. It is clear now that the standards for 5G are not yet available. Therefore, it is another jump in developing technology which will lead the entire biosphere and civilization to be exposed to new levels of electromagnetic pollution that are not defined and for which there are no standards and methods of control.

This was the reason that I started this project—to emphasize the necessity of terminology clarification, the specific absorption rate (SAR) use, and the thermal versus nonthermal effects.

Due to the courtesy of Drs. Rainer Nyberg and Lennart Hardell, I am able to open this book with the petition to the European Union that nearly 200 scientists from three continents signed asking that the 5G generation of mobile communications not be allowed before the standards for protection of the human population are developed and introduced.

This book would not be possible without the contribution of scientists from Europe and North America. Igor Belyaev and Carl Blackman helped in clarification of biological issues, Peter Gajšek, Jolanta Karpowicz, Dina Šimunić and Krzysztof Gryz wrote about the engineering problems. Biomedical engineer Lucas A. Portelli reported the recent advances in studying low-level thermal signals, while Henry Lai offered the readers a summary of recent literature on the neurobiological effects of radio frequency radiation. Martin Pall proposed a possible mechanism explaining how cancer can be caused by microwave frequency EMF exposures. Yury Grigoriev and Natalia Khortzeva reported Russian experience in setting standards and the investigations of the RF EMF effects on children in Russian schools.

Dear reader, please do not forget that we are at the bottom of the ocean of electromagnetic waves. The mobile communication industry is creating newer and newer tools in order to eventually increase the speed of communications. Smartphones and smart meters significantly change the electromagnetic environment not only for occupational conditions, but in every home. Billions of people are even not informed about the fact that their homes and their organisms are subjected to the "new and advanced" technological development. This cohort includes babies and elderly people, schoolboys and professionals.

It is our duty, we biologists, physicists, engineers, and medical professionals need to help today and future generations in the creation of standards for healthy life. **It is time to ring the bell.** Please help.

Editor

Marko S. Markov earned his BS, MS, and PhD from Sofia University, Bulgaria. He has been professor and chairman of the Department of Biophysics and Radiobiology of Sofia University for 22 years. He has been an invited professor and lecturer in a number of European and American academic and industry research centers.

Dr. Markov is well recognized as one of the world's premier experts in clinical applications of electromagnetic fields. He has given 288 invited and platform presentations at more than 70 international meetings. His list of publications includes 196 papers and 18 books.

Dr. Markov has more than 45 years' experience in basic science research and more than 40 years' experience in the clinical application of electromagnetic fields for treatment of bone and soft tissues pathologies and injuries.

His commercial affiliation started in Bulgaria with a series of contractual appointments and continued in the USA in his capacity as vice president of three companies involved in manufacturing and distribution of devices for magnetic field therapy. The spectrum of the signals ranges from static magnetic fields to 27.12 MHz. The clinical targets are in the area of bone and soft tissue problems, pain control, and innovation of the low frequency range for inhibition of angiogenesis and tumor growth. Recently, he introduced an analytical method for designing signals and devices for bioelectromagnetics research.

In 1981, Dr. Markov wrote his first book *Professions of Laser*. In 1988, he coedited with Martin Blank *Electromagnetic Fields and Biomembranes* published by Plenum Press. In 2004, he coedited a work published by Marcel Dekker, *Bioelectromagnetic Medicine*, together with Paul Rosch, President of the American Institute of Stress. In 2006, together with Sinerk Ayrapetyan, he coedited *Bioelectromagnetics: Current Concepts*. In 2010, he coedited with Damijan Miklavcic and Andrei Pakhomov *Advanced Electroporation Techniques in Biology and Medicine*, published by CRC Press. His latest book, also published by CRC Press in 2015, *Electromagnetic Fields in Biology and Medicine*, is currently being translated in China.

Dr. Markov has edited seven special issues of two journals, *The Environmentalist* and *Electromagnetic Biology and Medicine* consisting of selected papers of biannual International Workshops on Biological Effects of Electromagnetic Fields.

Dr. Markov is cofounder of the International Society of Bioelectricity, the European Bioelectromagnetic Association (EBEA), and the International Society of Bioelectromagnetism. He has been a member of the Board of Directors of Bioelectromagnetics Society and an organizer of several NATO research meetings.

Contributors

Igor Belyaev
Department of Radiobiology
Cancer Research Institute
Biomedical Research Center
Slovak Academy of Science
Bratislava, Slovak Republic

and

Laboratory of Radiobiology
General Physics Institute
Russian Academy of Science
Moscow, Russia
Email: Igor.Beliaev@savba.sk

Carl Blackman
Department of Cancer Biology
Wake Forest Baptist Medical Center
Winston-Salem, North Carolina
Email: carl.blackman@gmail.com

Peter Gajšek
Institute of Nonionizing Radiation (INIS)
Ljubljana, Slovenia
Email: peter.gajsek@inis.si

Yury G. Grigoriev
Russian National Committee on
Non-ionizing Radiation Protection
Scientific Council of RAS on
Radiobiology
Moscow, Russia
Email: profgrig@gmail.com

Krzysztof Gryz
Laboratory of Electromagnetic
Hazards
Central Institute for Labour
Protection – National Research
Institute (CIOP-PIB)
Warszawa, Poland
Email: krgry@ciop.pl

Jolanta Karpowicz
Laboratory of Electromagnetic Hazards
Central Institute for Labour
Protection – National Research
Institute (CIOP-PIB)
Warszawa, Poland
Email: jokar@ciop.pl

Natalia I. Khorseva
N.M. Emanuel Institute of Biochemical
Physics
Russian Academy of Sciences
and
Space Research Institute
Russian Academy of Sciences
Moscow, Russia
Email: sheridan1957@mail.ru

Henry Lai
Department of Bioengineering
University of Washington
Seattle, Washington
Email: hlai@u.washington.edu

Marko S. Markov
Research International
Williamsville, New York
Email: msmarkov@aol.com

Martin L. Pall
Professor Emeritus of Biochemistry and Basic Medical Sciences
Washington State University
Working from home in Portland, Oregon
Email: martin_pall@wsu.edu

Lucas A. Portelli
Kirsus Institute
Zürich, Switzerland
Email: lucasportelli@gmail.com

Dina Šimunić
Faculty of Electrical Engineering and Computing
University of Zagreb
Zagreb, Croatia
Email: dina.simunic@fer.hr

5G Appeal

The following text is a reproduction of the Appeal for Moratorium of 5G technology sent to the European Union and Council of Europe from more than 190 scientists and doctors worldwide.

To: ***The Council of the European Union***

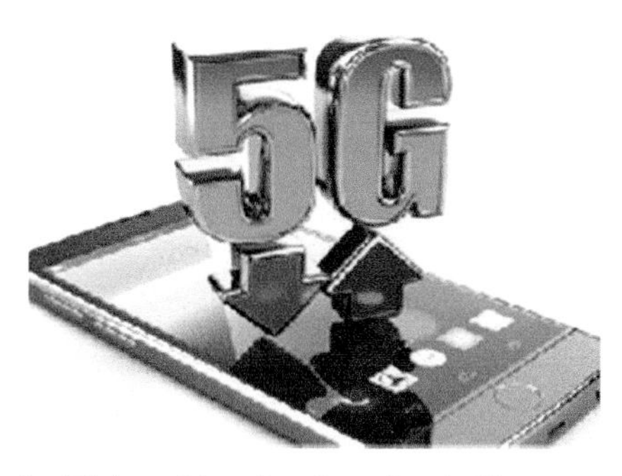

Scientists Call For Moratorium on 5G

Over 190 scientists and doctors have signed a 5G-Appeal (see Attachment) to the European Union and Council of Europe seeking a moratorium on the deployment of 5G (Fifth Generation of Telecommunication) using super-high 10–100 GigaHz frequencies, so new that they are not scientifically proven safe. However, the signatories determined that the microwave radiation emitted by lower frequency wireless technology is "*harmful to humans and the environment.*" Deployment of 5G will substantially increase the total exposure to wireless radiation. We refer to the EU Council recommendation (1999/519/EC) of 12 July 1999: *(4)* "***It is imperative to protect members*** *of the general public within the Community against established adverse health effects that may result as a consequence of exposure to electromagnetic fields.*"

The current safety guidelines only recognize heating effects. The independent scientists are in agreement that science has shown that wireless radiation "*affects living organisms at levels well below* most *international and national guidelines.*" These effects are seen at non-thermal radiation levels and cannot be explained by heating. Thus, the current guidelines based on tissue heating do not protect against health hazards.

The scientists who signed the Appeal demand the EU and Council of Europe – instead of massively *increasing* total exposure – now apply the Parliamentary Assembly of the Council of Europe PACE Resolution 1815 and "*take* ***all reasonable measures necessary to reduce exposure*** *to electromagnetic fields*" and to halt the 5G expansion until an **expert group** of truly independent scientists can assure that 5G and the increased sum of radiation levels caused by 5G wireless technology added to 2G, 3G, 4G, Wi-Fi[1]) etc. will be safe.

October 24, 2017

Respectfully submitted

Rainer Nyberg

Rainer Nyberg
EdD, Professor Emeritus
Vasa, Finland
NRNyberg@abo.fi

Lennart Hardell

Lennart Hardell
MD, PhD, Oncologist
Örebro, Sweden
lennart.hardell@regionorebrolan.se

[1] EU decided 29/05/2017: "Free public Wi-Fi hotspots...across the EU" will be installed for **€120** million before 2020

5G Appeal

Scientists and doctors warn of potential serious health effects of 5G

September 13, 2017

We the undersigned, more than 180 scientists and doctors from 36 countries, recommend a moratorium on the roll-out of the fifth generation, 5G, for telecommunication until potential hazards for human health and the environment have been fully investigated by scientists independent from industry. 5G will substantially increase exposure to radiofrequency electromagnetic fields (RF-EMF) on top of the 2G, 3G, 4G, Wi-Fi, etc. for telecommunications already in place. RF-EMF has been proven to be harmful for humans and the environment.

(Note: Underlined links below are references.)

5G leads to massive increase of mandatory exposure to wireless radiation

5G technology is effective only over short distance. It is poorly transmitted through solid material. Many new antennas will be required and full-scale implementation will result in antennas every 10 to 12 houses in urban areas, **thus massively increasing mandatory exposure.**

With "the ever more extensive use of wireless technologies," nobody can avoid to be exposed. Because on top of the increased number of 5G-transmitters (even within housing, shops and in hospitals) according to estimates, "10 to 20 billion connections" (to refrigerators, washing machines, surveillance cameras, self-driving cars and buses, etc.) will be parts of the Internet of Things. All these together can cause a substantial increase in the total, long term RF-EMF exposure to all EU citizens.

Harmful effects of RF-EMF exposure are already proven

Over 230 scientists from more than 40 countries have expressed their "serious concerns" regarding the ubiquitous and increasing exposure to EMF generated by electric and wireless devices already before the additional 5G roll-out. They refer to the fact that "numerous recent scientific publications have shown that *EMF affects living organisms at levels well below most international and national guidelines*". Effects include increased cancer risk, cellular stress, increase in harmful free radicals, genetic damages, structural and functional changes of the reproductive system, learning and memory deficits, neurological disorders, and negative impacts on general well-being in humans. Damage goes well beyond the human race, as there is growing evidence of harmful effects to both plants and animals.

After the scientists' appeal was written in 2015 additional research has convincingly confirmed serious health risks from RF-EMF fields from wireless technology. The world's largest study (25 million US dollar) National Toxicology Program (NTP), shows statistically significant increase in the incidence of *brain and heart cancer* in animals exposed to EMF below the ICNIRP (International Commission on Non-Ionizing Radiation Protection) guidelines followed by most countries. These results support results in human epidemiological studies on RF radiation and brain tumour risk. A large number of peer-reviewed scientific reports demonstrate harm to human health from EMFs.

The International Agency for Research on Cancer (IARC), the cancer agency of the World Health Organization (WHO), in 2011 concluded that EMFs of frequencies 30 KHz – 300 GHz are possibly carcinogenic to humans (Group 2B). However, new studies like the NTP study mentioned above and several epidemiological investigations including the latest studies on mobile phone use and brain cancer risks confirm that RF-EMF radiation is carcinogenic to humans.

5G Appeal

The EUROPA EM-EMF Guideline 2016 states that "there is strong evidence that *long-term exposure to certain EMFs is a risk factor for diseases* such as certain cancers, Alzheimer's disease, and male infertility...Common EHS (electromagnetic hypersensitivity) symptoms include headaches, concentration difficulties, sleep problems, depression, lack of energy, fatigue, and flu-like symptoms."

An increasing part of the European population is affected by ill health symptoms that have for many years been linked to exposure to EMF and wireless radiation in the scientific literature. The International Scientific Declaration on EHS & multiple chemical sensitivity (MCS), Brussels 2015, declares that: "In view of our present scientific knowledge, we thereby stress all national and international bodies and institutions...to recognize EHS and MCS as true medical conditions which acting as sentinel diseases may create a *major public health concern in years to come worldwide* i.e. in all the countries implementing unrestricted use of electromagnetic field-based wireless technologies and marketed chemical substances...***Inaction is a cost to society*** and is not an option anymore...we unanimously acknowledge this serious hazard to public health...that major primary *prevention measures are adopted and prioritized, to face this* ***worldwide pan-epidemic*** *in perspective."*

Precautions

The **Precautionary Principle** (UNESCO) was adopted by EU 2005: *"When human activities may lead to morally unacceptable harm that is scientifically plausible but uncertain,* actions shall be taken to *avoid or diminish that harm."*

Resolution 1815 (Council of Europe, 2011): *"Take all reasonable measures to reduce exposure to electromagnetic fields,* especially to radio frequencies from mobile phones, and particularly the exposure to children and young people who seem to be most at risk from head tumours...Assembly strongly recommends that the ALARA (as low as reasonably achievable) principle is applied, covering both the so-called thermal effects and the athermic [non-thermal] or biological effects of electromagnetic emissions or radiation" and to "improve risk-assessment standards and quality".

The **Nuremberg code** (1949) applies to all experiments on humans, thus including the roll-out of 5G with new, higher RF-EMF exposure. All such experiments: "should be based on previous knowledge (e.g., an expectation derived from animal experiments) that justifies the experiment. No experiment should be conducted, *where there is an a priori reason to believe that death or disabling injury will occur*; except, perhaps, in those experiments where the experimental physicians also serve as subjects." (Nuremberg code pts 3-5). Already published scientific studies show that there is "a priori reason to believe" in real health hazards.

The **European Environment Agency** (EEA) is warning for "Radiation risk from everyday devices" in spite of the radiation being below the WHO/ICNIRP standards. EEA also concludes: "There are many examples of the failure to use the precautionary principle in the past, which have *resulted in serious and often irreversible damage to health and environments*...harmful exposures can be widespread before there is both 'convincing' evidence of harm from long-term exposures, and biological understanding [mechanism] of how that harm is caused."

"Safety guidelines" protect industry — not health

The current ICNIRP "safety guidelines" are obsolete. All proofs of harm mentioned above arise although the radiation is below the ICNIRP "safety guidelines". Therefore new safety standards are necessary. The reason for the misleading guidelines is that "conflict of interest of ICNIRP members due to their *relationships with telecommunications or electric companies* undermine the impartiality that should govern the

5G Appeal

regulation of Public Exposure Standards for non-ionizing radiation...To evaluate cancer risks it is necessary to include scientists with competence in medicine, especially oncology."

The current ICNIRP/WHO guidelines for EMF are based on the obsolete hypothesis that "The critical effect of RF-EMF exposure relevant to human health and safety is heating of exposed tissue." However, scientists have proven that many different kinds of *illnesses and harms are* caused without heating ("non-thermal effect") at radiation levels well below ICNIRP guidelines.

We urge EU:

1) To take all reasonable measures to halt the 5G RF-EMF expansion until independent scientists can assure that 5G and the total radiation levels caused by RF-EMF (5G together with 2G, 3G, 4G, and WiFi) will not be harmful for EU-citizens, especially infants, children and pregnant women, as well as the environment.

2) To recommend that all EU countries, especially their radiation safety agencies, follow Resolution 1815 and inform citizens, including, teachers and physicians, about health risks from RF-EMF radiation, how and why to avoid wireless communication, particularly in/near e.g., daycare centers, schools, homes, workplaces, hospitals and elderly care.

3) To appoint immediately, without industry influence, an EU task force of independent, truly impartial EMF-and-health scientists with no conflicts of interest[1] to re-evaluate the health risks and:
a) To decide about new, safe "maximum total exposure standards" for all wireless communication within EU.
b) To study the total and cumulative exposure affecting EU-citizens.
c) To create rules that will be prescribed/enforced within the EU about how to avoid exposure exceeding new EU "maximum total exposure standards" concerning all kinds of EMFs in order to protect citizens, especially infants, children and pregnant women.

4) To prevent the wireless/telecom industry through its lobbying organizations from persuading EU-officials to make decisions about further propagation of RF radiation including 5G in Europe.

5) To favor and implement wired digital telecommunication instead of wireless.

***We expect an answer** from you no later than **October 31, 2017** to the two first mentioned signatories about what measures you will take to protect the EU-inhabitants against RF-EMF and especially 5G radiation. This appeal and your response will be publicly available.*

Respectfully submitted,

Rainer Nyberg, EdD, Professor Emeritus (Åbo Akademi), Vasa, Finland (NRNyberg@abo.fi)

Lennart Hardell, MD, PhD, Professor (assoc) Department of Oncology, Faculty of Medicine and Health, University Hospital, Örebro, Sweden (lennart.hardell@regionorebrolan.se)

[1] Avoid similar mistakes as when the Commission (2008/721/EC) appointed industry supportive members for SCENIHR, who submitted to EU a misleading SCENIHR report on health risks, giving telecom industry a clean bill to irradiate EU-citizens. The report is now quoted by radiation safety agencies in EU.

1 Mobile Communications and Public Health

Marko S. Markov

CONTENTS

1.1 INTRODUCTION

Recent research on the distribution of mobile devices indicated that at present their number surpasses 7.5 billion users especially with increasing distribution of smartphones and electronically driven utility meters. Tighter integration between the mobile devices and smart home environments will ultimately provide the infrastructure with a wide range of applications, further personalizing consumer and citizen interaction with the world around them. The emerging advances in mobile phone technology, including recent 4G and 5G modalities, open the discussions on the potential hazard for the biosphere and mankind.

Unfortunately, the scientific, medical, and public health communities at present (after more than a quarter of a century of discussions) do not have a common opinion on the issue if, and to what extent, the EMF from mobile communications represent a hazard for public health, including identification of the conditions and parameters at which the exposure of the population to these microwaves became chronic. The clarification had been basically searched for the signal emitted by base stations and practically no attention was paid to the mobile devices themselves. The base stations operate 24/7 and expose the entire biosphere (including the human population) to various electromagnetic signals. The problem here is that the population is exposed to this radiation with no knowledge of the exposure or of the parameters of the received EMF. It would probably be correct to say that the international system for control and regulation has failed. In order to get a license, the manufacturers need to follow some artificially created guidelines which are basically far away from the care for the health of users of mobile devices, for the entire population, and even for the biosphere. Every discussion starts with "thermal effects" and the possibility to create overheating of the critical organs in human organisms, mainly the brain.

The influence of radio frequency electromagnetic fields (RF EMF) on the brain when mobile phones are in use could vary with periodicity, carrier frequency, and modulation. Thus, it is difficult, if not impossible, to evaluate the daily, monthly, and yearly rate of use, including the total value of the absorbed energy. Therefore, even the epidemiological studies performed with a large cohort of participants could not provide reliable information. The other problem is connected to the gender and age of the user, the life style use, and the business use of mobile phones. Therefore, mobile phones should be relegated to the sources of EMF that cannot be properly characterized, despite the already proven potential hazard of this emission.

Several specific problems have arisen in respect to the health of a small, but very important fraction of the human population: children. (IARC, 2002; WHO, 2003; Markov, 2012; Markov and Grigoriev, 2013; Grigoriev and Khorseva, 2014; Grigoriev and Grigoriev, 2013). This is even more important because mobile devices and cell phones may be seen in the hands of children as young as 1–3 years in age. It is already recognized that children have a unique vulnerability to external adverse factors of the environment (WHO, 2003). There is no way to assess and predict the potential damage to children's brains exposed to RF radiation. The industry is offering now new toys and various electronic games based upon Internet access and these toys are now in the hands of 1-year old children. A recent report of the National Toxicology Program (NTP) provides more information about the possibility of cancer promotion as result of exposure to the microwave EMF of cellular communications.

1.2 EVOLUTION OF THE SMARTPHONE

The use of mobile communications started in the late 1980s with bulky devices that quickly became popular; the public demand and industry interest led to transfer of the bulky telephone to small devices and later to smartphones. Today, smartphones are difficult to simply call "phones." They are portable, powerful computers which are "on" immediately after the battery is installed. When the user switches the phone "off," it basically means nothing. The unit is "on" 24/7 receiving and emitting information, data, etc. In less than 10 years, simple mobile phones became smartphones with increasing capacity, frequency range, number of users, and so on. They have changed the way of communications between individuals in their everyday and business uses. They became the universal controller of household and business facilities. A new term was created, IoT (Internet of Things), bringing the business people, retirees, and even small children into this miracle world of wireless communication.

It is clear now that the future of mobile communications belongs to the smartphones. If in 2015 there were 3.5 billion subscribers, the prediction for 2022 shows 6.8 billion users. It is expected that the data used by a single smartphone will rise by 8 times up to 1 GB/month (Gillenwater, 2017). To handle this increase of the mobile data network, providers offer 2G, 3G, 4G, and the coming 5G generations which elevate the carrier frequency bands. Not going into technicalities, I should point out that the peak to average power ratio will exceed 4.5 dB and will be introduced as a new power standard (Power class 2) that doubles the output power to 26 dBm to overcome the greater losses at high frequency bands. Thermal performance becomes critical at this higher power and the dissipation of the additional heat becomes very important (Gillenwater, 2017). So far, the industry does not speak about the extent to which this technical issue will potentially elevate biological importance and hazards.

As wireless broadband technology has evolved from generation to generation, the manufacturers were able to upgrade and adapt to necessary changes in the products. Today, the situation is different—the problem is not to upgrade—any new generation is basically new technology, especially 5G which is a step deeper in the millimeter range of the electromagnetic spectrum. In addition to the new frequency range, the distribution of the signal requires a large number of antenna elements which need to be integrated into advanced device packaging. It is clear now that the standards for 5G are not yet available. Therefore—it is another jump in developing technology which will lead the entire biosphere and civilization to be exposed to new levels of electromagnetic pollution which are not defined, which have no standard, and have no methods of control. As with the entire development of wireless communication, the industry is pushing to first develop mobile devices and networks and then to further develop the standards (Oltman, 2017).

We have been on this avenue for about a quarter of a century. Did we not learn something? For me, it is not clear as why the 5G generation is called the Internet of Things. Looks intriguing, doesn't it? Consequently, smart operators and providers are learning all they can about 5G now to understand how they will need to evolve their backhaul strategy to create more effective and financially viable business models.

The industry is pushing for development of controversial legislation to expedite the distribution of this new technology. This new legislation is related to the fact that local governments and private citizens can not oppose the dense installations of antennas (at every 20 houses in urban areas). As result, the potential health risk for the population is ignored. Since the distribution of millimeter waves is blocked by buildings and even walls, it may be that at any school or office building, several transmitters will need to be placed on each floor of the building.

The FCC (Federal Communication Commission in USA) in 1996 introduced a limit for thermal effects from EMF of 1.5–100 GHz to be 1 mW/cm^2 for 30 min of use. This limit was set 20 years ago and is related only to thermal effects. The engineering community of today continues claiming that nonthermal effects of EMF do not exist. This statement is absolutely incorrect and negates hundreds of publications reporting the nonthermal effects of EMF. I would emphasize here that most of the reports of the effects of millimeter waves have reported on short term exposure, while there is practically no information about long term exposure. Even short exposure to millimeter waves was reported to cause significant nonthermal effects (Betskii and Lebedeva, 2004).

The writings of more than 160 scientists with experience in the evaluation of the hazards of wireless communications (published in this book) demonstrate that scientific assessment of the development of this new way of communication has been learned from past experience. (See "5G Appeal" Introduction in front section of this book.)

1.3 DEFINITIONS: BIOLOGICAL EFFECTS, HEALTH EFFECTS, HEALTH HAZARD

These three terms need special attention from any point of view: physics, engineering, biology, and medicine. Something here is wrong. Although a number of institutions assume the privilege of setting guidelines and standards, we do not have proper definitions of these categories. Moreover, by misusing the words, the scientific community has created havoc in discriminating what is a biological effect, what is a health effect, and what is a hazardous effect. Unfortunately, this was further transferred to the language and terminology of the policy, standard, and regulation bodies.

The industry publications as well as the papers from the engineering community have time and time again promoted the notion that the only harm might be the thermal effect. The "experts" claimed that there is no hazard from mobile phone radiation since the intensity levels are low and there is no thermal effect reported. Moreover, Nikita and Kiourri (2011) defined three types of physical effects: thermal, athermal, and nonthermal. The introduction of the term "athermal" is nonsense. By definition, athermal means the absence of temperature, which is impossible for any living system. The authors continue in this wrong direction with the statement of an athermal effect because even though the energy is capable of heating the tissue, the temperature does not increase because of tissue thermoregulation mechanisms. (In parallel, there are number of publications referring to "hot spots.")

On the other hand, the WHO policy is that "**not every biological effect is a health effect**." This is not a correct definition. Obviously, by saying "health effect," WHO is considering the adverse effects in the sense of diseases, pathologies, and injuries. If the action of EMF is to be evaluated, the correct WHO statement should be "**Not every biological effect initiated by EMF is a health hazard**." There is at least one reason for such a statement: the worldwide development of bioelectromagnetic medicine clearly indicates that properly chosen EMF/magnetic field (MF)/electric field (EF) and electric current may be beneficial in the treatment of various diseases and injuries, even when all other known medical treatments dramatically failed (Rosch and Markov, 2004; Barnes and Greenebaum, 2007; Markov, 2015).

There is an abundance of publications pointing out that some biological effects of EMF are reversible, while others are transient. "Transient" indicates biological effects which quickly disappear once the application is terminated. Reversible effects require a longer time to disappear.

So, the term "hazard" should be kept for irreversible effects caused by short or prolonged exposure to EMF. In the 1990s, the hazard was associated with the EMF of power and distribution lines. Lately, the power lines have been forgotten and discussions within the scientific community, policy makers, medical establishment, news media, and general public are mostly oriented toward cellular communications, mainly cell phones and base stations.

There are several international (International commission of non-ionization radiation protection [ICNIRP], International committee of electromagnetic safety [ICES]) and American (Institute of Electrical and Electronic Engineering [IEEE], American National Standard Institution [ANSI]) committees which more or less attempt to direct the world standards. However, even the simple fact of the existence of several committees indicates the existence of a problem. There should be only one recognized and largely accepted standard institution which should develop various national and international standards. Following this idea, in the late 1990s, WHO initiated a project involving different laboratories, standard organizations, and countries called "EMF Project of Harmonization of Standards." Basically, nobody opposes such an action, but everybody wants his standard to be in use. This, however, is the smallest problem.

The big problem is: Which standard should be used; that based on SAR which is the USA approach, or the ones based on the biological response as many scientists from Eastern Europe and the former Soviet Union requested? This is a problem with several faces: East versus West; Biophysics versus Engineering; Thermal versus NonThermal. What is curious is that all three basically reflect the last possibility. Why is this so?

Eastern standards are based upon biophysics (biological response) which assumes nonthermal mechanism(s). In contrast to the ICNIRP, the Russian safety standards for example, which are based on nonthermal effects, do not use SAR values but instead limit the duration of exposure and power flux density (PD, W/cm^2) (SanPiN, 1996). Western standards are based on engineering/computation and assume thermal mechanisms only.

As pointed out earlier, heat based mechanisms exclude the possibility for the occurrence of nonthermal effects. In a document adopted by the International Committee of Electromagnetic Safety (ICES) cited by Cho and D'Andrea (2003), "Nonthermal RF biological effects **have not been established** and none of the reported nonthermal effects are proven adverse to health. Thermal effect is the only established adverse effect." Interestingly enough, the same document started with, "**The RF safety standards should be based on science**." There is no doubt that the standards should be based on science, but what science is this that neglects hundreds and hundreds of published results on the nonthermal effects of RF EMF?

It is interesting to know that the value of 100 W/m^2 (10 mW/cm^2) was proposed by the late Herman Schwan in his letter to the US Navy in 1953 as a safe limit for human exposure to microwave energy based on calculations (Foster, 2005).

Let me remind the reader, too, of the early statement of Becker (1990) that "Based solely on calculations, the magic Ture of 10 milliWatts per square centimeter was adopted by the air force as the standard for safe exposure. **Subsequently the thermal effects concept has dominated policy decisions to the complete exclusion of nonthermal effects. While the 10 mW/cm^2 standard was limited to microwave frequencies, the thermal concept was extended to all other parts of the electromagnetic spectrum. This view led to the policy of denying any nonthermal effects from any electromagnetic usage, whether military or civilian**." The majority of the international and national guidelines for the exposure limits of health protection are still based on the recommendations by the International Commission on Non-Ionizing Radiation Protection (ICNIRP) taking into account only the thermal effects resulting in tissue heating (ICNIRP, 1998). On the other hand, many studies in humans and animals have reported the biological and physiological effects of microwave radiation at levels of exposure below the thermal limits. The effects include cellular stress, increase in free radicals, changes in DNA, functional changes in the reproductive system, alterations in the brain bioelectrical activity, and learning and memory deficits in humans and animals (Valentini et al., 2007;

Blank and Goodman, 2009; De Iuliis et al., 2009; Juutilainen et al., 2011; Leszczynski et al., 2012; Lerchl et al., 2015). As Belyaev (2018) pointed out in this book "At chronic conditions, exposure to mobile phones may reproduce a number of real signals even during the same exposure session and thus provide a better possibility to assess detrimental effects from mobile telephony than experiments with fixed frequencies/frequency bands/modulations, which evaluate only a minor part of real signals." In addition, mobile phones emit not only MW but also extremely low frequency magnetic (ELF) EMF, which have also been shown to produce detrimental health effects and to interfere with MW effects (IARC, 2002; Belyaev, 2010). Szmigielski (2013) reviewed studies on the impacts of weak RF/MW fields, including cell phone radiation on various immune functions, both *in vitro* and *in vivo*. The bulk of available evidence clearly indicated that various shifts in the number and/or activity of immunocompetent cells are possible, although the results were inconsistent. In particular, a number of lymphocyte functions have been found to be either enhanced or weakened based on exposure to similar MW intensities although the other important variables of the experiments were different. The author concluded that, in general, short-term exposure to weak MW radiation may temporarily stimulate certain humoral or cellular immune functions, while chronic irradiation inhibits the same functions.

The ICNIRP guidelines for high frequency EMF (covering 100 kHz–300 GHz) was established in 1988—just at the time of the start of the development of mobile communications. Since this time, research on the GHz frequency region has started. The question arises—what are the scientific bases for such standards? Moreover, in 2014, ICNIRP announced that a revision of the guidelines would be made then on December 7, 2017, the deadline was reset to the middle of 2018. Four years are needed for the revision of guidelines? It is not surprising that in the same note, ICNIRP declares that "...the 1998 guidelines remain protective..." and "...still provide protection against all known health effects of high frequency radiation...". What will happen with 4G and 5G technologies that the industry aggressively distributes if the ICNIRP comes up with a revision and they are pronounced as hazardous? Will the standardization bodies follow the industry rules?

It is strange that on November 27, 2017, the EMF portal announced that "due to the lack of financial resources the site had to suspend import of any new radio-frequency and mobile phone-related articles as of now. The portal will continue to import other EMF papers." **To me, there is something suspicious here.**

The problem here is that for ICNIRP, the only possible effects of high frequency EMF are thermal. Also, ICNIRP does not see any thermal effects possible. Period. Therefore, any non-ionizing radiation will possibly be applied over the human population.

Because they are well-funded and respond to the interests of influential political, military, and business circles, the supporters of the thermal mechanisms of action prevail so far. **For how long will this continue?**

1.3.1 SAR

We should emphasize the lack of clear understanding and use of the terminology, especially the **specific absorption rate** (SAR). It is obvious that the SAR is a useful criterion and the only criterion which attempts to estimate the energy absorbed by the body. However, the name clearly indicates **absorption** and I personally wonder why for so many decades we, the entire bioelectromagnetics community, has used the SAR to clarify the energy **delivered** by the generating system, no matter how far the source is from the target, nor what the specific structure of this target is.

Up until today, SAR has more often been used to describe the energy delivered by the source of the electromagnetic field (EMF). One can only wonder how a device may be characterized by SAR. Let me repeat, the **SAR identifies the amount of energy that is absorbed** in a gram of tissue. The use of the SAR should be a measure of the absorbed energy, and this will result in a serious debate among researchers, since that would mean the safety standards would need to be restated in terms of internal energy absorption in addition to power density at the surface.

For more than half a century, a very serious group of policy makers and even scientists have been playing around with the term SAR. Let me repeat, SAR given in terms of Watts per Kilogram (W/Kg) or milliWatts per gram (mW/g) is assumed to provide a measure of absorbed energy in a given tissue. **Once again, absorption, not delivery.**

The aim of SAR is to assess the probability of temperature increase as result of the exposure of a biological body to EMF. This parameter is introduced in some "artificial" way. The problem is that it assumes homogeneous tissue, which biological bodies certainly are not. Basically, even from the point of equilibrium thermodynamics, such an approach is not appropriate. It is well known that the penetration of EMF is a function of the body size and dielectric properties as well as the parameters of the "arriving" field, not to mention energy dispersion and thermoregulation. Thus, by performing external measurement of EMF, it is hard to accept the estimation and spatial distribution of SAR (Bienkowski and Trzaska, 2015).

1.4 EMF INTERACTIONS WITH LIVING SYSTEMS

It would be plausible to start this section with the statement that "**Life is a set of electromagnetic events performed in an aqueous medium**." This did not happen yesterday. It is a product of a long evolution of the physical conditions on our planet and adaptation of the electromagnetic nature of life to these conditions. Take as an example bird and fish navigation along a geomagnetic field and the "suffering" of microorganisms when deprived of the usual ambient magnetic and electric fields.

It is clear now that the whole biology and physiology of living creature(s) are based upon three types of transfer:

- Energy
- Matter
- Information

While the first two processes might be described in terms of classical (equilibrium) thermodynamics, the information transfer obviously needs another approach and this may be found in nonequilibrium thermodynamics. As the late Ross Adey (2004) wrote in his last paper, "**Current equilibrium thermodynamics models fail to explain**

an impressive spectrum of observed bioeffects at non-thermal exposure levels. Much of this signaling within and between cells may be mediated by free radicals of the oxygen and nitrogen species." Cell signaling, signal transduction cascades, and conformational changes are events and processes that may be explained only by nonequilibrium thermodynamics.

For unicellular organisms, the cellular membrane is both detector and effector of physical and chemical signals. As a sensor, it detects altered conditions in the environment and further provides pathways for signal transduction. As an effector, the membrane may also transmit a variety of electrical, magnetic, and chemical signals to the neighboring cells with an invitation to "whisper together" as suggested by Ross Adey (2004). One condition is necessary here, that cells are tuned to the same signal. In general, this leads to resonance or a window hypothesis. What does this hypothesis actually mean? Exactly that a given tissue, organ or organism needs to be tuned to a given EMF signal. When the applied EMF has the parameters (amplitude or frequency, for example), the biological object will respond. If these parameters are beyond the resonance parameters, the target may not respond at all or the response will be not optimal/maximal.

It was shown that selected exogenous, weak, low frequency electric or magnetic fields can modulate certain important biochemical and physiological processes (Todorov, 1982; Detlavs, 1987; Carpenter and Ayrapetyan, 1994; McLean et al., 2003; Rosch and Markov, 2004, Barnes and Greenebaum, 2007; Markov, 2015). An estimate of detectable EMF exposure can, therefore, only be made if the amplitude and spatial dosimetry of the induced EMF at the target site are evaluated for each exposure system and condition (Markov, 2015). The electrostatic interactions involving different proteins are assumed to result primarily from polarization and reorientation of dipolar groups as well as changes in the concentrations of charged species in the vicinity of charges and dipoles. These effects could be well characterized for interactions in isotropic, homogeneous media. However, biological structures represent complex inhomogeneous systems for which the ionic and dielectric properties are difficult to predict. In these cases, factors such as the shape and composition of the surface and presence/absence of charged or dipolar groups appear to be especially important. The problem of the sensitivity of living cells and tissues to exogenous EMF is principally related to the ratio of the signal amplitude to that of thermal noise at the target site (Markov, 2006). It is clear now that in order for electric and/or electromagnetic field bioeffects to be possible, the applied signal should not only satisfy the dielectric properties of the target, but also induce sufficient voltage to be detectable above thermal noise (Markov and Pilla, 1995). Such an approach relies on conformational changes and transfer of information (Markov, 2004).

It appears useful to point out some features of the information transfer:

- Static EMF, time varying EMF, and pulsed EMF affect biological systems via information transfer.
- This information transfer can trigger various biochemical processes, ion binding, and signal transduction.
- The EMF information may be detected in an ion binding pathway via Larmor precession in the presence of thermal noise.

- For oscillating or pulsed signals, MF information is encoded in the frequency/amplitude spectrum of the signal.
- Signal decoding occurs via the impedance of electrochemical processes at a cell surface subject to signal/noise ratio requirements.

1.4.1 Thermal Effects

There is a classical thermodynamics dogma, "You get energy, you will have heating." Even if one accepts this statement, several questions remain to be answered:

- How does EMF heating occur within complex biological structures?
- Do we have a flow of heat?
- What happens at the interface between tissues with different dielectric properties?

These questions, which interpret the physics of interactions, should be complemented with at least two biological questions:

- What are the biological implications of heat generation?
- What is the cascade of events and the alterations in the signal transduction and in the enzyme reaction rate?

I would ask what heat is expected in elementary biochemical processes, such as the transport of ions through membranes or blood flow? Yes, energy is needed, but heating (or more precisely overheating) had never been observed. Why do we need to accept that the chemical factors can modulate biological activity, but forbid this for physical factors?

When the effects of magnetic fields are discussed, the issue of an induced electric field immediately appears on the scene. Although basically correct, this improperly shifts the emphasis from the primary to a secondary factor. The acting factor is the incident magnetic field and the biological effects should be analyzed from that point of view. One should not forget that when EMF is applied to a biological body, the electric component is shielded by the surface of the body creating surface electric current, while the magnetic component is capable of penetrating inside the body volume and will be distributed within the target without a change in the intensity (Otano-Lata et al., 1996).

Another problem is that engineers often (if not always) apply models that do not consider the fact that biological systems are heavily nonlinear systems and in such cases, nonlinear thermodynamics must be applied.

Material and ionic fluxes are territories that magnetobiology avoids. Energy interactions are always the focus of the research. However, transfer of information is constantly neglected in bioelectromagnetics, even though communication technologies are based upon modulation. Nobody is capable of estimating the SAR alteration inside the human brain that results from EMF modulation. This is not and cannot be a thermal effect. Here, one should introduce nonequilibrium thermodynamics in order to search for mechanisms of action, instead of classical, heat based thermodynamics.

The occurrence of hot spots in which the temperature increase is significantly higher than in a neighboring cell cannot be explain by equilibrium thermodynamics. It is strange that the thermal approach accepts some features from classical thermodynamics, but neglects others. For example, the classical "kT" criterion is always used to deny the possibility of occurrence of biological responses to static and low frequency MF.

It is hard to understand why the papers on thermal mechanisms of high frequency EMF do not consider a set of parameters which more than 29 years ago had been pointed as important EMF characteristics (Markov, 1994; Valberg, 1995), such as vector, gradient, component, modulation, etc., but instead only emphasize the SAR values.

In addition, in order to understand the biological consequence of RF exposure, one must know whether the effect is cumulative, whether compensatory responses result, and if or when homeostasis will break down.

1.4.2 Nonthermal Effect

There is a whole series of biologically important modifications that appear under weak static or alternating EMF action that could be explained only from the view point of nonthermal mechanisms. The spectrum includes changes at various levels: alterations in membrane structure and function and changes in a number of subcellular structures such as proteins and nucleic acids, protein phosphorylation, cell proliferation, free radical formation, ATP synthesis, etc. (Basset, 1994; Adey, 2004). Another important evidence in favor of the nonthermal character of EMF interaction could be found in the systemic effects (Markov et al., 2004; Barnes and Greenebaum, 2007; Markov, 2015). The wide range of reported beneficial effects of using electric current or EMF/EF/MF therapy worldwide shows that more than 3 million patients received relief from their medical problems. From bone unification (Detlavs, 1987; Basset, 1994), pain relief (Holcomb et al., 2003; Markov, 2004; Rosch and Markov, 2004; Barnes and Greenebaum, 2007; Pilla, 2007) and wound healing (Vodovnik and Karba, 1992; Markov and Pilla, 1995; Pilla, 2007, 2015; Mayrovitz, 2015) to relatively new applications for victims of multiple sclerosis (Lapin, 2004), Parkinson's, and Alzheimer's diseases (Richter and Lozano, 2004), bioelectromagnetic medicine has an important place in twenty-first century medicine (Rosch and Markov, 2004; Markov, 2015).

Continuing with the review of nonthermal biological effects, I would point to the fact that the EMF effects are better seen within the systems out of equilibrium. The observation showed a kind of "**pendulum effect**"—the larger the deviation from equilibrium, the stronger the response is. Such regularity may be seen in changes in the cell cycle, signal transduction, free radical formation, and performance, as well as in therapeutic modalities.

It should be remembered that during evolution, living organisms developed specific mechanisms for perception of natural electric and magnetic fields. These mechanisms require specific combinations of physical parameters of the applied field to be detected by biological systems. In other words, the "windows" are means by which discrete MF/EMF are detected by biological systems. Depending on the level of structural organization, these mechanisms of detection and response may be seen at different levels, for example, at membrane, cellular or tissue levels. Sometimes the "windows" function via signal transduction cascade, brain activity or the central nervous system (Markov, 2004). Neither of the above effects and mechanisms requires thermal contributions, but the biological response is evident. The sensitivity of the biological systems to weak MF has been described elsewhere, mainly in respect to the dependence of bioeffects on the amplitude or frequency of applied fields. It may be interesting to know that all early publications made a link between "windows" and information transfer (Adey, 1981, 1989; Markov, 1979, 1984, 1994).

Such "windows of opportunities" are very successfully used in magnetic and electromagnetic field therapies. This is sometimes based upon systematic research, but more often, selected magnetic/electromagnetic fields used for therapy are based upon the intuition of the inventor of the device and the medical staff. Why "selected?" Because these selected values of the physical characteristics of the MF/EMF correspond to the "windows of opportunities." Living systems are ready to detect, absorb, and utilize signals with specific characteristics and remain "silent" or unresponsive for the rest of the amplitude and/or frequency spectrum.

Resonance mechanisms, frequency, and intensity windows, as well as reports of modulated fields producing stronger or different effects than continuous wave fields, and the presence of effects that occur at very low intensities could be indications of nonthermal effects and cannot be explained by SAR or thermal effects.

An interesting approach to the mechanism of low-level microwave radiation was proposed by Hinrikus and his team (Hinrikus et al., 2008, 2011, 2015, 2017a,b). This model considers the microwave radiation as a physical stressor. Therefore, the physical approach is applied as a primary factor in this analysis. The basic physical model can be extended for further interpretation of biological effects. The content of water in various living tissue is high, about 80% (Foster and Schwan, 1995). Therefore, the water model has been frequently used for describing the properties of tissues. Without a doubt, low-level microwave radiation can rotate dipolar molecules and causes dipolar polarization of water and other dielectric materials. This is the fundamental starting point of the model. Foster and Schwan (1995) provide exhaustive information about the frequency-dependent dielectric properties of water. The calculations by the Debye model show that the relaxation time of free water at 20°C is picoseconds. A corresponding peak in ε'' occurs around 16 GHz. Experimental data confirm that ε'' keeps its value of around 80 up to GHz, decreases to around 40 at 10 GHz, and the rotation-related part of permittivity becomes negligible at frequencies close to 100 GHz. The upper response frequency is set by intermolecular forces that produce a rotational time constant of a few picoseconds. At greater frequencies, the orientational polarization becomes negligible and the dielectric constant has the frequency independent value of 1.8 determined only by the molecular polarization (Hasted, 1973). The values of relative permittivity measured at different frequencies showed a decrease with frequency for the major types of tissues: muscle, liver, lung, kidney, brain white and gray matter, blood, etc. (Foster and Schwan, 1995; Gabriel et al., 1996a,b). The measured relative permittivity of tissues is about 80–50 at frequencies of about 100 MHz–3 GHz and reaches values of 18–23 at the frequency of 35 GHz.

Recently, the results of the US National Toxicology Program Carcinogenesis Studies of Cell Phone Radio Frequency Radiation confirmed an increased cancer risk in rats and mice. In the cases of confirmed low-level microwave radiation effects, a mechanism other than tissue heating should be involved. There is justified demand for the clarification of the nonthermal mechanisms of low-level microwave radiation effects.

1.5 MOBILE COMMUNICATIONS AND PUBLIC HEALTH

I want to make clear that the potential hazard of mobile communication is related more to the nonthermal effects of this physical factor (RF EMF), which was unknown to mankind until half a century ago. The cellular telephone delivers a power density of RF radiation that is 2 billion times greater than occurs naturally in the environment. The absorbed energy potentially could cause dangerous and damaging biological effects within the human brain. Biological effects initiated by non-ionizing radiation could be achieved via conformational changes of important biological molecules (proteins, nucleic acids) and structures (as biological membranes) directly or via signal transduction pathways.

The small cellular telephones effectively deposit large amounts of energy into small areas of the user's head and brain. The major guidelines and standards established by the engineering community provide an approach and terminology which are not accepted by the physics and biological communities, but nevertheless remain the guiding rules (mainly for the industry). One can only wonder how it is possible to speak about the potential "health effects" of RF EMF instead of a "health hazard." The misuse of the term "health effect" completely neglects the fact that physical/chemical factors could have either positive (beneficial) or negative (hazardous) effects (Markov, 2012). We are suspicious that this is done on purpose in order to not alarm the general public about the hazards of the use of microwave radiation in close proximity to the human brain.

It has been pointed out elsewhere (Markov, 2006) that when the engineering committees stated "Nonthermal RF biological effects have not been established," they were basically guiding science and society in the wrong direction. To deny the possibility of nonthermal effects is not reasonable, but more important is that they mixed "effect" and "hazard." If nonthermal effects do not exist, why do societies such as Bioelectromagnetics society (BEMS) and European bioelectromagnetic association (EBEA) exist? What is discussed at any yearly meeting of BEMS? Why has the journal *Bioelectromagnetics* existed for 38 years? Why, since 1984, has another journal, *Electromagnetic Biology and Medicine*, published hundreds and hundreds of papers?

One of the first papers on the absorption of electromagnetic energy was published by Schwan and Piersol (1978), in which absorption was connected to the tissue composition. It is important to note once again that the composition of living tissues is very complex and varies from organ to organ and from person to person. From a biophysics point of view, the energy absorption also depends on the depth of penetration for the specific frequency range (for 825–845 MHz the penetration depth into brain tissue is from 2 to 3.8 cm) (Polk and Postow, 1986; Kane, 1995).

Forty-five years ago, Michaelson (1972) wrote, "It should be understood that a cumulative effect is the accumulation of damages resulting from repeated exposures each of which is individually capable of producing some small degree of damage." In other words, the repeated irritation of a particular biological area, such as a small region of the brain, can lead to irreparable damage.

The EMF effects on human tissues and the human brain specifically are strongly related to the tissue dielectric properties. However, these dielectric properties are basically not well known for the human brain, and especially for children's brains. To better understand the problem of the hazard of RF EMF for the human brain, it will be useful to consider the structure of the human head. It is known that the human head is a complex structure of many different tissue types. Each of the tissues—skin, bone, cerebrospinal fluid, fat, brain, dura, etc., absorbs and reflects RF energy in its own way. In addition, the human head is far from having a uniform shape, volume or structure. Therefore, the RF EMF interacts with the human head in a nonuniform way depending on the specific location of the brain areas/volumes. Sage (2012) presented a remarkable review of the similarity of low dose effects of ionizing and non-ionizing radiation on the initiation of genotoxic effects, which are nonthermal.

Interestingly enough, the Parliamentary Assembly, Council of Europe, in its Resolution 1815 from 2011 recommends to "reconsider the scientific basis for the present electromagnetic fields exposure standards set by the ICNIRP, which have serious limitations and apply 'as low as reasonably achievable' (ALARA) principles, covering both the thermal effects and the nonthermal or biological effects of electromagnetic emissions or radiation" (Parliamentary Assembly, 2011).

1.5.1 "Hot Spots"

It is clear that "hot spot" is a term that scientists have introduced to describe exactly what is happening at specific locations within the brain or other tissues. Which regions of the brain will be subjected to "hot spot" absorption depend on a number of factors related to head size, shape, curvature, subcutaneous fat layer thickness, and internal skull structures as well as the parameters of the applied signal (especially frequency, pulsing, and modulation).

Some of the interior "hot spots" in the brain are related to the radius of curvature of the human head. First, one should recognize that human head is far from the ideal spherical shape that is used in the modeling. It is easy to assume that the radius of the curvature is different for a baby, a little child, a teenager or an adult individual. The energy absorption within the brain tissue was found to be about 20 times greater than in the skull and subcutaneous fat. RF EMF energy can be concentrated into very high-intensity spots just as sunlight may be concentrated with a magnifying glass. The same effect occurs within living tissue at RF radiation "hot spot" locations. Please keep in mind that most, if not all of the biological effects, are nonlinear. Importantly, during short exposures from a few seconds to a few minutes, very little heat accumulation could take place. This is important in view of "hot spot" absorptions. If a "hot spot" was formed, a rapid energy absorption would have a maximum destructive effect because, as shown by Lin (1977), very little of the absorbed heat will have an opportunity to dissipate. "Because, microwave absorption occurs in a very short time, there will be little chance for heat conduction to take place."

At these "hot spots," however, the heating is rapid and the cooling is slow. The inability of biological tissue to get rid of excess heat quickly and efficiently may be the mechanism leading to destructive exposure. If "hot spots" occur at microscopic regions within the brain, where there are no thermal or sensory receptors, there is no reason to expect that the body will attempt to compensate for the overheating. The human brain simply does not have the capacity to prevent the damage. Human brain tissue is the most sensitive to any change in the physical parameters of the environment. There is evidence that with an increase in temperature of only 0.5°C in specific locations, various adverse effects might occur, the most important of which are (1) increase in membrane permeability; (2) modification of normal cell metabolism through changes in the enzyme activity; and (3) tissue destruction and death.

Consider now the same structural features on the heads of children and smaller adults. The curved area behind and above the ears is more arched and the total width of the head is correspondingly reduced. Since "hot spot" absorption is a function of head curvature, children and some adults are more susceptible to this type of "hot spot" formation. Long before the introduction of cellular telephones, scientists obtained data indicating that children absorb approximately 50% more radiation within their heads than adults (Durney et al., 1979). Lin in 1976 placed the increased absorption effect into a better perspective when he reported that "hot spot" energy absorption can be as much as ten times higher at certain areas within the brain. From experiments performed using models of the human head, he reported energy absorptions in the center of the head that were even higher than absorption levels near the surface. This is a prime example of "hot spot" energy deposition.

The presence of nonuniform energy absorption that indicated the new type of "hot spot" was initially characterized by Schwan in 1972 (Schwan, 1972a,b). He suggested that when the diameter is smaller, the energy absorbing "hot spots" become more pronounced. The research found that for heads significantly smaller than that of a mature man, the "hot spot" effects increase and so does the amount of energy that is absorbed into the interior of the brain. Clearly, this indicates an increased risk of "hot spot" absorption within the brains of women and children, with small children being at maximum risk for "hot spot" absorption within their brains. It had also been reported by Schwan (1972a,b) that maximum "hot spot" energy absorption occurs in the frequency region around the cellular telephone frequencies. **There were no cellular telephones on the market at that time.**

Johnson and Guy (1972) report that "for human brain exposed to 918 MHz power, the absorption at a depth 2.3 times the depth of penetration (depth of penetration = 3.2 cm) is twice the absorption at the surface. This corresponds to a factor greater than 200 times that expected." This means that at a depth within the human brain of about 7 cm, "hot spots" have energy absorption 200 times greater than would be the case if no "hot spot" existed.

During the past several decades, the absorption of RF energy in various body tissues has been investigated by homogeneous and/or heterogeneous models. Looking at these models, we were impressed that the most serious review of the models was done in 1978 by Durney et al. (1978). Interestingly enough, nearly 40 years later, this manual is the most comprehensive document on modeling RF absorption.

1.5.2 Protect Children

For the first time during the whole period of civilization, massive electromagnetic radiation reaches the most critical system of the body—the brain and nervous system structures of the inner ear of the child and adolescent. Children and adolescents are exposed to conditions analogical with professionals and are at risk of being in the zone of constantly determining the impact of a harmful type of radiation, which makes the potential risk to the health of children very high (Grigoriev, 2012; Grigoriev and Khortzeva, 2018). At the 2001 WHO meeting on harmonization of standards, **I made a statement that allowing little children to use the cell phones is a crime against humanity** (Markov, 2001). I think that it is still a valid statement.

Despite the large number of reports on the effects of RF EMF on human organisms, the publications on the potential hazard for the organisms of children are a relatively small fraction in the world literature. In most cases, the publications are based on epidemiological data collected by some surveys and quite frequently without having direct contact with children or their parents. Therefore, this approach passes the issues to statistics, not to science. One needs to operate with huge numbers in order to evaluate the presence or absence of an effect. But these numbers basically do not go to the biology, to the process of occurrence of one or another modification of the living tissue. Following this approach they state, "there is no conclusive and consistent evidence that nonionizing radiation emitted by cell phone is associated with cancer risk" (Boice and Tarone, 2011).

In the international meetings organized mainly by the WHO (Seol, 2001; Istanbul, 2004; Sanct Petersburg, 2005; London, 2008; Brussel, 2013), there were special sessions related to the hazards of RF EMF for children. However, the approach of engineering and standard creation authorities to the evaluation of RF hazards for children using cellular phones does not account for the specifics of the developing brain.

We would like to point to the study of Wiart et al. (2008) that utilized MRI data obtained in different French hospitals for the creation of six child head models at different ages (5, 6, 8, 9, 12, 15 years). In publication 66 of the ICNIRP (1998, 2009), an adult human model was scaled for reference to that of a 10-year old child. The most widely accepted database of human tissue (Gabriel et al., 1996a,b) lacks data for children. Not only is there a lack of information for children's brains, but for children's tissues in general.

There are several models scaling adult models down to children heads, which appears to be wrong. This approach does not account for geometrical differences, and what is more important, the anatomical and physiological differences between an adult brain and a developing brain of a child. Nikita and Kiourri (2011) published barograms that express 37% difference in local SAR for adult and child brains. If the data really present SAR for the brain of adults and children—in accordance with the engineering approach, these values should be similar. If not—as the case is—it means that the scaling exercises should be forgotten and forbidden.

The same authors stated that "in the case of canonical models, the child model is perfectly proportional to an adult model." This is possible only in theoretical (more likely mathematical) modeling when no one take into account the specifics of geometry, composition, and development of children's heads and brains. It is even written that Koulouridis and Nikita (2004) obtained a children's model through uniform deformation of spherical adult head models. I should remind the authors that an adult head is spherical, nor is the brain composition of adults and children homogeneous.

Several publications on cell phone dosimetry in children (ICNIRP, 2009; Christ et al., 2010a,b) reported a higher SAR for children's brains which is correctly attributed to the geometrical difference in the heads of children and adults. Scientists working in the dosimetry areas proposed different explanations for the fact that different laboratories concluded that SAR in children's brains is higher, smaller or equal to the SAR in adult brains.

More than 40 years ago, Joines and Spiegel (1974) analyzed human head models composed of six layers: skin, subcutaneous fat, skull, dura, cerebrospinal fluid, and brain tissue. The total thickness of the five layers that surround the brain is assumed to be 1.10 cm. However, we must keep in mind that the layers could vary significantly from one human head to another. What is more important, the proportion of these five layers changes during a child's aging. As the models become more complex and increasingly representative of an actual human head, the findings continue to indicate that the energy absorption is much higher than previously thought.

The range of sizes includes almost all human heads. It is clear that what was first observed as a danger to those with smaller cranial structures, most notably including children, has been extended by additional studies to include nearly all humans. Of course, the most dramatic "hot spot" peaks are within the smaller heads.

It would be plausible to point out the Russian experience in studying the hazards of the RF EMF for children and the legislation in this direction. In 2001, the Russian National Committee for protection from non-ionizing radiation recommended that children under the age of 18 as well as pregnant women not use mobile phones. These recommendations had further been incorporated into the Hygienic Norms for EMF of mobile communications (SanPiN 2.1.8/2.2.4.1190-03, valid from 2003). In 2004, Grigoriev suggested that a **precautionary principle** must be applied for evaluation of hazards for children. Beginning in 2006, a number of studies of RF EMF effects on children have been conducted in Russia. These longitudinal studies of effects of microwave radiation were oriented mainly toward the evaluation of the cognitive functions of different aged children by using a complex of psychophysiological tests. It has been detected that an increase in the time of the reaction to light or sound signals, disturbances in the phonematic association, decrease of the work ability, faster occurrence of fatigue, and increase of time for completion of the task has been associated with a simultaneous decrease of accuracy (Grigoriev and Khorseva, 2014; Grigoriev and Khorseva, 2018).

Since the industry and unfortunately, the scientific community, do not have appropriate care for the health of children, the responsibility is on parents. Look what has happened: Children in kindergarten or primary school are considering a mobile phone as a nice toy and play with it for hours and hours. At that age, their body and more importanty their brain is not yet developed. Who may be so brave as to claim that the use of a mobile phone at that age is not dangerous? Who may predict what would happen with these "users" 20–30–50 years later?

As WHO postulated, we should know that children are more sensitive to all factors of the environment than adults: "Children differ from adults. Children are uniquely vulnerable when they grow and develop, they have 'windows of susceptibility': periods when their organs and systems may be particularly sensitive to the effect of certain environmental threats" (WHO, Backgrounder, 2003). Therefore, it should not be doubted that the developing brain is exposed to increasing irradiation during the formation of higher nervous activity. Society, in general, and scientists, in particular, should not forget this.

One thing that I think about when I listen to or read the epidemiologists papers on children's exposure to RF radiation is that they do not take into account the fact that the cancer does not occur overnight and that there is a slow accumulation of damages that after a certain time may turn in a dangerous direction.

"These studies have not provided any sign that RF EMF emitted by cellular phones increases the chance for carcinogenesis" (Nikita and Kiourri, 2011). I certainly do not think that this statement is correct. At the risk of being confronted by epidemiologists, I should say that they do not do science, they do statistics. Look at any study performed by epidemiologists—it operates with huge numbers in order to evaluate the presence or absence of an effect. But these numbers basically do not go to biology, to the process of occurrence of one or another modifications of the living tissue. Then the epidemiological team claims "there isn't consistent evidence for occurrence of the modification." They also state "there is no conclusive and consistent evidence that nonionizing radiation emitted by cell phone is associated with cancer risk" (Boice and Tarone, 2011). It is remarkable that this paper was published after IARC defined RF as "possible cancerogenic for humans." In another paper, (Markov, 2012), the fact that the long-delayed publication of the INTERPHONE data resulted in a strange situation is discussed: two groups of participants in the project published papers that basically contradict each other. In addition, some epidemiologists wrote that the rates of tumor incidence in Swedish children decrease (over 50%) in the presence of increasing and substantial usage of cell phones (Aydin et al., 2011). This is another confirmation that the conclusion of epidemiological studies should not be trusted, especially since in most cases, the investigators are funded by the industry. The epidemiological community was separated in publications of the results of the INTERPHONE project. But they became surprised by the IARC classification of the RF microwave as possibly carcinogenic. The quick publication of Swerdlow et al. (2011) attempted to negate the classification and continue guiding the general public and scientific community.

The thermal approach to the absorbance of RF energy assumes that the energy is converted to heat, and the resulting heat, when sufficient, "cooks" the brain cells. Since nobody reported such a "cooking" effect it does not exist—this is the general conclusion of the epidemiology and industry supported papers.

However, a number of studies had pointed out that electromagnetic energy in the 900 MHz region may be more harmful because of its greater penetrating capability compared to 2,450 MHz, therefore, more energy in the 900 MHz frequency range is deposited deep within biological tissue. In 1976, Lin concluded that 918 MHz energy constitutes a greater health hazard to the human brain than does 2,450 MHz energy for a similar incident power density.

It is not difficult to envision that even one cubic centimeter of brain tissue (corresponding to 1 g) includes billions of molecules and interconnecting bonds. Each of these molecules or bonds may be susceptible to extremely high energy absorption under certain conditions even while other molecules, only a short distance away, might receive lower energy levels.

Let me remind the reader that studies of diathermy applications consistently show that electromagnetic energy at frequencies near and below 900 MHz is best suited for deep penetration into brain tissue. The depth of penetration is noticeably greater at this frequency range, which includes the cellular phone frequencies as compared with higher frequencies. What is also important is the proven fact that deep tissue heating is obtained without detecting significant heating in the surface tissues. By their nature, the frequencies that provide the best therapeutic heating would also be frequencies that could be the most hazardous to man in an uncontrolled situation. High absorption in inner tissue such as the brain occurs while fat and bone absorption is many times less (Johnson and Guy, 1972).

Aside from the thermal issues, I should point out that the nonlinear properties of biological tissues could provide conditions for conformational changes in various important biological molecules via nonthermal effects (Markov, 2006). These changes could modify the entire signal transduction cascade.

I could agree that the first step in modeling the thermal effects should be the creation and building of tissue models. However, it sounds strange that this first step is addressed in papers published in 2011 (Nikita and Kiourri, 2011). Various models have been created in the decades before now, and surprisingly, they are neglected by the engineering community. More amazing is that these head models consist of only three layers: skin, fat, and muscle.

In addition, the dielectric properties of brain tissues are still not known with the degree of precision that would allow the accurate prediction of the absorbance of RF energy. If this is correct, how one can estimate the SAR? Despite the claims of IEEE and ICNIRP members, the experimental dosimetry is very insufficient for creating safety conditions for the users of mobile communications.

In 1994, I was planning to build a tissue phantom for evaluating the temperature effects caused by A 27.12 MHz pulsed electromagnetic field, approved by the food and drug administration (FDA) for therapeutic use. Richard Olsen, who was known to me as an expert in dosimetry of EMF, informed me that even placing a cadaver bone inside a liquid/gel model would not be accurate enough in respect to real tissues. Why in 2017 are we discussing the models without taking into account the complexity of the biological tissues, especially the human brain? From the physics and thermodynamics view point, biological tissues represent nonlinear systems (see White et al., 2011). The occurrence of a "hot spot" in response to RF radiation to a great extent corresponds to this nonlinearity.

Let me point to one very important fact: the manufacturers of diathermy devices should indicate the maximum safe distances and directions that must be maintained by therapists. Of course, if there must be defined some safe distance to be maintained from devices emitting 5.0 mW/cm^2, then certainly we might expect some safe distance to be kept from devices emitting higher levels of RF radiation—portable cellular telephones. This should be especially true when suggesting the spacing between the portable device and a human head, and respectively, to the human brain.

Since the human brain has little, if any, sensory capability, damage or trauma occurring internally will not be felt until the effects, such as heating, are so severe that they work their way outward. If tissue damage occurs within a localized region of the brain, it may be completely unnoticed. The threshold for irreversible skin damage is about 45°C which is also the temperature at which pain is felt. So, by the time a person exposed to RF radiation feels pain at the skin, that skin is irreversibly damaged as is the deeper tissue beneath the skin. Similarly, internal heating of brain tissue would not be sensed as a burning sensation. Likely, there would be no sensation at all. Interest in the ability to "sense" the presence of high levels of RF radiation motivated researchers to determine threshold levels for detecting heat sensations due to radiation exposure (Justesen, 1982).

Considering the lack of sensory detectors in the brain, we can expect that no warning of brain tissue destruction would be provided to a cellular telephone user until the damage was so extensive that the scalp, which absorbs very little energy, sensed heating. There is value in the research as they observed and documented an energy absorption "hot spot" associated with high electric fields at the tip of their antenna (Balzano et al., 1978a,b). One of the problems that needs to be stressed is that the brain did not absorb the energy uniformly.

In conclusion, today the entire biosphere and mankind are subjected to signals from space and terrestrial sources, unknown by numbers and by their physical characteristics. We are at the bottom of the ocean of electromagnetic waves. What is worse—this global "experiment" is conducted without protocol, monitoring, and the possibility to produce any protections. The mobile communication industry is creating newer and newer tools in order to eventually increase the speed of communications. Smartphones and smart meters significantly change the electromagnetic environment not only for occupational conditions, but in every home. Billions of people are not informed about the fact that their homes and they themselves are subjected to the "new and advanced" technological developments. This cohort includes babies and elderly people, schoolboys and professionals.

What is even worse, the new 5G mobile technology is being introduced even before the development of industrial standards. No health hazard estimation is planned, no guidance for protection and standards are developed. **It is time to ring the bell.**

REFERENCES

Adey WR. 1981. Tissue interactions with nonionizing electromagnetic fields. *Physiol Review* 61:435–514.

Adey WR. 1989. The extracellular space and energetic hierarchies in electromagnetic signaling between cells. In Allen MJ, Cleary S and Howkridge F (eds) *Charge and Field Effects in Biosystems*. Plenum Press, NY, 263–290.

Adey WR. 2004. Potential therapeutic applications of nonthermal electromagnetic fields: Ensemble organization of cells in tissue as a factor in biological field sensing. In Rosch PJ and Markov MS (eds) *Bioelectromagnetic Medicine*. Marcell Dekker, NY, 1–14.

Aydin D et al. 2011. Mobile phone use and brain tumors in children and adolescence: A multicenter case-control study. *J Natl Cancer Inst* 103(16):1264–1276.

Balzano G et al. 1978a. Energy deposition in simulated human operators of 800 MHz portable transmitters. *IEEE Trans Vehicular Technol* VT-27(4):174–181.

Balzano Q et al. 1978b. Heating of biological tissue in the induction field of VHF portable radio transmitters. *IEEE Trans Biomed Eng May* 1978:49–53.

Barnes F, Greenebaum B (eds). 2007. *Handbook of Biological Effects of Electromagnetic Fields*. CRC Press, Boca Raton FL, volumes 1 and 2.

Basset CAL. 1994. Therapeutic uses of electric and magnetic fields in orthopaedics. In Carpenter D and Ayrapetyan S (eds) *Biological Effects of Electric and Magnetic Fields*. Academic Press, San Diego CA, 13–18.

Becker R. 1990. *Cross Current*. Jeremy Tarcher Inc., New York, 32.

Belyaev IG. 2018. Health effects of chronic exposure to radiation from mobile communications. In Markov MS (ed) *Mobile Communications and Public Health*. CRC Press, Boca Raton FL. In press.

Belyaev IY. 2010. Dependence of non-thermal biological effects of microwaves on physical and biological variables: Implications for reproducibility and safety standards. *European Journal of Oncology—Library* 5:187–218.

Betskii OV, Lebedeva NN. 2004. Low-intensity millimeter waves in biology and medicine. In Rosch PJ and Markov MS (eds) *Bioelectromagnetic Medicine*. Marcel Dekker, NY, 741–760.

Bienkowski P, Trzaska H. 2015. Quantifying in Bioelectromagnetics. In Markov M (ed) *Dosimetry in Bioelectromagnetics*. CRC Press, Boca Raton FL, 269–284.

Blank M, Goodman R. 2009. Electromagnetic fields stress living cells. *Pathophysiology* 16:71–78.

Boice J, Tarone RE. 2011. Cell phone, cancer and children. *J Natl Inst Cancer* 103(16):1211–1213.

Carpenter DO, Ayrapetyan S. 1994. *Biological Effects of Electric and Magnetic Fields*. Academic Press, New York, v. 1 (362 p.), v. 2 (357 p.).

Cho CK, D'Andrea JA. 2003. Review of effects of RF fields on various aspects of human health. *Bioelectromagnetics*. 24:S5–S6.

Christ A et al. 2010a. Age-dependent tissue specific exposure of cell phone users. *Phys Med Biol* 55:1763–1783.

Christ A et al. 2010b. Impact of pinna compression on the RF absorption in the head of adults and juvenile cell phone users. *Bioelectromagnetics* 31:406–412.

De Iuliis GN, Newey RJ, King BV, Aitken RJ. 2009. Mobile phone radiation induces reactive oxygen species production and DNA damage in human spermatozoa *in vitro*. *PLoS One*. 4:e6446. doi: 10.1371/journal.pone.0006446.

Detlavs I (ed). 1987. *Electromagnetic Therapy in Traumas and Diseases of Support-Apparatus*. RMI, Riga, 198 p.

Durney CH, Massodi E, Iskander MF. 1978. *Radiofrequency Radiation Dosimetry Handbook*, Rep. SAM-TR-78-22, 1978. USAF School of Aerospace Medicine, Brooks Air Force Base, Texas.

Durney CH et al. 1979. An empirical formula for broad-band SAR calculations of prolate spheroidal models of humans and animals. *IEEE Trans Microw Theory Tech* MTT-27(8):758–763.

Foster K. 2005. Bioelectromagnetics pioneer Herman Schwan passed away at age 90. *Bioelectromagnetics Newsletter* 2:1–2.

Foster KR, Schwan H. 1995. Dielectric properties of tissues. In Polk C and Postow E (eds) *Handbook of Biological Effects of Electromagnetic Fields*. CRC Press, Boca Raton FL, 25–102.

Gabriel C, Gabriel S, Corthout E. 1996a. The dielectric properties of biological tissues: Literature survey. *Phys Med Biol* 41:2231–2249.

Gabriel S, Law RW, Gabriel C. 1996b. The dielectric properties of biological tissues: Measurements in the frequency range 10 Hz–20 GHz. *Phys Med Biol* 41:2251–2269.

Gillenwater T. 2017. Evolution of the smartphone. *Microwave Journal* February:40–48.
Grigoriev Y, Khortzeva N. 2018. A longitudinal study of psychophysiological indicators of pupils—User mobile communication in Russia (2006–2017) Children are at the group of risk. In Markov MS (ed) *Mobile Communications and Public Health*. CRC Press, Boca Raton FL. In press.
Grigoriev YG. 2012. Mobile communications and health of population: The risk assessment, social and ethical problems. *The Environmentalist* 32(2):193–200.
Grigoriev YG, Grigoriev OA. 2013. Cellular communication and health. *The electromagnetic environment. Radiobiology and hygiene problems. Forecast of danger.* M.: Economy, 567 p (in Russian).
Grigoriev YG, Khorseva NI. 2014. Mobile communications and health of children. *Risk assessment of the use of mobile communication by children and adolescents.* Recommendations to children and parents M.: Economics, 230 p (in Russian).
Hasted JB. 1973. *Aqueous Dielectrics*. Chapman and Hall, London, 302 p.
Hinrikus H, Bachmann M, Karai D, Lass J. 2017a. Mechanism of low-level microwave radiation effect on nervous system. *Electromagn Biol Med* 36:202–212.
Hinrikus H, Bachmann M, Lass J. 2011. Parametric mechanism of excitation of the electroencephalographic rhythms by modulated microwave radiation. *Int J Rad Biol* 87:1077–1085.
Hinrikus H, Bachmann M, Lass J. 2017b. Mechanism of low-level microwave radiation effect on brain: Frequency limits. *EMBEC & NBC 2017 Joint Conference of the European Medical and Biological Engineering Conference (EMBEC) and the Nordic-Baltic Conference on Biomedical Engineering and Medical Physics (NBC)*, Tampere, Finland, June 2017, IFMBE Proceedings, 65:647–650.
Hinrikus H, Bachmann M, Lass J, Tomson R, Tuulik V. 2008. Effect of 7, 14 and 21 Hz modulated 450 MHz microwave radiation on human electroencephalographic rhythms. *Int J Rad Biol* 84:69–79.
Hinrikus H, Lass J, Karai D, Pilt K, Bachmann M. 2015. Microwave effect on diffusion: A possible mechanism for non-thermal effect. *Electromagn Biol Med* 34:327–333.
Holcomb RR, McLean MJ, Engstrom S, Williams D, Morey J, McCullough B. 2003. Treatment of mechanical low back pain with static magnetic fields. In McLean MJ, Engstrom S and Holcomb RR (eds) *Magnetotherapy: Potential Therapeutic Benefits and Adverse Effects*. TFG Press, New York, pp. 169–190.
IARC Working Group on the Evaluation of Carcinogenic Risks to Humans. 2002. Non-ionizing radiation part 1: Static and extremely low-frequency (ELF) electric and magnetic fields. *IARC Monogr Eval Carcinog Risks Hum* 80:1–395.
ICNIRP Guidelines. 1998. Guidelines for limiting exposure to time-varying electric, magnetic, and electromagnetic fields (up to 300 GHz). *Health Physics* 74:484–522.
ICNIRP (International Commission on Non-Ionizing Radiation Protection). 2009. Exposure to high frequency electromagnetic fields, biological effects and health consequences (100 kHz–300 GHz).
Johnson CC, Guy AW. 1972. Nonionizing electromagnetic wave effects in biological materials and systems. *Proceedings of the IEEE* 60(6): 692–718.
Joines WT, Spiegel RJ. 1974. Resonance absorption of microwaves by the human skull. *IEEE Trans Biomed Eng* January 1974:46–48.
Justesen DR. 1982. A comparative study of human sensory thresholds: 2450-MHz microwaves vs far-infrared radiation. *Bioelectromagnetics* 3:117–125.
Juutilainen J, Höytö A, Kumlin T, Naarala J. 2011. Review of possible modulation-dependent biological effects of radiofrequency fields. *Bioelectromagnetics* 32:511–534.
Kane R. 1995. *Cellular Telephone Russian Roulette*. Vantage Press Inc., New York, p. 241.
Koulouridis S, Nikita KS. 2004. Study of the coupling between human head and cellular phone helical antennas. *IEEE Trans Electrom Compat* 46:62–71.

Lapin MS. 2004. Noninvasive pulsed electromagnetic therapy for migraine and multiple sclerosis. In Rosch PJ and Markov MS (eds) *Bioelectromagnetic Medicine*. Marcel Dekker, NY, 277–292.

Lerchl A, Klose M, Grote K, Wilhelm AF, Spathmann O, Fiedler T, Streckert J, Hansen V, Clemens M. 2015. Tumor promotion by exposure to radiofrequency electromagnetic fields below exposure limits for humans. *Biochem Biophys Res Commun* 459:585–90.

Leszczynski D, de Pomerai D, Koczan D, Stoll D, Franke H, Albar JP. 2012. Review Five years later: The current status of the use of proteomics and transcriptomics in EMF research. *Proteomics* 12:2493–2509.

Lin JC. 1976. Interaction of two cross-polarized electromagnetic waves with mammalian cranial structures. *IEEE Trans Biomed Eng BME* 23(5):371–375.

Lin JC. 1977. On microwave-induced hearing sensation. *IEEE Trans Microw Theory Tech* MTT-25(7):605–613.

Markov MS. 1979. Informational character of magnetic field action on biological systems. In Jensen K and Vassileva YU (eds) *Biophysical and Biochemical Information Transfer in Recognition*. Plenum Press, NY, 496–500.

Markov MS. 1984. Influence of constant magnetic field on biological systems. In Allen M (ed) *Charge and Field Effects in Biosystems*. Abacus Press, Kent, 319–329.

Markov MS. 1994. Biophysical estimation of the environmental importance of electromagnetic fields. *Review of Environmental Health* 10(2):75–83.

Markov MS. 2001. Magnetic and electromagnetic field dosimetry—Necessary step in harmonization of standards. *Proceedings of WHO Meeting*, Varna, April 2001, http://www.who.int/peh-emf/publications/Varna

Markov MS. 2004. Magnetic and electromagnetic field therapy: Basic principles of application for pain relief. In Rosch PJ and Markov MS (eds) *Bioelectromagnetic Medicine*. Marcel Dekker, NY, 251–264.

Markov MS. 2006. Thermal vs. nonthermal mechanisms of interactions between electromagnetic fields and biological systems. In Markov M and Ayrapetyan (eds) *Bioelectromagnetics: Current Concepts*, Springer, 1–16.

Markov MS. 2012. Impact of physical factors on the society and environment. Environmentalist. doi: 10.1007/s10669-012-9386-5.

Markov MS (ed). 2015. *Electromagnetic Fields in Biology and Medicine*. CRC Press, Boca Raton FL.

Markov MS, Grigoriev YG. 2013. WiFi technology—An uncontrolled experiment on human health. *Electromagnetic Biology and Medicine* 32(2):200–208.

Markov MS, Hazlewood CF, Ericsson AD. 2004. Systemic effect—A plausible explanation of the benefit of magnetic field therapy: A hypothesis. *3rd International Workshop on Biological Effects of EMF—Kos*, Greece, October 4–8, 2004, 673–682, ISBN 960-233-151-158.

Markov MS, Pilla AA. 1995. Electromagnetic field stimulation of soft tissue: Pulsed radiofrequency treatment of post-operative pain and edema. *Wounds* 7(4):143–151.

Mayrovitz H. 2015. Electromagnetic fieldsfor soft tissue wound healing. In Markov MS (ed) *Electromagnetic fields in biology and medicine*. CRC Press, Boca Raton, F1231–F252.

McLean MJ, Engstrom S, Holcomb RR (eds). 2003. *Magnetotherapy: Potential Therapeutic Benefits and Adverse Effects*. TFG Press, New York, 279 p.

Michaelson SM. 1972. Human exposure to nonionizing radiant energy—potential hazards and safety standard's. *Proceedings of the IEEE* April 1972:389–421.

Nikita KS, Kiourri A. 2011. Mobile communication field in biological systems. In: Lin J (ed) *Electromagnetic Fields in Biological Systems*. CRC Press, Boca Raton, 261–329.

Oltman R. 2017. 5G is coming. *Microwave Journal* October:40–42.

Otano-Lata S, Markov M, Iyer V. 1996. Biophysical dosimetry as a function of body target. In Daskalov I (ed) *Proceedings of the Seventh Conference of Biomedical Physics and Engineering*, Sofia, Bulgaria, October 17–19, 1996, 66–72.

Parliamentary Assembly. Council of Europe. 2011. Resolution 1815. *The potential dangers of electromagnetic fields and their effect on the environment.* http://assembly.coe.int/nw/xml/XRef/Xref-XML2HTML-en.asp?fileid=17994

Pilla AA. 2007. Mechanisms and therapeutic applications of time varying and static magnetic fields. In Barnes F and Greenebaum B (eds) *Biological and Medical Aspects of Electromagnetic Fields.* CRC Press, Boca Raton FL, 351–411.

Pilla AA. 2015. Pulsed electromagnetic fields; from signaling to healing. In Markov MS (ed) *Electromagnetic Fields in Biology and Medicine.* CRC Press, Boca Raton FL, 29–48.

Polk C, Postow E. 1986. *Handbook of Biological Effects of Electromagnetic Fields.* CRC Press, Boca Raton, FL.

Richter EO, Lozano AM. 2004. Deep brain stimulation for Parkinson's disease and movement disorders. In Rosch PJ and Markov MS (eds) *Bioelectromagnetic Medicine.* Marcel Dekker, New York, 265–276.

Rosch PJ, Markov MS (eds). 2004. *Bioelectromagnetic Medicine.* Marcel Dekker, New York, 850 p.

Sage C. 2012. The similar effects of low-dose ionizing radiation and non-ionizing radiation from background environmental levels of exposure. *Environmentalist* 32:144–156.

SanPiN. 1996. Radiofrequency electromagnetic radiation (RF EMR) under occupational and living conditions Moscow: Minzdrav; (in Russian).

Schwan HP. 1972a. Microwave radiation; hot spots in conducting spheres by electromagnetic waves and biological implications. *IEEE Trans Biomed Eng BME* 19(1):53–58.

Schwan HP. 1972b. Microwave radiation; biophysical considerations and standards criteria. *IEEE Trans Biomed Eng BME* 19(4):304–312.

Schwan HP, Piersol GM. 1978. The absorption of electromagnetic energy in body tissues. *Int Rev Phys Med Rehabil* December 1954:371–404. *IEEE Transactions on Vehicular TechnologyVT-27*, no. 2 (May 1978):51–56.

Swerdlow AJ et al. 2011. Mobile phone, brain tumors and theinterphone study: Where we are now? *Environ Health Persp* 119:1534–1538.

Szmigielski S. 2013. Reaction of the immune system to low-level RF/MW exposures. *Sci Total Environ* 454–455:393–400.

Todorov N. 1982. *Magnetotherapy.* Medicina and Physcultura Publishing House, Sofia.

Valberg. 1995. How to plan EMF experiments. *Bioelectromagnetics* 16:396–401.

Valentini E, Curcio G, Moroni F, Ferrara M, De Gennaro L, Bertini M. 2007. Neurophysiological effects of mobile phone eletromagnetic fields on humans: A comprehensive review. *Bioelectromagnetics* 28:415–432.

Vodovnik L, Karba R. 1992. Treatment of chronic wounds by means of electric and electromagnetic fields. *Med Biol Eng Comp* 30:257–266.

White GN, Egot-Lamaire SJP, Baclavage WX. 2011. A novel view of biologically active electromagnetic fields. *The Environmentalist* 31(2):107–113.

WHO Healthy Environment for Children. Backgrounder No 3, April 2003, 3 p.

Wiart J, Hadjem A, Wong M, Bloch I. 2008. Analysis of RF exposure in the head tissues of children and adults. *Phys Med Biol* 53:3681–3695.

2 Cell Phone Radiation

*Evidence From ELF and RF Studies Supporting More Inclusive Risk Identification and Assessment**

Carl Blackman

CONTENTS

* Reprinted from Pathophysiology 16 (2009) 205–216, "Cell phone radiation: Evidence from ELF and RF studies supporting more inclusive risk identification and assessment", Copyright 2009, with permission from Elsevier.

2.1 INTRODUCTION

It is universally accepted that radio frequency radiation (RFR) can cause tissue heating (thermal effects, TE) and that extremely low-frequency (ELF) fields, for example, 50 and 60 Hz, can cause electrical current flows that shock and even damage or destroy tissues [1]. These factors alone are the underlying bases for present exposure standards. EMF exposures that cause biological effects at intensities that do not cause obvious thermal changes, that is, non-thermal effects (NTE), have been widely reported in the scientific literature since the 1970s, including beneficial applications in development and repair processes. The current public safety limits do not take modulation into account and thus are no longer sufficiently protective of public health where chronic exposure to pulsed or pulse-modulated signal is involved, and where sub-populations of more susceptible individuals may be at risk from such exposures.

2.1.1 Modulation as a Critical Element

Modulation signals are one important component in the delivery of EMF signals to which cells, tissues, organs, and individuals can respond biologically. At the most basic level, modulation can be considered a pattern of pulses or repeating signals which have specific meaning in defining that signal apart from all others. Modulated signals have a specific 'beat' defined by how the signal varies periodically or aperiodically over time. Pulsed signals occur in an on–off pattern, which can be either smooth and rhythmic or sharply pulsed in quick bursts. Amplitude and frequency modulation involves two very different processes where the high frequency signal, called the carrier wave, has a lower frequency signal that is superimposed on or 'rides' on the carrier frequency. In amplitude modulation, the lower frequency signal is embedded on the carrier wave as changes in its amplitude as a function of time, whereas in frequency modulation, the lower frequency signal is embedded as slight changes in the frequency of the carrier wave. Each type of low-frequency modulation conveys specific 'information,' and some modulation patterns are more effective (more bioactive) than others depending on the biological reactivity of the exposed material. This enhanced interaction can be a good thing for therapeutic purposes in medicine, but can be deleterious to health where such signals could stimulate disease-related processes, such as increased cell proliferation in precancerous lesions. Modulation signals may interfere with normal, nonlinear biological functions. More recent studies of modulated RF signals report changes in human cognition, reaction time, brain-wave activity, sleep disruption, and immune function. These studies have tested the RF and ELF-modulated RF signals from emerging wireless technologies (cell phones) that rely on pulse-modulated RF to transmit signals. Thus, modulation can be considered as information content embedded in the higher frequency carrier wave that may have biological consequences beyond any effect from the carrier wave directly.

In mobile telephony, for example, modulation is one of the underlying ways to categorize the radio frequency signal of one telecom carrier from another (time division multiple access [TDMA] from code division multiple access [CDMA] from global system for mobile communications [GSM]). Modulation is likely a key factor in determining whether and when biological reactivity might be occurring, for example, in the new technologies which make use of modulated signals, some modulation (the packaging for delivery for an EMF 'message') may be bioactive, for example, when frequencies are similar to those found in brain wave patterns. If a new technology happens to use brain wave frequencies, the chances are higher that it will have effects, in comparison, for example, to choosing some lower or higher modulation frequency to carry the same EMF information to its target.

This chapter will show that other EMF factors may also be involved in determining if a given low-frequency signal directly, or as a modulation of a radiofrequency wave, can be bioactive. Such is the evolving nature of information about modulation. It argues for great care in defining standards that are intended to be protective of public health and well-being. This chapter will also describe some features of exposure and physiological conditions that are required in general for non-thermal effects to be produced, and specifically *to illustrate how modulation is a fundamental factor which should be taken into account in public safety standards.*

2.2 LABORATORY EVIDENCE

Published laboratory studies have provided evidence for more than 40 years on bioeffects at much lower intensities than cited in the various widely publicized guidelines for limits to prevent harmful effects. Many of these reports show EMF-caused changes in processes associated with cell growth control, differentiation, and proliferation that are biological processes of considerable interest to physicians for potential therapeutic applications and for scientists who study the molecular and cellular basis of cancer. EMF effects have been reported in gene induction, transmembrane signaling cascades, gap junction communication, immune system action, rates of cell transformation, breast cancer cell growth, regeneration of damaged nerves, and recalcitrant bone fracture healing. These reports have cell growth control as a common theme. Other more recent studies on brain-wave activity, cognition, and human reaction time lend credence to modulation (pulsed RF and ELF-modulated RF) as a concern for wireless technologies, most prominently from cell phone use.

In the process of studying nonthermal biological effects, various exposure parameters have been shown to influence whether or not a specific EMF can cause a biological effect, including intensity, frequency, the coincidence of the static magnetic field (both the natural earth's magnetic field and anthropogenic fields), the presence of the electrical field, and the magnetic field, or their combination and whether EMF is sinusoidal, pulsed or in more complex wave forms. These parameters will be discussed below.

Experimental results will be used to illustrate the influence of each EMF parameter, while also demonstrating that it is highly unlikely the effects are due to EMF-caused current flow or heating.

2.2.1 Initial Studies That Drew Attention to NTE

Several papers in the 1960s and early 1970s reported that ELF fields could alter circadian rhythms in laboratory animals and humans. In the latter 1960s, a paper by Hamer [2] reported that the EMF environment in planned space capsules could cause human response time changes, that is, the interval between a signal and the human response. Subsequent experiments by a research group led by Adey were conducted with monkeys and showed similar response time changes and also electroencephalogram (EEG) pattern changes [3,4]. The investigators shifted the research subject to cats and decided they needed to use a radio frequency field to carry the ELF signal into the cat brain, and observed EEG pattern changes, ability to sense and behaviorally respond to the ELF component of RFR, the ability of minor electric current to stimulate the release of an inhibitory neurotransmitter, gamma amino-butyric acid (GABA), and simultaneous release of a surrogate measure, calcium ions, from the cortex [5,6]. At this time Bawin, a member of the research group, adopted newly hatch chickens as sources of brain tissue and observed changes in the release of calcium ions from *in vitro* specimens as a function of ELF frequency directly or as amplitude modulation ('AM') of RFR (RFRAM) [7–11]. Tests of both EMF frequency and intensity dependences demonstrated a single sensitive region (termed 'window') over the range of frequency and intensity examined. This series of papers showed that EMF-induced changes could occur in several species (human, monkey, cat, and chicken), that calcium ions could be used as surrogate measures for a neurotransmitter, that ELF fields could produce effects similar to RFRAM (note: without the 'AM', there was no effect although the RFR intensity was the same), and that the dose and frequency response consisted of a single sensitivity window.

Subsequent, independent research groups published a series of papers replicating and extending this earlier work. Initial studies by Blackman, Joines, and colleagues [12–25] used the same chick brain assay system as Bawin and colleagues. These papers reported multiple windows in intensity and in frequency within which calcium changes were observed in the chick brain experimental systems under EMF exposure. Three other independent groups offered confirmation of these results by reporting intensity and frequency windows for calcium, neurotransmitter or enolase release under EMF exposure of human and animal nervous system-derived cells *in vitro* by Dutta et al. [26–29], of rat pancreatic tissue slices by Albert et al. [30], and of frog heart by Schwartz et al. [31], but not frog heart atrial strips *in vitro* [32]. This series of papers showed that multiple frequency and intensity windows were a common phenomenon that required the development of new theoretical concepts to provide a mechanism of action paradigm.

2.2.2 Refined Laboratory Studies Reveal More Details

Additional aspects of the EMF experiments with the chick brain described by Blackman and colleagues above, also revealed critical co-factors that influenced the action of EMF to cause changes in calcium release, including the influence of the local static magnetic field, and the influence of physico-chemical parameters, such as pH, temperature, and the ionic strength of the bathing solution surrounding the brain tissue during exposure. This information provides clues for and constraints on any theoretical mechanism that is to be developed to explain the phenomenon. Most current theories ignore these parameters that need to be monitored and controlled for EMF exposure to produce NTE. These factors demonstrate that the current risk assessment paradigms, which ignore them, are incomplete and thus may not provide the level of protection currently assumed.

2.2.3 Sensitivity of Developing Organisms

An additional study was also conducted to determine if EMF exposure of chicken eggs while the embryo was developing could influence the response of brain tissue from the newly hatched chickens. The detailed set of frequency and intensity combinations under which effects were observed were all obtained from hatched chickens whose eggs were incubated for 21 days in an electrically heated chamber containing 60-Hz fields. Thus, tests were performed to determine if the 60-Hz frequency of ELF fields (10 V/m in air) during incubation, that is, during embryogenesis and organogenesis, would alter the subsequent calcium release responses of the brain tissue to EMF exposure. The reports of Blackman et al. [19] and Joines et al. [25] showed that the brain tissue response was changed when the field during the incubation period was 50 Hz rather than 60 Hz. This result is consistent with an anecdotal report of adult humans institutionalized because of chemical sensitivities, who were also responsive to the frequency of power line EM fields that were present in the countries where they were born and raised [33]. This information indicates there may be animal and human exposure situations where EMF imprinting during development could be an important factor in laboratory and epidemiological situations. EMF imprinting, which may only become manifest when a human is subjected to chemical or biological stresses, could reduce the ability to fight disease and toxic insult from environmental pollution, resulting in a population in need of more medical services, with resulting lost days at work.

2.3 FUNDAMENTAL EXPOSURE PARAMETERS: TO BE CONSIDERED WHEN ESTABLISHING A MODE (OR MECHANISM) OF ACTION FOR NONTHERMAL EMF-INDUCED BIOLOGICAL EFFECTS

2.3.1 Intensity

There are numerous reports of biological effects that show intensity "windows," that is, regions of intensity that cause changes surrounded by higher and lower intensities that show no effects from exposure. One very clear effect by Blackman and colleagues is 16-Hz, sine wave-induced changes in calcium efflux from brain tissue in a test tube because it shows two very distinct and clearly separated intensity windows of effects surrounded by regions of intensities that caused no effects [17]. There are other reports for similar multiple windows of intensity in the radio frequency range [22,26,29,31]. Note that calcium ions are a secondary signal transduction agent active in many cellular pathways. These results show that intensity windows exist and they display an unusual and unanticipated "nonlinear" (nonlinear and non-monotonic) phenomenon that has been ignored in all risk assessment and standard setting exercises, save the NCRP 1986 publication [1]. Protection from multiple intensity windows has never been incorporated into any risk assessment; to do so would call for a major change in thinking. These results mean that lower intensity is not necessarily less bioactive or less harmful.

Multiple intensity windows appeared as an unexpected phenomenon in the late 1970s and 1980s. There has been one limited attempt to specifically model this phenomenon by Thompson et al. [34], which was reasonably successful. This modeling effort should be extended because there are publications from two independent research groups showing multiple intensity windows for 50, 147, and 450 MHz fields when amplitude modulated at 16 Hz using the calcium ion release endpoint in chicken brains *in vitro*. The incident intensities (measured in air) for the windows at the different carrier frequencies do not align at the same values. However, Joines et al. [23,24] and Blackman et al. [20] noted the windows of intensity align across different carrier frequencies if one converts the incident intensity to the intensity expected within the sample at the brain surface. This conversion was accomplished by correcting for the different dielectric constants of the sample materials due to the different carrier frequencies. The uniqueness of this response provides a substantial clue to theoreticians, but it is interesting and disappointing that no publications have appeared attempting to address this relationship. It is obvious that this phenomenon is one that needs further study.

2.3.2 Frequency

Frequency-dependent phenomena are common occurrences in nature. For example, the human ear only hears a portion of the sound that is in the environment, typically from 20 to 20,000 Hz, which is a frequency "window." Another biological frequency window can be observed for plants grown indoors. Given normal indoor lighting, the plants may grow to produce lush vegetation but not produce flowers unless illuminated with a lamp that emits a different spectrum of light partially mimicking the light from the sun. Thus, frequency windows of response to various agents exist in biological systems from plants to *homo sapiens*.

In a similar manner, there are examples of EMF-caused biological effects that occur in a frequency-dependent manner that cannot be explained by current flow or heating. The examples include reports of calcium ion efflux from brain tissue *in vitro* by Blackman and Joines and colleagues at low frequency [15,19] and at high frequency modulated at low frequency [20,35,24]. An additional example of an unexpected result is by Liboff [36].

In addition, two apparently contradictory multiple-frequency exposure results provide examples of the unique and varied nonthermal interactions of EMF with biological systems. Litovitz and colleagues showed that an ELF sinusoidal signal could induce a biological response in a cell culture preparation, and that the addition of a noise signal of equal average intensity could block the effect caused by the sinusoidal signal, thereby negating the influence of the sinusoidal signal [37]. Similar noise canceling effects were observed using chick embryo preparations [38,39]. It was also shown that the biological effects caused by microwave exposures imitating cell phone signals could be mitigated by ELF noise [40]. However, this observation should not be generalized; a noise signal is not always benign. Milham and Morgan [41] showed that a sinusoidal ELF (60-Hz) signal was not associated with the induction of cancer in humans, but when that sinusoidal signal was augmented by a noise signal, basically transients that added higher frequencies, an increase in cancer was noted in humans exposed over the long-term. Thus, the addition of noise in this case was associated with the appearance of a health issue. Havas [42–44] has described other potential health problems associated with these higher frequency transients, termed "dirty power." The bioactive frequency regions observed in these studies have never been explicitly considered for use in any EMF risk assessments, thus demonstrating the incomplete nature of current exposure guideline limits.

There are also EMF frequency-dependent alterations in the action of nerve growth factor (NGF) to stimulate neurite outgrowth (growth of primitive axons or dendrites) from a peripheral nerve-derived cell (PC-12) in culture shown by Blackman et al. [45,46] and by Trillo et al. [47]. The combined effect of frequency and intensity is also a common occurrence in both the analogous sound and the light examples given above. Too much or too little of either frequency or intensity shows either no or undesirable effects. Similarly, Blackman et al. [15] has reported EMF responses composed of effect "islands" of intensity and frequency combinations, surrounded by a "sea" of intensity and frequency combinations of null effects. Although the mechanisms responsible for these effects have not been established, the effects represent a here-to-fore unknown phenomenon that may have complex ramifications for risk assessment and standard setting. Nerve growth and neurotransmitter release that can be altered by different combinations of EMF frequencies and intensities, especially in developing organisms like children, could conceivably produce over time a subsequent altered ability to successfully or fully respond behaviorally to natural stressors in the adult environment; research is urgently needed to test this possibility in animal systems.

Nevertheless, this phenomenon of frequency-dependence is ignored in the development of present exposure standards. These standards rely primarily on biological responses to intensities within arbitrarily defined engineering-based frequency bands, not biologically based response bands, and are solely based on energy deposition determinations.

2.4 STATIC MAGNETIC FIELD: A COMPLETELY UNEXPECTED COMPLEXITY

The magnetic field of the earth at any given location has a relatively constant intensity as a function of time. However, the intensity value, and the inclination of the field with respect to the gravity vector, varies considerable over the face of the earth. More locally, these features of the earth's magnetic field can also vary by more than 20% inside manufactured structures, particularly those with steel support structures.

At the Bioelectromagnetics Society annual meeting in 1984 [48], Blackman revealed his group's discovery that the intensity of the static magnetic field could establish and define those oscillatory frequencies that would cause changes in calcium ion release in his chick brain preparation. This result was further discussed at a North Atlantic Treaty Organization (NATO) Advanced Research workshop in Erice, Italy, in the fall of 1984 and by publications from that meeting and subsequent research: Blackman et al. [14,18] and Liboff et al. [36,49,50]. Substantial additional research on this feature was reported by Liboff and colleagues [50–52]. Blackman et al. also reported on the importance of the relative orientation of the static magnetic field vector to the oscillating magnetic field vector [21] and demonstrated a reverse biological response could occur depending on parallel or perpendicular orientations of the static and oscillating magnetic fields [53].

There have been many attempts to explain this phenomenon by a number of research teams led by Smith [49], Blackman [15], Liboff [36,54], Lednev [55], Blanchard [56], Zhadin [57], del Giudice [58], Binhi [59–62], and Matronchik [63], but none has been universally accepted. Nevertheless, experimental results continued to report static and oscillating field dependencies for nonthermally induced biological effects in studies led by Zhadin [64,65], Vorobyov [66], Baureus Koch [67], Sarimov [68], Prato [69,70], Comisso [71], and Novikov [72].

With this accumulation of reports from independent, international researchers, it is now clear that if a biological response depends on the static magnetic field intensity and even its orientation with respect to an oscillating field, then the conditions necessary to reproduce the phenomenon are very specific and might easily escape detection (see e.g., Blackman and Most [73]). The consequences of these results are that there may be exposure situations that are truly detrimental (or beneficial) to organisms, but that are insufficiently common on a large scale that they would not be observed in epidemiological studies; they need to be studied under controlled laboratory conditions to determine impact on health and well-being.

2.5 ELECTRIC AND MAGNETIC COMPONENTS: BOTH BIOLOGICALLY ACTIVE WITH DIFFERENT CONSEQUENCES

Both the electric and the magnetic components have been shown to directly and independently cause biological changes. There is one report that clearly distinguishes the distinct biological responses caused by the electric field and by the magnetic field. Marron et al. [74] show that electric field exposure can increase the negative surface charge density of an amoeba, *Physarum polycephalum*, and that magnetic field exposure of the same organism causes changes in the surface of the organism to reduce its hydrophobic character. Other scientists have used concentric growth surfaces of different radii and vertical magnetic fields perpendicular to the growth surface to determine if the magnetic or the induced electric component is the agent causing biological change. Liburdy et al. [75], examining calcium influx in lymphocytes, and Greene et al. [76], monitoring ornithine decarboxylase (ODC) activity in cell culture, showed that the induced electric component was responsible for their results. In contrast, Blackman et al. [77,78], monitoring neurite outgrowth from two different clones of PC-12 cells and using the same exposure technique used by Liburdy and by Greene, showed the magnetic component was the critical agent in their experiments. EMF-induced changes on the cell surface where it interacts with its environment, can dramatically alter the homeostatic mechanisms in tissues, whereas changes in ODC activity are associated with the induction of cell proliferation, a desirable outcome if one is concerned about wound healing, but undesirable if the concern is tumor cell growth. This information demonstrates the multiple, different ways that EMF can affect biological systems. Present analyses for risk assessment and standard setting have ignored this information, thus making their conclusions of limited value.

2.6 SINE AND PULSED WAVES: LIKE DIFFERENT PROGRAMS ON A RADIO BROADCAST STATION

Important characteristics of pulsed waves that have been reported to influence biological processes include the following: (1) frequency, (2) pulse width, (3) intensity, (4) rise and fall time, and (5) the frequency, if any, within the pulse ON time. Chiabrera et al. [79] showed that pulsed fields caused de-differentiation of amphibian red blood cells. Scarfi et al. [80] showed enhanced micronuclei formation in lymphocytes of patients with Turner's syndrome (only one X chromosome), but no change in micronuclei formation when the lymphocytes were exposed to sine waves (Scarfi et al. [81]). Takahashi et al. [82] monitored thymidine incorporation in Chinese hamster cells and explored the influence of pulse frequency (two windows of enhancement reported), pulse width (one window of enhancement reported), and intensity (two windows of enhancement reported followed by a reduction in incorporation). Ubeda et al. [83] showed the influence of different rise and fall times of pulsed waves on chick embryo development.

2.6.1 Importance for Risk Assessment

It is important to note that the frequency spectrum of pulsed waves can be represented by a sum of sine waves which, to borrow a chemical analogy, would represent a mixture of chemicals, any one of which could be biologically active. Risk assessment and exposure limits have been established for specific chemicals or chemical classes of compounds that have been shown to cause undesirable biological effects. Risk assessors and the general public are sophisticated enough to recognize that it is impossible to declare all chemicals safe or hazardous; consider the difference between food and poisons, both of which are chemicals. A similar situation occurs for EMF; it is critical to determine which combinations of EMF conditions have the potential to cause biological harm and which do not.

Obviously, pulse wave exposures represent an entire genre of exposure conditions, with additional difficulty for exact independent replication of exposures, and thus of results, but with increased opportunities for the production of biological effects. Current standards were not developed with explicit knowledge of these additional consequences for biological responses.

2.7 MECHANISMS

Two papers have the possibility of advancing understanding in this research area. Chiabrera et al. [84] created a theoretical model for EMF effects on an ion's interaction with protein that includes the influence of thermal energy and of metabolism. Before this publication, theoreticians assumed that biological effects in living systems could not occur if the electric signal is below the signal caused by thermal noise, in spite of experimental evidence to the contrary. In this paper, the authors show that this limitation is not absolute, and that different amounts of metabolic energy can influence the amount and parametric response of biological systems to EMF. The second paper, by Marino et al. [85], presents a new analytical approach to examine endpoints in systems exposed to EMF. The authors, focusing on exposure-induced lymphoid phenotypes, report that EMF may not cause changes in the mean values of endpoints, but by using recurrence analysis, they capture exposure-induced, statistically significant nonlinear movements of the endpoints to either side of the mean endpoint value. They provide further evidence using immunological endpoints from exposed and sham treated mice [86–88]. Additional research has emerged from this laboratory on EMF-induced animal and human brain activity changes that provides more evidence for the value of their research approach (Marino et al. [89–92], Kolomytkin et al. [93] and Carrubba et al. [94–98]). Further advanced theoretical and experimental studies of relevance to nonthermal biological effects are emerging; see, for example, reports by Binhi et al. [59–62], Zhadin et al. [64,65,99], and Novikov et al. [72]. *It is apparent that much remains to be examined and explained in EMF biological effects research through more creative methods of analysis than have been used before. The models described above need to be incorporated into risk assessment determinations.*

2.8 PROBLEMS WITH CURRENT RISK ASSESSMENTS: OBSERVATIONS OF EFFECTS ARE SEGREGATED BY ARTIFICIAL FREQUENCY BANDS THAT IGNORE MODULATION

One fundamental limitation of most reviews of EMF biological effects is that exposures are segregated by the physical (engineering/technical) concept of frequency bands favored by the engineering community. This is a default approach that follows the historical context established by the incremental addition of newer technologies that generate increasingly higher frequencies. However, this approach fails to consider unique responses from biological systems that are widely reported at various combinations of frequencies, modulations, and intensities.

When common biological responses are observed without regard for the particular, engineering-defined EMF frequency band in which the effects occur, this reorganization of the results can highlight the commonalities in biological responses caused by exposures to EMF across the different engineering-defined frequency bands. An attempt to introduce this concept to escape the limitations of the engineering-defined structure occurred with the development of the 1986 NCRP radio frequency exposure guidelines because published papers from the early 1970s to the mid 1980s (to be discussed below) demonstrated the need to include amplitude modulation as a factor in setting of maximum exposure limits. The 1986 NCRP guideline [1] was the one and only risk evaluation that included an exception for modulated fields.

The current research and risk assessment attempts are no longer tenable. The 3-year delay in the expected report of the 7-year Interphone study results has made this epidemiological approach a 10-year long effort, and the specific exposure conditions, due to improved technology, have changed so that the results may no longer be applicable to the current exposure situation. It is unproductive to continue to fund epidemiological studies of people who are exposed to a wide variety of diversified, uncontrolled, and poorly characterized EMF in their natural and work environments.

In place of the funding of more epidemiological studies should be funding to support controlled laboratory studies to focus on the underlying processes responsible for the NTE described above, so that mechanisms or modes of action can be developed to provide a theoretical framework to further identify, characterize, and unify the action of the here-to-fore ignored exposure parameters shown to be important.

2.8.1 Potential Explanation for the Failure to Optimize Research in EMF Biological Effects

Unfortunately, risk evaluations following the 1986 NCRP example [1] returned to the former engineering-defined analysis conditions, in part because scientists who reported nonthermal effects were not placed on the review committees, and in the terms of Slovic [100] "Risk assessment is inherently subjective and represent a blend of science and judgment with important psychological, social, cultural, and political factors....Whoever controls the definition of risk controls the rational solution to the problem at hand....Defining risk is thus an exercise in power." It appears that by excluding scientists experienced with producing nonthermal biological effects, the usually sound judgment by the selected committees was severely limited in its breadth-of-experience, thereby causing the members to retreat to their own limited areas of expertise when forced to make judgments, as described by Slovic [100], "Public views are also influenced by worldviews, ideologies, and values; so are scientists' views, particularly when they are working at limits of their expertise." The current practice of segregating scientific investigations (and resulting public health limits) by artificial divisions of frequency dramatically dilutes the impact of the basic science results, thereby reducing and distorting the weight of evidence in any evaluation process (see evaluations of bias by Havas [101], referring to NRC 1997 [102] compared to NIEHS 1998 [103] and NIEHS 1999 [104]).

2.9 SUGGESTED RESEARCH

Are there substitute approaches that would improve on the health effects evaluation situation? As mentioned above, it may be useful in certain cases to develop a biologically based clustering of the data to focus on and enrich understanding of certain aspects of biological responses. Some examples to consider for biological clustering include: (1) EMF features, such as frequency and intensity interdependencies, (2) common cofactors, such as the earth's magnetic field or coincident application of chemical agents to perturb and perhaps sensitize the biological system to EMF, or (3) physiological state of the biological specimen, such as age or sensitive subpopulations, including genetic predispositionas described by Fedrowitz et al. [105,106], and for human populations recently reported by Yang et al. [107].

To determine if this approach has merit, one could combine reports of biological effects found in the ELF (including sub-ELF) band with effects found in the RF band when the RF exposures are amplitude modulated (AM) using frequencies in the ELF band. The following data should be used: (a) human response time changes under ELF exposure [2], (b) monkey response time and EEG changes under ELF exposure [3,4], (c) cat brain EEG, GABA, and calcium ion changes induced by ELF and AM-RF [5–11,108], (d) calcium ion changes in chick brain tissue under ELF and AM-RF [7–25,35], and (e) calcium changes under AM-RF in brain cells in culture [26–28] and in frog heart under AM-RF [31]. The potential usefulness of applying biological clustering in the example given above even though AM is used is that the results may have relevance to assist in the examination of some of the effects reportedly caused by cellular phone exposures which include more complex types of modulation of RF. This suggestion is reasonable because three groups later reported human responses to cell phone emissions that include changes in reaction times—Preece et al. [109,110], Koivisto et al. [111,112], and Krause et al. [113,114] – or to brain wave potentials that may be associated with reaction time changes—Freude et al. [115,116].

Subsequently, Preece et al. [117] tested cognitive function in children and found a trend, but not a statistically significant change in simple reaction time under exposure, perhaps because they applied a Bonferroni correction to the data (alpha for significance was required to be less than 0.0023). It would appear that a change in the experimental protocol might provide a more definitive test of the influence of exposure on simple reaction time because it is known that a Bonferroni correction is a particularly severe test of statistical significance, or as the author observed, "a particularly conservative criterion."

Krause et al. [118] examined cognitive activity by observing oscillatory EEG activity in children exposed to cell phone radiation while performing an auditory memory task and reported exposure related changes in the ~4–8 Hz EEG frequencies during memory encoding, changes in that range, and also ~15 Hz during recognition. The investigators also examined cognitive processing, an auditory memory task or a visual working memory task in adults exposed to continuous wave (CW) or pulsed cell phone radiation on either the right or left side of the head, and reported modest changes in brain EEG activity in the ~4–8 Hz region compared to CW exposure, but with caveats that no behavior changes were observed, and that the data were varying, unsystematic, and inconsistent with previous reports (Krause et al. [119]). Haarala and colleagues conducted an extensive series of experiments examining reaction time [120], short-term memory [121], short-term memory in children [122], and right versus left hemisphere exposure [123]. Although these studies did not support the positive effects from exposure reported by others, they provided possible explanations for the apparent lack of agreement.

Other research groups have also examined the effects of cell phone radiation on the central nervous system, including Borbely et al. [124], Huber et al. [125], Loughran et al. [126], and D'Costa et al. [127], who found changes in sleep EEG patterns and other measures during or after short-term exposures, while others, such as Fritzer et al. [128], who studied exposures for longer time periods, found no changes in sleep parameters, EEG power spectra, correlation dimension nor cognitive function. The work of Pritchard [129] served as the basis to examine correlation dimensions, which is opening a potentially fertile avenue for investigation. Although this approach provides more in depth information on ongoing processes and function, it has not yet been used to address potential consequences associated with long-term cell phone use.

The papers published in the 1960s through 1991, described in earlier sections of this paper, foreshadowed the more recent publications in 1999 through 2008 showing response time changes or associated measures in human subjects during exposure to cell phone-generated radiation. It is unfortunate that essentially none of the earlier studies was acknowledged in these recent reports on cognition, reaction time, and other measures of central nervous system processes. Without guidance from this extensive earlier work, particularly those demonstrating the variety of exposure parameter spaces that must be controlled to produce repeatable experiments, the development of the mechanistic bases for nonthermal effects from EMF exposures will be substantially delayed. The omission of the recognition of the exposure conditions that affect the biological outcomes continues as recently as the National Academy of Science 2009 publication [130] of future directions for research, which emphasizes the modest perspective in the results from committee members working at the limits of expertise, as anticipated by Slovic [100].

Let us hope that subsequent national and international committees that consider future directions for EMF research include members who have performed and reported nonthermal effects in order to provide a broader perspective to develop programs that will more expeditiously address potential health problems as well as to provide guidance to industry on prudent procedures to establish for their technologies.

At present, we are left with a recommendation voiced in 1989 by Abelson [131] in an editorial in Science Magazine that addressed electric power-specific EMF, but is applicable to higher frequency EMF as well, to "adopt a prudent avoidance strategy" by "adopting those which look to be 'prudent' investments given their cost and our current level of scientific understanding about possible risks."

2.10 CONCLUSIONS

There is substantial scientific evidence that some modulated fields (pulsed or repeated signals) are bioactive, which increases the likelihood that they could have health impacts with chronic exposure even at very low exposure levels. Modulation signals may interfere with normal, nonlinear biological processes. Modulation is a fundamental factor that should be taken into account in new public safety standards; at present it is not even a contributing factor. To properly evaluate the biological and health impacts of exposure to modulated RFR (carrier waves), it is also essential to study the impact of the modulating signal (lower frequency fields or ELF-modulated RF). Current standards have ignored modulation as a factor in human health impacts, and thus are inadequate in the protection of the public in terms of chronic exposure to some forms of ELF-modulated RF signals. The current Institute of Electrical and Electronic Engineers (IEEE) and International Commission on Non-Ionizing Radiation Protection (ICNIRP) standards are not sufficiently protective of public health with respect to chronic exposure to modulated fields (particularly new technologies that are pulse-modulated and heavily used in cellular telephony). The collective papers on modulation appear to be omitted from consideration in the recent World Health Organization (WHO) and IEEE science reviews. This body of research has been ignored by current standard setting bodies that rely only on traditional energy-based (thermal) concepts. More laboratory as opposed to epidemiological research is needed to determine which modulation factors and combinations are bioactive and deleterious at low intensities, and are likely to result in disease-related processes and/or health risks; however, this should not delay preventative actions supporting public health and wellness. If signals need to be modulated in the development of new wireless technologies, for example, it makes sense to use what existing scientific information is available to avoid the most obviously deleterious exposure parameters and select others that may be less likely to interfere with normal biological processes in life. The current membership on Risk Assessment committees needs to be made more inclusive by adding scientists experienced with producing nonthermal biological effects. The current practice of segregating scientific investigations (and resulting public health limits) by artificial, engineering-based divisions of frequency needs to be changed because this approach dramatically dilutes the impact of the basic science results and eliminates consideration of modulation signals, thereby reducing and distorting the weight of evidence in any evaluation process.

REFERENCES

1. National Council for Radiation Protection and Measurements, Biological Effects and Exposure Criteria for Radiofrequency Electromagnetic Fields, National Council for Radiation Protection and Measurements, 1986, 400 pp.
2. J. Hamer, Effects of low level, low frequency electric fields on human reaction time, *Communications in Behavioral Biology* 2(5 part A), 1968, 217–222.
3. R.J. Gavalas, D.O. Walter, J. Hamer, W.R. Adey, Effect of low-level, low-frequency electric fields on eeg and behavior in macaca nemestrina, *Brain Research* 18(3), 1970, 491–501.
4. R. Gavalas-Medici, S.R. Day-Magdaleno, Extremely low frequency, weak electric fields affect schedule-controlled behaviour of monkeys, *Nature* 261(5557), 1976, 256–259.
5. L.K. Kaczmarek, W.R. Adey, The efflux of 45ca2+ and (3 h)gamma-aminobutyric acid from cate cerebral cortex, *Brain Research* 63, 1973, 331–342.
6. L.K. Kaczmarek, W.R. Adey, Weak electric gradients change ionic and transmitter fluxes in cortex, *Brain Research* 66(3), 1974, 537–540.
7. S.M. Bawin, L.K. Kaczmarek, W.R. Adey, Effects of modulated vhf fields on the central nervous system, *Annals of the New York Academy of Sciences* 247, 1975, 74–81.
8. S.M. Bawin, W.R. Adey, Sensitivity of calcium binding in cerebral tissue to weak environmental electric fields oscillating at low frequency, *Proceedings of the National Academy of Sciences of the United States of America* 73(6), 1976, 1999–2003.
9. S.M. Bawin, W.R. Adey, I.M. Sabbot, Ionic factors in release of 45ca2+ from chicken cerebral tissue by electromagnetic fields, *Proceedings of the National Academy of Sciences of the United States of America* 75(12), 1978, 6314–6318.
10. S.M. Bawin, A.R. Sheppard, W.R. Adey, Possible mechanism of weak electromagnetic field coupling in brain tissue, *Bioelectrochemistry & Bioenergetics* 5, 1978, 67–76.
11. A.R. Sheppard, S.M. Bawin, W.R. Adey, Models of long-range order in cerebral macromolecules: Effects of sub-elf and of modulated vhf and uhf fields, *Radio Science* 14(6S), 1979, 141–145.
12. C.F. Blackman, J.A. Elder, C.M. Weil, S.G. Benane, D.C. Eichinger, D.E. House, Induction of calcium ion efflux from brain tissue by radio-frequency radiation: Effects of modulation-frequency and field strength, *Radio Science* 14(6S), 1979, 93–98.
13. C.F. Blackman, S.G. Benane, J.A. Elder, D.E. House, J.A. Lampe, J.M. Faulk, Induction of calcium-ion efflux from brain tissue by radiofrequency radiation: Effect of sample number and modulation frequency on the power-density window, *Bioelectromagnetics* 1(1), 1980, 35–43.

14. C.F. Blackman, The biological influences of low-frequency sinusoidal electromagnetic signals alone and superimposed on rf carrier waves, in: A. Chiabrera, C. Nicolini, H.P. Schwan (Eds.), *Interaction between Electromagnetic Fields and Cells*, Erice, Italy, Plenum, New York, 1984, North Atlantic Treaty Organization Advanced Study Institute (NATO ASI) Series A97, pp. 521–535.
15. C.F. Blackman, S.G. Benane, D.J. Elliott, D.E. House, M.M. Pol-lock, Influence of electromagnetic fields on the efflux of calcium ions from brain tissue *in vitro*: A three-model analysis consistent with the frequency response up to 510 hz, *Bioelectromagnetics* 9(3), 1988, 215–227.
16. C.F. Blackman, S.G. Benane, W.T. Joines, M.A. Hollis, D.E. House, Calcium-ion efflux from brain tissue: Power-density versus internal field-intensity dependencies at 50-mhz rf radiation, *Bioelectromagnetics* 1(3), 1980, 277–283.
17. C.F. Blackman, S.G. Benane, L.S. Kinney, W.T. Joines, D.E. House, Effects of elf fields on calcium-ion efflux from brain tissue *in vitro*, *Radiation Research* 92(3), 1982, 510–520.
18. C.F. Blackman, S.G. Benane, J.R. Rabinowitz, D.E. House, W.T. Joines, A role for the magnetic field in the radiation-induced efflux of calcium ions from brain tissue *in vitro*, *Bioelectromagnetics* 6(4), 1985, 327–337.
19. C.F. Blackman, D.E. House, S.G. Benane, W.T. Joines, R.J. Spiegel, Effect of ambient levels of power-line-frequency electric fields on a developing vertebrate, *Bioelectromagnetics* 9(2), 1988, 129–140.
20. C.F. Blackman, W.T. Joines, J.A. Elder, Calcium-ion efflux in brain tissue by radiofrequency radiation, in: K.H. Illinger (Ed.), *Biological Effects of Nonionizing Radiation*, vol. 157, American Chemical Society, Washington, DC, 1981, pp. 299–314.
21. C.F. Blackman, S.G. Benane, D.E. House, D.J. Elliott, Importance of alignment between local dc magnetic field and an oscillating magnetic field in responses of brain tissue *in vitro* and *in vivo*, *Bioelectromagnetics* 11(2), 1990, 159–167.
22. C.F. Blackman, L.S. Kinney, D.E. House, W.T. Joines, Multiple power-density windows and their possible origin, *Bioelectromagnetics* 10(2), 1989, 115–128.
23. W.T. Joines, C.F. Blackman, Equalizing the electric field intensity within chick brain immersed in buffer solution at different carrier frequencies, *Bioelectromagnetics* 2(4), 1981, 411–413.
24. W.T. Joines, C.F. Blackman, M.A. Hollis, Broadening of the rf power-density window for calcium-ion efflux from brain tissue, *IEEE Transactions on Bio-Medical Engineering* 28(8), 1981, 568–573.
25. W.T. Joines, C.F. Blackman, R.J. Spiegel, Specific absorption rate in electrically coupled biological samples between metal plates, *Bioelectromagnetics* 7(2), 1986, 163–176.
26. S.K. Dutta, K. Das, B. Ghosh, C.F. Blackman, Dose dependence of acetylcholinesterase activity in neuroblastoma cells exposed to modulated radio-frequency electromagnetic radiation, *Bioelectromagnetics* 13(4), 1992, 317–322.
27. S.K. Dutta, B. Ghosh, C.F. Blackman, Radiofrequency radiation-induced calcium ion efflux enhancement from human and other neuroblastoma cells in culture, *Bioelectromagnetics* 10(2), 1989, 197–202.
28. S.K. Dutta, A. Subramoniam, B. Ghosh, R. Parshad, Microwave radiation-induced calcium ion efflux from human neuroblastoma cells in culture, *Bioelectromagnetics* 5(1), 1984, 71–78.
29. S.K. Dutta, M. Verma, C.F. Blackman, Frequency-dependent alterations in enolase activity in escherichia coli caused by exposure to electric and magnetic fields, *Bioelectromagnetics* 15(5), 1994, 377–383.
30. E. Albert, C. Blackman, F. Slaby, Calcium dependent secretory protein release and calcium efflux during rf irradiation of rat pancreatic tissue slices, in: A.J. Berteaud, B. Servantie (Eds.), *Ondes Electromagnetiques et Biologie, URSI International Symposium*

on Electromagnetic Waves and Biology, June 30–July 4. Jouy-en-Josas, France, Centre National de la Recherche Scientifique, 2 rue Henry Dunant, 94320 Thiais, France: A.J. Berteaud, 1980, pp. 325–329.
31. J.L. Schwartz, D.E. House, G.A. Mealing, Exposure of frog hearts to cw or amplitude-modulated vhf fields: Selective efflux of calcium ions at 16 hz, *Bioelectromagnetics* 11(4), 1990, 349–358.
32. J.L. Schwartz, G.A. Mealing, Calcium-ion movement and contractility in atrial strips of frog heart are not affected by low-frequency-modulated, 1 ghz electromagnetic radiation, *Bioelectromagnetics* 14(6), 1993, 521–533.
33. C.F. Blackman, Can EMF exposure during development leave an imprint later in life? *Electromagnetic Biology and Medicine* 25(4), 2006, 217–225.
34. C.J. Thompson, Y.S. Yang, V. Anderson, A.W. Wood, A cooperative model for ca(++) efflux windowing from cell membranes exposed to electromagnetic radiation, *Bioelectromagnetics* 21(6), 2000, 455–464.
35. W.T. Joines, C.F. Blackman, Power density, field intensity, and carrier frequency determinants of rf-energy-induced calcium-ion efflux from brain tissue, *Bioelectromagnetics* 1(3), 1980, 271–275.
36. A.R. Liboff, Cyclotron resonance in membrane transport, in: A. Chiabrera, C. Nicolini, H.P. Schwan (Eds.), *Interaction between Electromagnetic Fields and Cells*, Erice, Italy, Plenum, New York, 1984, North Atlantic Treaty Organization Advanced Study Institute (NATO ASI) Series A97, pp. 281–296.
37. T.A. Litovitz, D. Krause, C.J. Montrose, J.M. Mullins, Temporally incoherent magnetic fields mitigate the response of biological systems to temporally coherent magnetic fields, *Bioelectromagnetics* 15(5), 1994, 399–409.
38. J.M. Farrell, M. Barber, D. Krause, T.A. Litovitz, The superposition of a temporally incoherent magnetic field inhibits 60 hz-induced changes in the odc activity of developing chick embryos, *Bioelectromagnetics* 19(1), 1998, 53–56.
39. T.A. Litovitz, C.J. Montrose, P. Doinov, K.M. Brown, M. Bar-ber, Superimposing spatially coherent electromagnetic noise inhibits field-induced abnormalities in developing chick embryos, *Bioelectromagnetics* 15(2), 1994, 105–113.
40. T.A. Litovitz, L.M. Penafiel, J.M. Farrel, D. Krause, R. Meister, J.M. Mullins, Bioeffects induced by exposure to microwaves are mitigated by superposition of elf noise, *Bioelectromagnetics* 18(6), 1997, 422–430.
41. S. Milham, L.L. Morgan, A new electromagnetic exposure metric: High frequency voltage transients associated with increased cancer incidence in teachers in a california school, *American Journal of Industrial Medicine* 51(8), 2008, 579–586.
42. M. Havas, Electromagnetic hypersensitivity: Biological effects of dirty electricity with emphasis on diabetes and multiple sclerosis, *Electromagnetic Biology and Medicine* 25(4), 2006, 259–268.
43. M. Havas, Dirty electricity elevates blood sugar among electrically sensitive diabetics and may explain brittle diabetes, *Electromagnetic Biology and Medicine* 27(2), 2008, 135–146.
44. M. Havas, A. Olstad, Power quality affects teacher wellbeing and student behavior in three Minnesota schools, *The Science of the Total Environment* 402(2–3), 2008, 157–162.
45. C.F. Blackman, S.G. Benane, D.E. House, Frequency-dependent interference by magnetic fields of nerve growth factor-induced neurite outgrowth in pc-12 cells, *Bioelectromagnetics* 16(6), 1995, 387–395.
46. C.F. Blackman, J.P. Blanchard, S.G. Benane, D.E. House, Experimental determination of hydrogen bandwidth for the ion parametric resonance model, *Bioelectromagnetics* 20(1), 1999, 5–12.
47. M.A. Trillo, A. Ubeda, J.P. Blanchard, D.E. House, C.F. Blackman, Magnetic fields at resonant conditions for the hydrogen ion affect neurite outgrowth in pc-12 cells: A test of the ion parametric resonance model, *Bioelectromagnetics* 17(1), 1996, 10–20.

48. L. Slesin, Highlights: Elf bioeffects studies at bems, *Microwave News* IV(Sept. 7), 1984, 2.
49. S.D. Smith, B.R. McLeod, A.R. Liboff, K. Cooksey, Calcium cyclotron resonance and diatom mobility, *Bioelectromagnetics* 8(3), 1987, 215–227.
50. J.R. Thomas, J. Schrot, A.R. Liboff, Low-intensity magnetic fields alter operant behavior in rats, *Bioelectromagnetics* 7(4), 1986, 349–357.
51. A.R. Liboff, B.R. McLeod, Kinetics of channelized membrane ions in magnetic fields, *Bioelectromagnetics* 9(1), 1988, 39–51.
52. A.R. Liboff, W.C. Parkinson, Search for ion-cyclotron resonance in an na(+)-transport system, *Bioelectromagnetics* 12(2), 1991, 77–83.
53. C.F. Blackman, J.P. Blanchard, S.G. Benane, D.E. House, Effect of ac and dc magnetic field orientation on nerve cells, *Biochemical and Biophysical Research Communications* 220(3), 1996, 807–811.
54. A.R. Liboff, Electric-field ion cyclotron resonance, *Bioelectromagnetics* 18(1), 1997, 85–87.
55. V.V. Lednev, Possible mechanism for the influence of weak magnetic fields on biological systems, *Bioelectromagnetics* 12(2), 1991, 71–75.
56. J.P. Blanchard, C.F. Blackman, Clarification and application of an ion parametric resonance model for magnetic field interactions with biological systems, *Bioelectromagnetics* 15(3), 1994, 217–238.
57. M.N. Zhadin, E.E. Fesenko, Ionic cyclotron resonance in biomolecules, *Biomedical Science* 1(3), 1990, 245–250.
58. E. Del Giudice, M. Fleischmann, G. Preparata, G. Talpo, On the "Unreasonable" Effects of elf magnetic fields upon a system of ions, *Bioelectromagnetics* 23(7), 2002, 522–530.
59. V.N. Binhi, Stochastic dynamics of magnetosomes and a mechanism of biological orientation in the geomagnetic field, *Bioelectromagnetics* 27(1), 2006, 58–63.
60. V.N. Binhi, A few remarks on 'combined action of dc and ac magnetic fields on ion motion in a macromolecule,' *Bioelectromagnetics* 28(5), 2007, 409–412, discussion 412–404.
61. V.N. Binhi, A.B. Rubin, Magnetobiology: The kt paradox and possible solutions, *Electromagnetic Biology and Medicine* 26(1), 2007, 45–62.
62. V.N. Binhi, A.V. Savin, Molecular gyroscopes and biological effects of weak extremely low-frequency magnetic fields, *Physical Review* 65(5 Pt 1), 2002, 519.
63. A.Y. Matronchik, I.Y. Belyaev, Mechanism for combined action of microwaves and static magnetic field: Slow non uniform rotation of charged nucleoid, *Electromagnetic Biology and Medicine* 27(4), 2008, 340–354.
64. M.N. Zhadin, Combined action of static and alternating magnetic fields on ion motion in a macromolecule: Theoretical aspects, *Bioelectromagnetics* 19(5), 1998, 279–292.
65. M.N. Zhadin, V.V. Novikov, F.S. Barnes, N.F. Pergola, Combined action of static and alternating magnetic fields on ionic current in aqueous glutamic acid solution, *Bioelectromagnetics* 19(1), 1998, 41–45.
66. V.V. Vorobyov, E.A. Sosunov, N.I. Kukushkin, V.V. Lednev, Weak combined magnetic field affects basic and morphine-induced rat's eeg, *Brain Research* 781(1–2), 1998, 182–187.
67. C.L. Baureus Koch, M. Sommarin, B.R. Persson, L.G. Salford, J.L. Eberhardt, Interaction between weak low frequency magnetic fields and cell membranes, *Bioelectromagnetics* 24(6), 2003, 395–402.
68. R. Sarimov, E. Markova, F. Johansson, D. Jenssen, I. Belyaev, Exposure to elf magnetic field tuned to zn inhibits growth of cancer cells, *Bioelectromagnetics* 26(8), 2005, 631–638.
69. F.S. Prato, M. Kavaliers, J.J. Carson, Behavioural evidence that magnetic field effects in the land snail, cepaea nemoralis, might not depend on magnetite or induced electric currents, *Bioelectromagnetics* 17(2), 1996, 123–130.

70. F.S. Prato, M. Kavaliers, A.P. Cullen, A.W. Thomas, Light-dependent and -independent behavioral effects of extremely low frequency magnetic fields in a land snail are consistent with a parametric resonance mechanism, *Bioelectromagnetics* 18(3), 1997, 284–291.
71. N. Comisso, E. Del Giudice, A. De Ninno, M. Fleischmann, L. Giuliani, G. Mengoli, F. Merlo, G. Talpo, Dynamics of the ion cyclotron resonance effect on amino acids adsorbed at the interfaces, *Bioelectromagnetics* 27(1), 2006, 16–25.
72. V.V. Novikov, I.M. Sheiman, E.E. Fesenko, Effect of weak static and low-frequency alternating magnetic fields on the fission and regeneration of the planarian dugesia (girardia) tigrina, *Bioelectromagnetics* 29(5), 2008, 387–393.
73. C.F. Blackman, B. Most, A scheme for incorporating dc magnetic fields into epidemiological studies of EMF exposure, *Bioelectromagnetics* 14(5), 1993, 413–431.
74. M.T. Marron, E.M. Goodman, P.T. Sharpe, B. Greenebaum, Low frequency electric and magnetic fields have different effects on the cell surface, *FEBS Letters* 230(1–2), 1988, 13–16.
75. R.P. Liburdy, Calcium signaling in lymphocytes and elf fields. Evidence for an electric field metric and a site of interaction involving the calcium ion channel, *FEBS Letters* 301(1), 1992, 53–59.
76. J.J. Greene, W.J. Skowronski, J.M. Mullins, R.M. Nardone, M. Penafiel, R. Meister, Delineation of electric and magnetic field effects of extremely low frequency electromagnetic radiation on transcription, *Biochemical and Biophysical Research Communications* 174(2), 1991, 742–749.
77. C.F. Blackman, S.G. Benane, D.E. House, Evidence for direct effect of magnetic fields on neurite outgrowth, *FASEB J* 7(9), 1993, 801–806.
78. C.F. Blackman, S.G. Benane, D.E. House, M.M. Pollock, Action of 50 hz magnetic fields on neurite outgrowth in pheochromocytoma cells, *Bioelectromagnetics* 14(3), 1993, 273–286.
79. A. Chiabrera, M. Hinsenkamp, A.A. Pilla, J. Ryaby, D. Ponta, A. Belmont, F. Beltrame, M. Grattarola, C. Nicolini, Cytofluorometry of electromagnetically controlled cell dedifferentiation, *The Journal of Histochemistry and Cytochemistry* 27(1), 1979, 375–381.
80. M.R. Scarfi, F. Prisco, M.B. Lioi, O. Zeni, M. Della Noce, R. Di Pietro, C. Fanceschi, D. Iafusco, M. Motta, F. Bersani, Cytogenetic effects induced by extremely low frequency pulsed magnetic fields in lymphocytes from Turner's syndrome subjects, *Bioelectrochemistry & Bioenergetics* 43, 1997, 221–226.
81. M.R. Scarfi, M.B. Lioi, O. Zeni, G. Franceschetti, C. Franceschi, F. Bersani, Lack of chromosomal aberration and micronucleus induction in human lymphocytes exposed to pulsed magnetic fields, *Mutation Research* 306(2), 1994, 129–133.
82. K. Takahashi, I. Kaneko, M. Date, E. Fukada, Effect of pulsing electromagnetic fields on DNA synthesis in mammalian cells in culture, *Experientia* 42(2), 1986, 185–186.
83. A. Ubeda, J. Leal, M.A. Trillo, M.A. Jimenez, J.M. Delgado, Pulse shape of magnetic fields influences chick embryogenesis, *Journal of Anatomy* 137(Pt 3), 1983, 513–536.
84. A. Chiabrera, B. Bianco, E. Moggia, J.J. Kaufman, Zeeman-stark modeling of the rf EMF interaction with ligand binding, *Bioelectromagnetics* 21(4), 2000, 312–324.
85. A.A. Marino, R.M. Wolcott, R. Chervenak, F. Jourd'Heuil, E. Nilsen, C. Frilot 2nd, Nonlinear response of the immune system to power-frequency magnetic fields, *American Journal of Physiology* 279(3), 2000, R761–768.
86. A.A. Marino, R.M. Wolcott, R. Chervenak, F. Jourd'heuil, E. Nilsen, C. Frilot 2nd, Nonlinear determinism in the immune system. In vivo influence of electromagnetic fields on different functions of murine lymphocyte subpopulations, *Immunological Investigations* 30(4), 2001, 313–334.

87. A.A. Marino, R.M. Wolcott, R. Chervenak, F. Jourd'heuil, E. Nilsen, C. Frilot 2nd, Nonlinear dynamical law governs magnetic field induced changes in lymphoid phenotype, *Bioelectromagnetics* 22(8), 2001, 529–546.
88. A.A. Marino, R.M. Wolcott, R. Chervenak, F. Jourd'heuil, E. Nilsen, C. Frilot 2nd, S.B. Pruett, Coincident nonlinear changes in the endocrine and immune systems due to low-frequency magnetic fields, *Neuroimmunomodulation* 9(2), 2001, 65–77.
89. A.A. Marino, E. Nilsen, A.L. Chesson Jr., C. Frilot, Effect of low-frequency magnetic fields on brain electrical activity in human subjects, *Clinical Neurophysiology* 115(5), 2004, 1195–1201.
90. A.A. Marino, E. Nilsen, C. Frilot, Localization of electroreceptive function in rabbits, *Physiology & Behavior* 79(4–5), 2003, 803–810.
91. A.A. Marino, E. Nilsen, C. Frilot, Nonlinear changes in brain electrical activity due to cell phone radiation, *Bioelectromagnetics* 24(5), 2003, 339–346.
92. A.A. Marino, E. Nilsen, C. Frilot, Consistent magnetic-field induced dynamical changes in rabbit brain activity detected by recurrence quantification analysis, *Brain Research* 964(2), 2003, 317–326.
93. O.V. Kolomytkin, S. Dunn, F.X. Hart, C. Frilot 2nd, D. Kolomytkin, A.A. Marino, Glycoproteins bound to ion channels mediate detection of electric fields: A proposed mechanism and supporting evidence, *Bioelectromagnetics* 28(5), 2007, 379–385.
94. S. Carrubba, C. Frilot, A. Chesson, A.A. Marino, Detection of non-linear event-related potentials, *Journal of Neuroscience Methods* 157(1), 2006, 39–47.
95. S. Carrubba, C. Frilot, A.L. Chesson, A.A. Marino, Nonlinear eeg activation evoked by low-strength low-frequency magnetic fields, *Neuroscience Letters* 417(2), 2007, 212–216.
96. S. Carrubba, C. Frilot 2nd, A.L. Chesson Jr., A.A. Marino, Evidence of a nonlinear human magnetic sense, *Neuroscience* 144(1), 2007, 356–367.
97. S. Carrubba, C. Frilot, A.L. Chesson Jr., A.A. Marino, Method for detection of changes in the eeg induced by the presence of sensory stimuli, *Journal of Neuroscience Methods* 173(1), 2008, 41–46.
98. S. Carrubba, C. Frilot, A.L. Chesson Jr., C.L. Webber Jr., J.P. Zbilut, A.A. Marino, Magnetosensory evoked potentials: Consistent nonlinear phenomena, *Neuroscience Research* 60(1), 2008, 95–105.
99. M.N. Zhadin, O.N. Deryugina, T.M. Pisachenko, Influence of combined dc and ac magnetic fields on rat behavior, *Bioelectromagnetics* 20(6), 1999, 378–386.
100. P. Slovic, Trust, emotion, sex, politics, and science: Surveying the risk-assessment battlefield, *Risk Analysis* 19(4), 1999, 689–701.
101. M. Havas, Biological effects of non-ionizing electromagnetic energy: A critical review of the reports by the US national research council and the us national institute of environmental health sciences as they relate to the broad realm of EMF bioeffects, *Environmental Reviews* 8, 2000, 173–253.
102. National Research Council (U.S.), *Committee on the Possible Effects of Electromagnetic Fields on Biologic Systems*, National Academy Press, Washington, DC, 1997, 356 pp.
103. National Institute of Environmental Health Science Working Group Report, *Assessment of health effects from exposure to power-line frequencyelectric and magnetic fields*, 1998, NIH Pub 98-3981, 508 pp.
104. National Institute of Environmental Health Science, Report on health effects from exposure to power-line frequency electric and magnetic fields, NIH Pub No 99-4493, 1999, 67 pp.
105. M. Fedrowitz, K. Kamino, W. Loscher, Significant differences in the effects of magnetic field exposure on 7, 12-dimethylbenz(a)anthracene-induced mammary carcinogenesis in two substrains of sprague-dawley rats, *Cancer Research* 64(1), 2004, 243–251.

106. M. Fedrowitz, W. Loscher, Power frequency magnetic fields increase cell proliferation in the mammary gland of female fischer 344 rats but not various other rat strains or substrains, *Oncology* 69(6), 2005, 486–498.
107. Y. Yang, X. Jin, C. Yan, Y. Tian, J. Tang, X. Shen, Case-only study of interactions between DNA repair genes (hmlh1, apex1, mgmt, xrcc1 and xpd) and low-frequency electromagnetic fields in childhood acute leukemia, *Leukemia & Lymphoma* 49(12), 2008, 2344–2350.
108. S.M. Bawin, R.J. Gavalas-Medici, W.R. Adey, Effects of modulated very high frequency fields on specific brain rhythms in cats, *Brain Research* 58(2), 1973, 365–384.
109. A.W. Preece, G. Iwi, A. Davies-Smith, K. Wesnes, S. Butler, E. Lim, A. Varey, Effect of a 915-mhz simulated mobile phone signal on cognitive function in man, *International Journal of Radiation Biology* 75(4), 1999, 447–456.
110. A.W. Preece, K.A. Wesnes, G.R. Iwi, The effect of a 50 hz magnetic field on cognitive function in humans, *International Journal of Radiation Biology* 74(4), 1998, 463–470.
111. M. Koivisto, C.M. Krause, A. Revonsuo, M. Laine, H. Hamalainen, The effects of electromagnetic field emitted by gsm phones on working memory, *Neuroreport* 11(8), 2000, 1641–1643.
112. M. Koivisto, A. Revonsuo, C. Krause, C. Haarala, L. Sillanmaki, M. Laine, H. Hamalainen, Effects of 902 mhz electromagnetic field emitted by cellular telephones on response times in humans, *Neuroreport* 11(2), 2000, 413–415.
113. C.M. Krause, L. Sillanmaki, M. Koivisto, A. Haggqvist, C. Saarela, A. Revonsuo, M. Laine, H. Hamalainen, Effects of electromagnetic field emitted by cellular phones on the eeg during a memory task, *Neuroreport* 11(4), 2000, 761–764.
114. C.M. Krause, L. Sillanmaki, M. Koivisto, A. Haggqvist, C. Saarela, A. Revonsuo, M. Laine, H. Hamalainen, Effects of electromagnetic fields emitted by cellular phones on the electroencephalogram during a visual working memory task, *International Journal of Radiation Biology* 76(12), 2000, 1659–1667.
115. G. Freude, P. Ullsperger, S. Eggert, I. Ruppe, Effects of microwaves emitted by cellular phones on human slow brain potentials, *Bioelectromagnetics* 19(6), 1998, 384–387.
116. G. Freude, P. Ullsperger, S. Eggert, I. Ruppe, Microwaves emitted by cellular telephones affect human slow brain potentials, *European journal of Applied Physiology* 81(1–2), 2000, 18–27.
117. A.W. Preece, S. Goodfellow, M.G. Wright, S.R. Butler, E.J. Dunn, Y. Johnson, T.C. Manktelow, K. Wesnes, Effect of 902 mhz mobile phone transmission on cognitive function in children, *Bioelectromagnetics* 26(Suppl. 7), 2005, S138–143.
118. C.M. Krause, C.H. Bjornberg, M. Pesonen, A. Hulten, T. Liesivuori, M. Koivisto, A. Revonsuo, M. Laine, H. Hamalainen, Mobile phone effects on children's event-related oscillatory eeg during an auditory memory task, *International Journal of Radiation Biology* 82(6), 2006, 443–450.
119. C.M. Krause, M. Pesonen, C. Haarala Bjornberg, H. Hamalainen, Effects of pulsed and continuous wave 902 mhz mobile phone exposure on brain oscillatory activity during cognitive processing, *Bioelectromagnetics* 28(4), 2007, 296–308.
120. C. Haarala, L. Bjornberg, M. Ek, M. Laine, A. Revonsuo, M. Koivisto, Emitted by mobile phones on human cognitive function: A replication study, *Bioelectromagnetics* 24(4), 2003, 283–288.
121. C. Haarala, M. Ek, L. Bjornberg, M. Laine, A. Revonsuo, M. Koivisto, H. Hamalainen, 902 mhz mobile phone does not affect short term memory in humans, *Bioelectromagnetics* 25(6), 2004, 452–456.
122. C. Haarala, M. Bergman, M. Laine, A. Revonsuo, M. Koivisto, H. Hamalainen, Electromagnetic field emitted by 902 mhz mobile phones shows no effects on children's cognitive function, *Bioelectromagnetics* 26(Suppl. 7), 2005, S144–150.

123. C. Haarala, F. Takio, T. Rintee, M. Laine, M. Koivisto, A. Revonsuo, H. Hamalainen, Pulsed and continuous wave mobile phone exposure over left versus right hemisphere: Effects on human cognitive function, *Bioelectromagnetics* 28(4), 2007, 289–295.
124. A.A. Borbely, R. Huber, T. Graf, B. Fuchs, E. Gallmann, P. Achermann, Pulsed high-frequency electromagnetic field affects human sleep and sleep electroencephalogram, *Neuroscience Letters* 275(3), 1999, 207–210.
125. R. Huber, J. Schuderer, T. Graf, K. Jutz, A.A. Borbely, N. Kuster, P. Achermann, Radio frequency electromagnetic field exposure in humans: Estimation of sar distribution in the brain, effects on sleep and heart rate, *Bioelectromagnetics* 24(4), 2003, 262–276.
126. S.P. Loughran, A.W. Wood, J.M. Barton, R.J. Croft, B. Thompson, C. Stough, The effect of electromagnetic fields emitted by mobile phones on human sleep, *Neuroreport* 16(17), 2005, 1973–1976.
127. H. D'Costa, G. Truemann, L. Tang, U. Abdel-rahman, W. Abdelrahman, K. Ong, I. Cosic, Human brain wave activity during exposure to radiofrequency field emissions from mobile phones, *Australasian Physical & Engineering Sciences in Medicine* 26, 2003, 162–167.
128. G. Fritzer, R. Goder, L. Friege, J. Wachter, V. Hansen, D. Hinze-Selch, J.B. Aldenhoff, Effects of short-and long-term pulsed radiofrequency electromagnetic fields on night sleep and cognitive functions in healthy subjects, *Bioelectromagnetics* 28(4), 2007, 316–325.
129. W.S. Pritchard, D.W. Duke, Measuring chaos in the brain: A tutorial review of nonlinear dynamical eeg analysis, *The International Journal of Neuroscience* 67(1–4), 1992, 31–80.
130. National Academy of Science: Identification of Research Needs Relating to Potential Biological or Adverse Health Effects of Wireless Communication, Washington, DC, 2009, http://www.nap.edu/catalog/12036.html.
131. P.H. Abelson, Effects of electric and magnetic fields, *Science* 245(4915), 1989, 241. Doi: 10.1126/science.245.4915.241.

3 Public Exposure to Radio Frequency Electromagnetic Fields

Peter Gajšek

CONTENTS

3.1 INTRODUCTION

The increasing use of various wireless devices and development of new telecommunication technologies has resulted in a fundamental change of radio frequency electromagnetic fields (RF-EMF) exposure in the everyday environment. In the last three decades, a large number of scientific studies on the exposure assessment of the general public to RF-EMF in different environments were completed. The results of numerous exposure assessment studies come to almost the same conclusions: that public RF-EMF exposures in different micro environments are only a small fraction of existing RF exposure standards.

In particular due to the continuous introduction of new technologies which enable faster data transfers, mobile telephony base stations are being introduced in our living environment. In addition to mobile telephony, other wireless systems, such as Wi-Fi, broadband Worldwide Interoperability for Microwave Access (WiMAX) or Digital Video Broadcasting-Terrestrial (DVB-T) digital TV, are being upgraded or implemented. The exposure from sources such as base stations, Wi-Fi systems, radio or TV, and microwave links, is considered much lower than from mobile phones. For instance, wireless systems typically emit ten times less peak power than mobile phones (0.1–0.2 W). Mobile phones use low power transmitters that are less than 2 W at peak. But the typical output power of a mobile phone ranges from 0.01 to 0.1 W, which takes into account the operation of adaptive power control.

Furthermore, the overall increase of the use of these systems implies a potentially higher exposure level. Thus, it is necessary to have a better knowledge of the real exposure pattern, taking into account all existing sources.

3.2 RF-EMF EXPOSURE ASSESSMENT

So far, various efforts have been made to determine the exposure of the general public to RF-EMFs due to broadcasting, wireless networks, and different RF-EMF emitting systems and devices in our daily environments. Different methods of exposure assessment have been used for RF-EMF including: characterization of exposure to RF-EMF based on activities and sources, personal exposure assessment, and spot or long-term RF-EMF measurements. This chapter is focused solely on personal exposure assessment and spot or long-term measurements in different environments that gained significant attention in the scientific community.

3.2.1 Personal Exposure Assessment

Although there have been considerable advances in exposure assessment in epidemiological studies carried out in recent years, further development of methods and techniques in this field remains key for the improvement of epidemiological studies investigating the effects of electromagnetic fields. Poorly characterized exposure reduces the conclusiveness of epidemiological studies, increasing the degree of uncertainty in risk estimates. Because people move, personal exposure assessment requires mobile measurements with a portable device (*personal monitor—PM*). This approach takes into consideration the behavior of individuals. All sources (fixed installations, mobile devices, indoor, outdoor) can be included. However, exposure from equipment used close to the body (Digital Enhanced Cordless Telecommunications [DECT], mobile phones, and other wireless consumer goods) cannot yet be reliably assessed. The statistical significance of personal exposure data strongly depends on the number of persons included in a measurement campaign.

The uncertainty analysis when using a PM is crucial and is mainly influenced by body shielding, residual uncertainties due to calibration, measurement errors due to true root mean square (RMS) response, and measurement artifacts (out-of-band pick-up). In addition, these PM measurements tend to underestimate or overestimate the actual RF-EMF exposure (Bolte et al., 2011; Iskra et al., 2011). A potential solution would be to determine correction factors based on the calibrations in order to correct the measurement results (Thielens et al., 2015). The total uncertainty can reach up to 25 dB (Neubauer et al., 2010). Röösli et al. (2008) have developed a method for estimating the mean field strength based on an assumption of log-normality in the distribution of the data. This regression on order statistics method seems to produce plausible estimates of the mean field exposure even when only a few values are above the detection threshold.

Many personal exposure assessment studies were performed in different micro environments such as schools, offices, homes or outdoor urban areas, to characterize typical personal exposure levels in these places (micro environmental studies) worldwide (Trček et al., 2007; Bolte et al., 2008; Joseph et al., 2008; Thuroczy et al.,

2008; Frei et al., 2009a; Viel et al., 2009a; Urbinello et al., 2014a; Bhatt et al., 2016; Sagar et al., 2018). Some studies were population surveys in which the personal exposure distribution in the population of interest was determined. The strategies for the recruitment of the study participants as well as the data analysis methods differed between these studies, therefore, a direct comparison of their results is rather difficult.

Moreover, Joseph et al. (2010) performed a comparison study among the above mentioned results of RF-EMF measurement campaigns in different urban areas using PMs. The comparison study found that the exposure in all countries was of the same order of magnitude. All studies concluded that wireless communications are the largest source of exposure. In all countries, the mean exposure levels were found to be well below the International Commission on Non-Ionizing Radiation Protection (ICNIRP) exposure guidelines, with the highest exposure levels measured in transport vehicles (trains, cars, and buses).

Another personal measurement campaign was carried out in Germany (Thomas et al., 2008) involving 3022 children and adolescents. Exposure to GSM 900 and GSM 1800 uplink and downlink, DECT phones, and wireless local area network (WLAN) were taken into consideration in the measurements. A 24-hour RF-EMF exposure profile was generated using a PM. The majority of measured exposure values were below the detection limit (0.05 V/m, 82% of the values during waking hours). The overall exposure to RF-EMF in the considered frequency ranges was very low and ranged from a mean of 0.13% (all measurement values below the detection limit) to a mean of 0.92% of the ICNIRP reference level.

In their study, Bolte and Eikelboom (2012) reported that mean personal exposure to electric fields over 24 hours, excluding own mobile phone use, was 0.26 V/m. Daytime exposures were similar, whereas nighttime exposures were about half the magnitude, and evening exposures were approximately double. The main contribution to environmental exposure (calls by participant not included) were calls with mobile phones (37.5%) from cordless DECT phones and their docking stations (31.7%), and from the base stations (12.7%). The mean total exposure largely depends on phone calls of a high exposure level and short duration.

A residential RF-EMF exposure assessment was performed by Breckenkamp et al. (2012) using PMs to measure the electric field in fixed positions in bedrooms in 1348 households in Germany. The measurements were performed in 12 frequency bands from 88 MHz to 2.50 GHz. They found that DECT and Wi-Fi account for more than 80% of the total exposure level and are the most important single-exposure sources. However, mean levels of exposure to these sources were 0.09 V/m. Exposure from mobile phone base stations adds only 6.3% to total exposure with a mean exposure level of 0.03 V/m.

The demands for increased mobile phone signal coverage and signal capacity largely contributed to measured increases in outdoor environmental exposures of 20%–57%. The multicenter study (Urbinello et al., 2014a) compared mean exposure levels in outdoor areas across four different European cities. Measurements using personal monitors were conducted in three different types of outdoor areas (central and noncentral residential areas and downtown). Measurements per urban environment were repeated 12 times during 1 year. Arithmetic mean values for mobile phone base station exposure ranged between 0.22 V/m (Basel) and 0.41 V/m (Amsterdam) in all outdoor areas combined. The 95th percentile for total RF-EMF exposure varied between 0.46 V/m (Basel) and 0.82 V/m (Amsterdam) and the 99th percentile between 0.81 V/m (Basel) and 1.20 V/m (Brussels).

Sagar et al. (2016) have conducted an RF-EMF personal exposure assessment study by walking through 51 different outdoor micro environments in 20 different municipalities in Switzerland. Mean RF-EMF exposure (sum of 15 main frequency bands between 87.5 and 5875 MHz) was 0.53 V/m in industrial zones, 0.47 V/m in city centers, 0.32 V/m in central residential areas, 0.25 V/m in noncentral residential areas, 0.23 V/m in rural centers and rural residential areas, 0.69 V/m in trams, 0.46 V/m in trains, and 0.39 V/m in buses. Major exposure contribution at outdoor locations was from mobile phone base stations (48% for all outdoor areas with respect to the power density scale).

In another review, Sagar et al. (2018) systematically reviewed the 21 published studies in peer review journals on the RF-EMF exposure assessment in different micro environments in Europe. The mean total RF-EMF exposures for spot measurements in "Homes" and "Outdoor" micro environments were 0.29 V/m and 0.54 V/m, respectively. In the personal measurements studies with trained researchers, the mean total RF-EMF exposure was 0.24 V/m in "Home" and 0.76 V/m in "Outdoor" micro environments. In the personal measurement studies with volunteers, the population weighted mean total RF-EMF exposure was 0.16 V/m in "Home" and 0.20 V/m in "Outdoor" micro environments.

Personal exposure data were collected across 34 micro environments located in urban, suburban, and rural areas in Australia and Belgium, and compared with that of similar micro environments in both countries (Bhatt et al., 2016). The personal exposure across urban micro environments was higher than in the rural or suburban micro environments. Likewise, exposure levels across the outdoor micro environments were higher than those for indoor micro environments. The five highest median exposure levels were: city center (0.248 V/m), bus (0.124 V/m), railway station (0.105 V/m), mountain/forest (rural) (0.057 V/m), and train (0.055 V/m) [Australia]; and bicycle (urban) (0.238 V/m), tram station (0.238 V/m), city centre (0.156 V/m), residential outdoor (urban) (0.139 V/m), and park (0.124 V/m) [Belgium]. Exposures in the GSM 900 MHz frequency band across most of the microenvironments in Australia were significantly lower than the exposures across the micro environments in Belgium.

In general, personal exposure assessment studies indicated that mobile phone base stations (downlink signals) are a major source of whole body exposure to RF-EMF. More specifically, mobile phone base stations are a dominant exposure source to the whole body in urban outdoor environments and on public transport.

The dominant source with respect to localized body exposure is, as expected, the mobile phone (uplink signal). Mobile phones are a dominant exposure source to the localized body on public transport (Viel et al., 2009b; Urbinello et al., 2014b; Gajšek et al., 2015; Sagar et al., 2018).

3.2.2 Exposure Assessment of Children: Slovenia Case

A survey of personal exposure to RF-EMF in children/adolescents and their parents, which is a part of a Geronimo European Union (EU) funded project within FP7 programme (7th Framework Programme for Research and Technological Development), was completed in Slovenia. The main focus of the survey was to characterize the levels and range of exposure to RF-EMF in children and their parents and to analyze different activities related to the observed exposure patterns. A recent study of personal RF-EMF exposure included 49 children and one parent per child (total n = 98). Subjects carried portable PMs "ExpoM" for approximately 3 days. The RF personal monitors measured 16 frequency bands between 87.5 MHz and 5.875 GHz, and each band corresponded to a source of RF-EMF with a measurement interval of 4 seconds. We defined 6 general frequency bands named total, DECT, broadcast, uplink, downlink, and Wi-Fi. (Dynamic range: 0.005–5 V/m; True-RMS measurement). The exposure meters also recorded the geographic location using the Global Positioning System (GPS).

The devices were calibrated before the start of the measurements and after the measurements. Additionally, the participants kept a time-activity diary installed as an application on a smartphone provided by the study managers. The smartphone was operating in flight mode to prevent it from influencing the measurements. The diary contained predefined locations categorized into home, school, outdoors, train, bus, car, and various locations. At the end of the personal measurements, the participants filled in a questionnaire about their smartphone use during the measurement days and other potentially exposure relevant factors. This data can later be used to estimate contributions from near field sources to the personal exposure.

The study participants consisted of families who were willing to participate in a personal measurement study and were living in urban as well as in rural areas. The children were between 7 and 16 years old. In Slovenia, 49 pairs of children and parents have been successfully measured. The gender distribution for the children was 23 male and 26 females whereas for the parents 27 were male and 22 females.

The results are presented in six categories as follows:

- *Uplink* (mobile phone handset exposure): uplink frequencies (LTE800 Uplink), (Uplink900), (Uplink1800), (Uplink1900), and (LTE2600 Uplink);
- *Downlink* (mobile phone base station exposure): downlink frequencies (LTE800 Downlink), (Downlink900), (Downlink1800), (Downlink2100), and (LTE2600 Downlink);
- *Broadcasting*: radio spectrum used for broadcasting (FM) and (DVB-T);
- *DECT*; frequency namely (DECT);
- *WLAN* (WLAN; ISM 2.4 GHz), and (WLAN; ISM 5.8 GHz);
- *Total RF-EMF* exposure: sum of mean E of all frequency bands.

Total mean electric field was 0.26 V/m, which is well below the international exposure limit. Exposure from downlink contributed most to the total exposure (46%) followed by broadcasting (32%) and mobile uplink signal (17%). Other signals (DECT, Wi-Fi, Wimax) consistently contributed very little to exposure across all studied cases (less than 2%).

Within exposure to general frequency bands, FM radio contributed the most to broadcast, while 900 MHz contributed the most to uplink and downlink. Mean personal RF-EMF exposure by technology was 0.11 V/m from uplink, 0.18 V/m from downlink (900 MHz—50%, 1800 MHz—27%, and 2100 MHz—18%), 0.15 V/m from broadcasting, 0.07 V/m from DECT, and 0.08 from WLAN. Mean personal RF-EMF exposure by activity was 0.21 V/m at home, 0.18 V/m at school,

0.31 V/m at work, 0.38 V/m outside, 0.32 V/m during travel, and 0.27 V/m during other miscellaneous activities.

In general, parents were exposed to roughly 20% higher total mean values than children in all bands. The main difference was observed for uplink signals (up to fourfold) while for other technologies the exposure was not substantially different. This observation was due to frequent use of mobile phones by parents during the time of our measurements.

There was no difference between day versus night mean of total exposure of children while a significant difference in day/night exposure was observed among parents (ratio 1.8). Again, this difference could be attributed to parents' frequent mobile phone use during the day. Uplink exposure was higher during weekends, downlink and Wi-Fi exposure was higher during weekdays, and exposure to the other frequency bands remained similar between weekdays and weekends. Within micro environments, uplink exposure was higher while children were traveling, broadcast and downlink exposure were higher while children were outside or travelling, and Wi-Fi was slightly higher while children were at home.

The mean of total exposure was slightly higher during weekends compared to weekdays, but there was variation between regions.

Mean exposures were highest while children were outside (0.43 V/m) or traveling (0.34 V/m), where downlink signals contributed most to the exposure over the measurement period (88%). Much lower mean exposures were found at home (0.24 V/m) or in school (0.21 V/m). However, total exposure at home contributed most to the total exposure over the measurement period. In addition, broadcasting was the second largest contributor to measurements, and this general frequency band was largely composed of the FM radio frequency band.

Figure 3.1 shows the distribution of the participants' average exposures for parents and children according to 6 general frequency bands and workdays/weekends. The

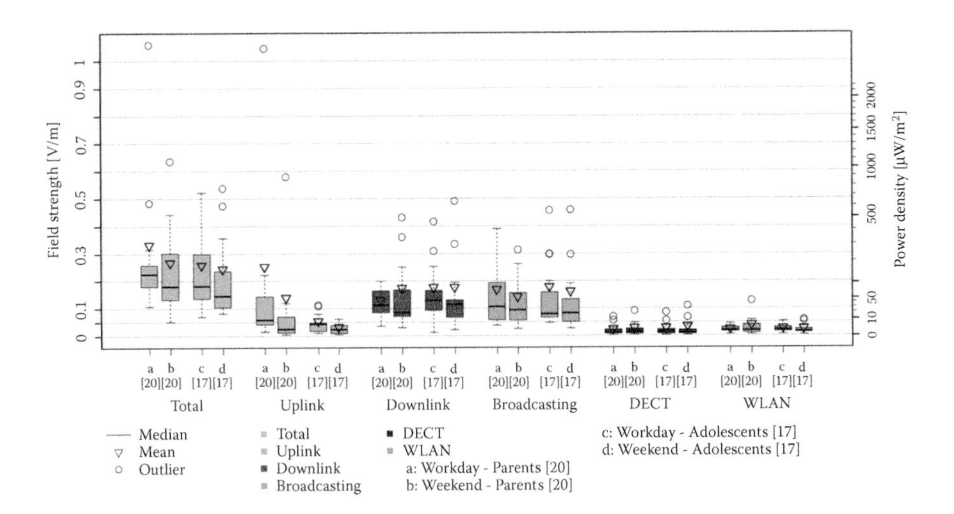

FIGURE 3.1 Distribution of the participants' average exposures (electric field strenghts of power density) for parents and children according to 6 general frequency bands and workdays/ weekends.

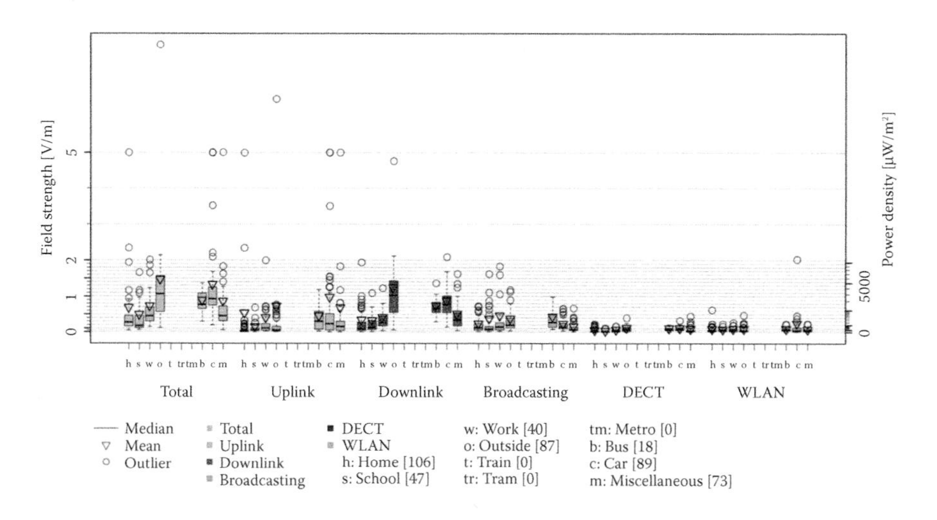

FIGURE 3.2 Distribution of the participants' average exposures (electric field strengths of power density) for parents and children according to different daily activities (h-Home; s-School; w-Work; o-Outside; t-Train, b-Bus, c-car; m-Miscellaneous) for different frequency bands.

arithmetic mean exposures of parents and children seem to be similar. The highest average personal exposures were found within the parents' group. It is mainly elevated Uplink exposure which is responsible for these "outliers."

Figure 3.2 shows the distribution of different frequency bands in different microenvironments.

3.2.3 Spot and Long Term RF-EMF Measurements

RF exposure measurement campaigns have been carried out in many countries since the mid-1990s. These onsite (spot and long term) RF-EMF measurement campaigns were performed either as part of the planning permission process or upon request by the public or local authorities.

Narrowband and broadband measurement methods of assessing exposure levels to RF-EMF fields have been applied in the range from several MHz to 10 GHz. Most of them were focused on exposure in the frequency range of broadcasting and mobile telecommunications (base stations).

Large-scale measurement campaigns (audits/spot measurements) were carried out and long-term RF-EMF monitoring systems have been installed in different countries (Gotsis et al., 2008; Troisi et al., 2008; Tomitsch et al., 2009; Rufo et al., 2011; Joseph et al., 2012). Spot measurements were conducted at one point in time at specific locations with stationary devices. The advantage of such exposure assessment is the use of sophisticated measurement devices according to strict standardized measurement protocols (international standards). The disadvantage of this method is limitation in the spatial resolution and in the variability of population exposure; it does not take into account the behavior of people. Analysis of temporal variability may be hampered by inaccuracy of the location of repeated spot measurements because RF-EMF may vary within a short distance.

A cross-sectional study in urban and rural areas close to base stations Hutter et al. (2006) have shown that total RF-EMF exposure, including mobile telecommunication signals, was far below recommended levels (maximum 1.24 V/m). The mean value of electric field strength was slightly higher in rural areas (0.13 V/m) than in urban areas (0.08 V/m). This discrepancy is because of the fact that only those households were selected that were close to mobile phone base stations, and base stations in rural areas typically transmit higher power as they are required to transmit over greater distances.

In another study (Tomitsch et al., 2009), spot measurements were taken in 226 households throughout Lower Austria. The overall RF-EMF electric field had an arithmetic mean of 0.39 V/m; 15% was due to indoor sources and 85% was attributed to outdoor sources. The highest values of RF-EMFs were caused by DECT telephone base stations (maximum 3.3 V/m) and mobile phone base stations (maximum 0.42 V/m).

Different locations close to the base stations and publicly accessible places (i.e., hospitals or schools) were investigated (Bornkessel et al., 2007). The maximum and minimum measured electric field strengths were 3.88 and 0.03 V/m, respectively. The mean values were 1.42 and 1.31 V/m when ignoring outliers.

An overall assessment of the nationwide monitoring networks measuring the RF spectrum in Greece showed that the mean electric field was 1.64 V/m. Gotsis et al. (2008) reported that this rather high value can be explained by the fact that the remote measurement stations were installed at sites near the base stations.

Similar national EMF monitoring network measurements were performed across all of Italy (Troisi et al., 2008). The overall results showed that 68.8% of recorded electric field strengths were <1 V/m, 22.6% were between 1 and 3 V/m, 6.3% were between 3 and 6 V/m, 2.2% were from 6 to 20 V/m, and <0.1% were >20 V/m.

On-site measurements in the frequency range between 0.5 MHz and 2200 MHz were also performed at 18 locations in Spain, where the median of electric field strength was found to be 0.17 V/m (Rufo et al., 2011). The mobile telephony frequency bands contributed most to total exposure (34.8%); radio broadcasting using frequency modulation (FM) technology and TV contributed to a lesser extent with 6.5% and 0.9%, respectively.

In situ exposure to base stations (downlink) serving emerging wireless technologies was assessed in three different countries at 311 locations, 68 indoor and 243 outdoor (Joseph et al., 2012) The highest total electric field value (3.9 V/m) was measured in a residential environment. The highest median exposures were measured in urban environments (0.74 V/m), followed by offices (0.51 V/m), industrial (0.49 V/m), suburban (0.46 V/m), residential (0.40 V/m), and rural (0.09 V/m) environments. The average contribution made to the total electric field by Global System for Mobile communications (GSMs) is >60%. With the exception of the rural environment, Universal Mobile Telecommunications System (UMTS) contributes on average 43%. Contributions of the emerging technologies Long Term Evolution (LTE) and WiMAX are on average <1%.

Rowley and Joyner (2012) reported a comparative analysis of data from surveys of mobile phone base stations in 23 countries worldwide. The analysis was based on more than 173,000 measurement results and covered the period from 2000 onward. The study shows that the global mean value was only 0.52 V/m, which is well below the international exposure limits.

Another comparative analysis of the results of spot or long-term RF-EMF measurements indicated that mean electric field strengths were between 0.08 and

1.8 V/m (Gajšek et al., 2015). The overwhelming majority of measured mean electric field strengths were <1 V/m. It is estimated that <1% were above 6 V/m and <0.1% were above 20 V/m. No exposure levels exceeded exposure limits.

Most population exposures from signals of broadcasting were observed to be weak because these transmitters are usually far away from exposed individuals and are spatially sparsely distributed. On the other hand, the contribution made to RF exposure from wireless telecommunications technology is continuously increasing and its contribution was above 60% of the total exposure.

3.2.4 Measurement Campaign in Slovenia

A nationwide RF-EMF measurement campaign was performed on 60 different locations in Slovenia between March and September 2017. For the selection of the measurement sample points, a variety of different outdoor urban and rural environments was considered. The location of mobile phone base stations was taken into account in the selection of the measurement points. The measurement locations can be grouped into three categories due to the population density: urban, suburban, and rural areas. For each category, we performed 20 independent measurements. Spot measurements were assessed using frequency-selective narrowband measurements. The setup consisted of a tri-axial isotropic antenna Narda 3501 in combination with a spectrum analyzer Narda SRM 3006 in the frequency range of 27 MHz to 6 GHz. The measurement uncertainty was ±2,5 dB for the considered setup according to the standard EN (European standard) 50492. This uncertainty represents the expanded uncertainty evaluated using a confidence interval of 95%. The location of the maximal total electric field value at the site under consideration is identified through sweeping the area.

The frequency-selective narrowband measurements were performed for the most used frequency bands that are summarized in Table 3.1.

TABLE 3.1
Investigated Systems/Technology with Corresponding Frequency Bands

System/Technology	Frequency Band (MHz)
FM radio broadcasting	87–108
Digital audio broadcasting (DAB) radio broadcasting	174–230
Link	380–470
DVB-T—broadcasting	470–790
800 base stations	790–862
GSM-R—railway	920–925
900 base stations	925–960
1800 base stations	1805–1880
2100 base stations	2110–2170
Wi-Fi	2400–2484
2600	2620–2690

3.3 RESULTS OF THE MEASURING CAMPAIGN

The results of the measurements in the whole RF spectrum show that the exposure to different wireless systems is quite low in different populated areas in Slovenia. An overall assessment of the measurement data showed that the mean total electric field in urban areas was 1.79 V/m, in suburban areas 1.08 V/m, and in rural areas 0.9 V/m, respectively. In Figure 3.3, the maximal, median, mean, and minimal values of the electric field measured in different micro environments (urban, suburban, rural) are shown.

Exposure from downlink signals in the 900 MHz frequency band contributed most to the mean total exposure (urban areas 31%, suburban areas 59%, and rural areas 53%). Also exposure from downlink signals in the 1800 MHz frequency band contributed significantly to mean total exposure (urban areas 36%, suburban areas 16%, and rural areas 10%).

In big cities (urban), the contribution of base stations in the 800 MHz frequency range to the total value of the electric field was 8%, in suburban areas 15%, and in rural areas 32%.

There are significant differences between different types of micro environments. In suburban and in rural areas, the contribution of base stations in the 1800 and 2100 MHz frequency bands is significantly lower than the contribution of the same system in urban areas (Figure 3.3).

It is noticeable that the average values of Wi-Fi signals are significantly higher in larger cities compared to values in suburban and rural areas, although in absolute terms, these values are extremely small. This is expected because public Wi-Fi

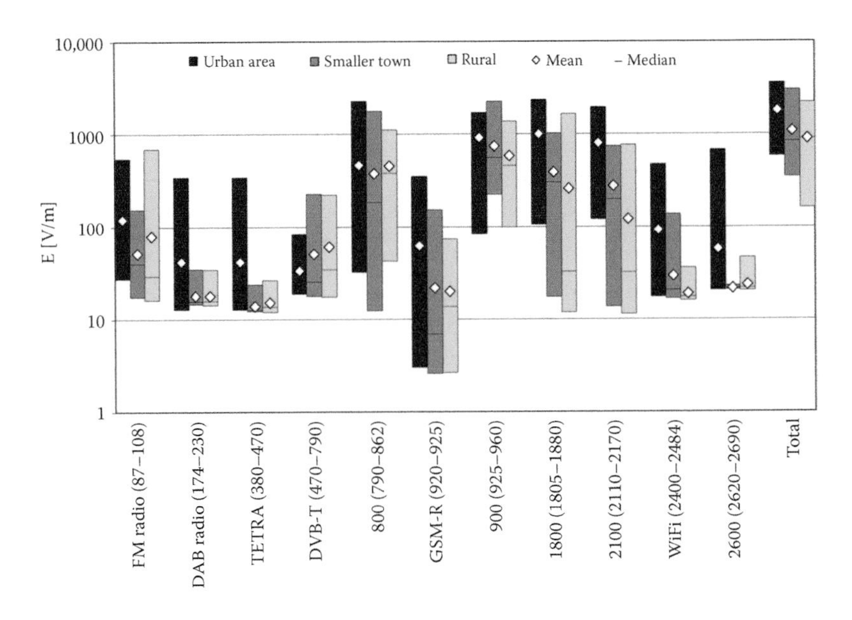

FIGURE 3.3 The maximal, median, mean, and minimal values of the electric field measured in different micro environments (urban, suburban, rural) according to different frequency bands.

networks that contribute significantly to exposure are usually employed in rural areas and only exceptionally in suburban areas, while Wi-Fi networks inside buildings contribute very little to the total exposure burden in different environments.

DVB-T technology causes higher exposures in rural and suburban areas than in larger cities, as DVB-T transmitters are usually located outside populated areas, therefore, are closer to the countryside than the larger city. Interestingly, the average values of FM radio transmitters are higher in urban areas, although it would be expected that the highest exposure would be identified in the countryside. These results indicate that the FM radio transmitters are also located closer to urban areas.

As already mentioned, the exposure from downlink signals in the 900 MHz frequency band contributed most to the mean total exposure (urban areas 81%, suburban areas 59%, and rural areas 53%). All base station systems in the 800, 900, 1800, 2100, and 2600 MHz frequency bands together contribute more than 90% to the total electric field in all types of micro environments.

For all mobile signals, the values of the electric field in urban areas are significantly higher than in the rural areas. Uplink signals in the 800 MHz range have better signal coverage, so they are often installed in rural areas; therefore, their contribution in rural areas is comparable to that in urban areas.

For Wi-Fi networks, the difference between the electric field in urban versus rural areas is noticeable. For urban areas, the average values of the electric field due to Wi-Fi are 0.09 V/m, for the suburban areas 0.03 V/m, and for the rural areas 0.02 V/m.

The total measured values of the electric field vary considerably for different types of micro environments. The total mean value of all measurements was 1.26 V/m, while in urban areas it was 1.80 V/m, in suburban areas 1.10 V/m, and in rural areas 0.90 V/m. On average, total exposure when taking into account all RF-EMF sources was twofold lower in rural areas in relation to urban areas. The main reason for this was the downlink signals from base stations which are numerous and densely installed in major cities (urban areas).

Measurements of RF-EMF in the wider area of Slovenia have shown that the typical values of the electric field due to the operation of wireless systems are low in all micro environments. For all 60 measurements made, the total average electric field was 1.3 V/m, which is a rather high value that can be explained by the fact that the measurements were selected at sites near the base stations.

3.4 PRECAUTIONARY MEASURES TO REDUCE EXPOSURES

With more and more research data available, it has become increasingly unlikely that exposure to RF-EMF, which is only a small fraction of the international guidelines, constitutes a serious health hazard, nevertheless, some uncertainty remains.

International guidelines are developed on the basis of the current scientific knowledge to ensure that the fields humans encounter are not harmful to health (ICNIRP, 1998). To compensate for uncertainties in knowledge (due, e.g., to experimental errors, extrapolation from animals to humans or statistical uncertainty), large safety factors are incorporated into the exposure limits. Because some studies suggest that that there may be health effects even if not supported by similar studies, this may be a cause of concern for some people. Among the reasons put forward are concerns about health risks related to RF-EMF classification as possibly carcinogenic to humans (2B).

Despite the scientific uncertainty related to health risk assessment, some societies introduce the *precautionary principle*, a recommendation to consider action to avoid a possible harm even if it is not certain to occur.

It has been suggested that taking additional precautions to cope with remaining uncertainties may be a useful policy to adopt while science improves knowledge on health consequences. However, the type and extent of the cautionary policy chosen critically depends on the strength of evidence for a health risk and the scale and nature of the potential consequences. The precautionary response should be proportional to the potential risk. In this regard, an analysis of the balance between cost and potential hazards is essential.

The precautionary principle is sometimes suggested if an uncertain but scientifically plausible risk is identified. It should be noted that involving the precautionary principle to manage exposure is not a simple matter and there are many important details to consider. A range of options and their consequences (including the option to take no action) should be considered. Measures should be proportional to the potential risk, and consistent with measures taken in similar circumstances for other risks. Moreover, measures should be subject to review as more scientific data become available.

Adopting a precautionary principle requires weighing potential costs against benefits (or disadvantages against advantages) of actions. It is important that any precautionary measures being advocated do not contradict the scientific basis of health guidance and safety regulations.

A range of precautionary measures could be considered, depending on the strength of evidence suggesting that there may be health effects and the severity of those effects:

- Numeric standards are formal steps to limit both the occurrence and consequences of potentially risky events.
- Communication and engagement programs can be used to help people voice their concern, understand the issues, become involved in the process, and make their own choices about what to do.
- A formal monitoring process provides transparency in monitoring the results of research and measurement and the decisions being made by standard setters, regulators, and others.
- A decision to take no formal action may be appropriate where the risk is considered very small or the scientific evidence is very weak.
- Research is an appropriate response to fill gaps in knowledge, help identify potential problems, and to allow for a better assessment of risk in the future.

An effective system of risk communication and risk management needs to be developed among scientists, administration, industry (mobile operators), and the public. Such a system could help raise the level of information about exposure and reduce mistrust and fears. It is advised that governmental authorities could implement inexpensive measures in the form of precautions to minimize public exposure to RF-EMF:

- The public should be transparently informed about state of science on health risks—especially on identified and confirmed health effects due to exposure to different technologies. Comprehensive information on EMF sources and exposure in the environment should be established on the national level. In this way, the public could be largely informed about the environmental burden and get an insight into the areas where RF-EMF exposure could exceed exposure limit values. Consequently, no additional RF-EMF sources would be permitted at such locations.
- Participation of local authorities and the public in the placement of new RF-EMF sources in the living environment (power lines and transformer stations, radars, base stations, broadcasting) must be permanent and constructive.
- When deciding on the place of installation of the RF-EMF source the spatial planning process, the visual impact and sensitivity of the public should be taken into account.
- Open communication during the planning process increases awareness of the public and its openness to such a placement.
- When designing wireless systems and issuing building permits, it is necessary for a new EMF source to determine its compliance zone according to the legally determined limit values and take into account all existing RF-EMF sources at the selected location in terms of total cumulative exposure.

Only frank communication between the owners of the EMS source, local authorities, and the public in the planning stages will help to understand the problem and will increase openness to installation of a new device. It is advised that mobile operators could also implement inexpensive measures in the form of precautions to minimize public exposure to RF-EMF:

- Mobile operators should take precautionary measures to optimize RF-EMF exposure through the optimization of the technical parameters of the individual base station: antenna height above the ground, output power, number of active channels, mechanical antenna tilt, gain, and radiation pattern of antenna.
- In the planning phase, special attention should be paid to areas of extended sensitivity (kindergartens, schools, daycare centers, etc.).
- It is necessary to increase the volume of information for the public, in particular on exposure assessment, health risks, risk management, and opportunities to reduce exposure in everyday life.
- The visual aspect and sensitivity of the public should also be taken into account.
- In their operation, operators should comply with the provisions of the relevant Code of Best Practice on Mobile Network Development including the sensitivity issues related to risk communication strategies.

- Therefore, the whole planning process should be based on dialog-based solutions between the investor, the local communities, and public.

And finally, what could an individual do to minimize his or her own exposure to RF-EMF while research continues?

The international guidelines recommended by ICNIRP provide protection for the population as a whole, however, uncertainties in the science suggest some additional level of precaution is warranted, particularly for sources such as mobile phones where simple measures can be taken to reduce exposure.

The precautionary steps to reduce mobile phone exposure:

- Use headphones or a low-power Bluetooth hands-free kit (Power Class 2 or 3) to reduce exposure to the head.
- Preferably use modern mobile networks such as LTE (4G) or UMTS (3G), whose radiation is lower than that of the old GSM technology. Telephoning with UMTS (3G) instead of GSM (2G) leads to significantly lower exposures in the head area.
- Inside or on a train, if possible, use a WLAN connection for telephoning or exchanging data.
- Using the phone in areas of good reception also decreases exposure as it allows the phone to transmit at reduced power.
- Moving the phone away from the body as when texting results in very much lower exposures than if a phone is held to the head.
- Excessive use of mobile phones by children should be discouraged.
- Keep calls short, making calls where the network signals are strong, and choose a phone with a low specific energy absorption rate (SAR) value quoted by the manufacturer.

At present, there is insufficient evidence in the science to substantiate the hypothesis that children may be more vulnerable to RF-EMF from mobile phones than adults. Irrespective of this, concerns have been raised about the possibility of greater vulnerability for children because of an increased susceptibility to health risks during developmental stages and because young people will use mobile phones for most of their lives. It is recommended that, due to the lack of any data relating to children and their long term use of mobile phones, parents encourage their children to limit their exposure by reducing call time, by making calls where reception is good, by using hands-free devices or speaker options or by texting.

3.5 CONCLUSION

In general, all the research studies related to exposure assessment of the general public to fixed RF-EMF sources in the environment including base stations, broadcasting, and wireless systems clearly demonstrated that the total mean value of the electric field was quite low and did not exceed 10% of the internationally recognized limit values.

It is expected that the strength and complexity of EMF exposures will increase continuously, especially in relation to expansion of the 5th generation of mobile telephony and other emerging technologies that will use different frequency bands. An increasing number of devices and processes employing these frequencies (household appliances, telecommunication, etc.) have already been introduced into everyday life. Almost nothing is known about these exposures and potential exposure levels.

It is expected that global mobile data traffic will grow at a compound annual rate of 45% in the coming years, which represents a tenfold increase between 2016 and 2022 (Ericsson, 2016). This increase is driven largely by the adoption of mobile video streaming. On top of that, the Internet of Things (IoT) is shifting from a vision to reality. The 29 billion connected devices by 2022 are expected to include 18 billion IoT or machine-to-machine (M2M) devices. Subsequently, the future 5G mobile networks will need to support new challenging and new use cases, which will demand more spectrum in ever higher frequency ranges.

Furthermore, emissions will continue to change in characteristics and levels due to new infrastructure deployments, smart environments, and novel wireless devices. Thus it is expected that the complexity of EMF exposures will increase in the future.

ACKNOWLEDGMENTS

The research leading to these results has received funding from the European Community's Seventh Framework Programme (FP7/2007-2013) under grant agreement no 603794—the GERONIMO project.

REFERENCES

Bhatt CR, Thielens A, Billah B, Redmayne M, Abramson MJ, Sim MR, Vermeulen R, Martens L, Joseph W, Benke G. Assessment of personal exposure from radiofrequency-electromagnetic fields in Australia and Belgium using on-body calibrated exposimeters. *Environ Res* 2016; 151: 547–563.

Bolte J, Pruppers M, Kramer J, Van der Zande G, Schipper C, Fleurke S et al. The Dutch exposimeter study: Developing an activity exposure matrix. *Epidemiology* 2008; 19: S78–S79.

Bolte J, Van der Zande G, Kamer J. Calibration and uncertainties in personal exposure measurements of radiofrequency electromagnetic fields. *Bioelectromagnetics* 2011; 32: 652–663.

Bolte JF, Eikelboom T. Personal radiofrequency electromagnetic field measurements in the Netherlands: Exposure level and variability for everyday activities, times of day and types of area. *Environ Int* 2012; 48: 133–142.

Bornkessel C, Schubert M, Wuschek M, Schmidt P. Determination of the general public exposure around GSM and UMTS base stations. *Radiat Prot Dosimetry* 2007; 124: 40–47.

Breckenkamp J, Blettner M, Schuz J, Bornkessel C, Schmiedel S, Schlehofer B et al. Residential characteristics and radiofrequency electromagnetic field exposures from bedroom measurements in Germany. *Radiat Environ Biophys* 2012; 51: 85–92.

Ericsson Mobility Report 2016. November 2016, available at: https://www.ericsson.com/assets/local/mobility-report/documents/2016/ericsson-mobility-report-november-2016.pdf

Frei P, Mohler E, Burgi A, Frohlich J, Neubauer G, Braun-Fahrlander C et al. A prediction model for personal radio frequency electromagnetic field exposure. *Sci Total Environ* 2009a; 408: 102–108.

Gajšek P, Ravazzani P, Wiart J, Grellier J, Samaras T, Thuróczy G. Electromagnetic field exposure assessment in Europe radiofrequency fields (10 MHz–6 GHz). *J Expo Sci Environ Epidemiol* 2015; 25: 37–44.

Gotsis A, Papanikolaou N, Komnakos D, Yalofas A, Constantinou P. Non-ionizing electromagnetic radiation monitoring in Greece. *Ann Telecommun* 2008; 63: 109–123.

Hutter H-P, Moshammer H, Wallner P, Kundi M. Subjective symptoms, sleeping problems and cognitive performance in subjects living near mobile phone base stations. *Occup Environ Med* 2006; 63: 307–313.

ICNIRP. Guidelines for limiting exposure to time-varying electric, magnetic, and electromagnetic fields (up to 300 GHz). *Health Physics* 1998; 74: 494–522.

Iskra S, McKenzie R, Cosic I. Monte Carlo simulations of the electric field close to the body in realistic environments for application in personal radiofrequency dosimetry. *Radiat Prot Dosimetry* 2011 Nov; 147(4): 517–527.

Joseph W, Frei P, Roosli M, Thuroczy G, Gajsek P, Trcek T et al. Comparison of personal radio frequency electromagnetic field exposure in different urban areas across Europe. *Environ Res* 2010; 110: 658–663.

Joseph W, Verloock L, Goeminne F, Vermeeren G, Martens L. Assessment of RF exposures from emerging wireless communication technologies in different environments. *Health Phys* 2012; 102: 161–172.

Joseph W, Vermeeren G, Verloock L, Heredia MM, Martens L. Characterization of personal RF electromagnetic field exposure and actual absorption for the general public. *Health Phys* 2008; 95: 317–330.

Neubauer G, Cecil S, Giczi W, Petric B, Preiner P, Fröhlich J, Röösli M. The association between exposure determined by radiofrequency personal exposimeters and human exposure: A simulation study. *Bioelectromagnetics* 2010; 31(7): 535–545.

Röösli M, Frei P, Mohler E, Braun-Fahrlander C, Burgi A, Frohlich J et al. Statistical analysis of personal radiofrequency electromagnetic field measurements with nondetects. *Bioelectromagnetics* 2008; 29: 471–478.

Rowley J, Joyner K. Comparative international analysis of radiofrequency exposure surveys of mobile communication radio base stations. *J Expo Sci Environ Epidemiol* 2012; 22: 304–315.

Rufo MM, Paniagua JM, Jimenez A, Antolın A. Exposure to high-frequency electromagnetic fields (100 kHz–2 GHz) in Extremadura (Spain). *Health Phys* 2011; 101: 739–745.

Sagar S, Dongus S, Schoeni A, Roser K, Eeftens M, Struchen B, Foerster M, Meier N, Adem S, Röösli M. Radiofrequency electromagnetic field exposure in everyday microenvironments in Europe: A systematic literature review. *J Expo Sci Environ Epidemiol* 2018; 28(2): 147–160.

Sagar S, Struchen B, Finta V, Eeftens M, Röösli M. Use of portable exposimeters to monitor radiofrequency electromagnetic field exposure in the everyday environment. *Environ Res* 2016; 150: 289–98.

SIST EN 50492:2009. Basic standard for the in-situ measurement of electromagnetic field strength related to human exposure in the vicinity of base stations, 2009.

Thielens A, Agneessens S, De Clercq H, Lecoutere J, Verloock L, Tanghe E, Aerts S, Puers R, Rogier H, Martens L, Joseph W. On-body calibration and measurements using a personal, distributed exposimeter for wireless fidelity. *Health Phys* 2015; 108(4): 407–418.

Thomas S, Kuhnlein A, Heinrich S, Praml G, Nowak D, von Kries R et al. Personal exposure to mobile phone frequencies and well-being in adults: A cross-sectional study based on dosimetry. *Bioelectromagnetics* 2008; 29: 463–470.

Thuroczy G, Molnar F, Janossy G, Nagy N, Kubinyi G, Bakos J et al. Personal RF exposimetry in urban area. *Ann Telecommun* 2008; 63: 87–96.

Tomitsch J, Dechant E, Frank W. Survey of electromagnetic field exposure in bedrooms of residences in lower Austria. *Bioelectromagnetics* 2009; 31: 200–208.

Trček T, Valic B, Gajsek P. Measurements of background electromagnetic fields in human environment. *IFMBE Proceedings 11th Mediterranean Conference on Medical and Biomedical Engineering and Computing*, vol. 16. MEDICON: Ljubljana, Slovenia, 2007, pp. 222–225.

Troisi F, Boumis M, Grazioso P. The Italian national electromagnetic field monitoring network. *Ann Telecommun* 2008; 63: 97–108.

Urbinello D, Huss A, Beekhuizen J, Vermeulen R, Röösli M. Use of portable exposure meters for comparing mobile phone base station radiation in different types of areas in the cities of Basel and Amsterdam. *Sci Total Environ* 2014a; 468: 1028–1033.

Urbinello D, Joseph W, Huss A, Verloock L, Beekhuizen J, Vermeulen R, Martens L, Röösli M. Radio-frequency electromagnetic field (RF-EMF) exposure levels in different European outdoor urban environments in comparison with regulatory limits. *Environ Int* 2014b; 68: 49–54.

Viel JF, Cardis E, Moissonnier M, de Seze R, Hours M. Radiofrequency exposure in the French general population: Band, time, location and activity variability. *Environ Int* 2009a; 35: 1150–1154.

Viel JF, Clerc S, Barrera C, Rymzhanova R, Moissonnier M, Hours M et al. Residential exposure to radiofrequency fields from mobile phone base stations, and broadcast transmitters: A population-based survey with personal meter. *Occup Environ Med* 2009b; 66: 550–556.

4 Health Effects of Chronic Exposure to Radiation From Mobile Communication

Igor Belyaev

CONTENTS

4.1 INTRODUCTION

Microwaves (MW, 300 MHz–300 GHz) or radio frequency (RF) radiation (3 kHz–300 GHz) induce a variety of biological and health effects which are commonly classified into thermal and nonthermal effects. Thermal effects are defined as those induced by elevation of temperature in the MW-exposed tissue. Thermal effects of acute exposure to MW are well characterized by the specific absorption rate (SAR, W/kg). Along with thermal MW effects, various biological responses to nonthermal (NT) MW, which are observed at the SAR values well below any measurable elevation of temperature, have been described by many research groups all over the world (1–6). Among many other variables, effects of NT MW strongly depend on frequency, modulation, polarization, and duration of exposure (7,8). It is generally accepted that all these parameters may be of importance for the effects of MW (4).

The SAR based safety limits adopted by the International Commission on Non-Ionizing Radiation Protection (ICNIRP), 2 W/kg, protecting from thermal MW effects only (9). In contrast to the ICNIRP, the Russian safety standards, which are based on nonthermal effects, do not use SAR values but instead limit the duration of exposure and power flux density (PD) (10).

Mobile phones emit a variety of MW signals (hundreds and even thousands, depending on location and type of mobile communication), which are different in carrier frequencies or frequency bands and modulations. The emitting signals, for example, GSM frequency channels, can be changed even within the same exposure session/talk. While one MW frequency/frequency band/modulation can induce detrimental effects, another one can be inactive (8). The studies with real mobile phones, given that the electromagnetic field (EMF) emitted by a phone is measured, represent the most valuable type of studies for assessment of various health effects including cancer risks from mobile telephony. Exposure to commercial or test mobile phones is close by all physical factors (carrier frequency, type of modulation, pulsed-field variables, near/far field, et cetera) to real exposure of the human brain and thus may provide valuable data for health risk assessment. At chronic exposures with longer duration, exposure to mobile phone may reproduce a number of real signals even during the same exposure session and thus provide a better possibility to assess detrimental effects from mobile telephony than experiments with fixed frequencies/frequency bands/modulations, which evaluate only a minor part of real signals. In addition, mobile phones emit not only MW, but also static and extremely low frequency (ELF) magnetic fields (11–16), which have also been shown to produce detrimental health effects and to interfere with MW effects (4,8,17).

There were many studies performed recently with chronic exposure to NT MW. While some studies with mobile phones did not provide measurements of EMF, only refereeing the SAR values from the manuals, EMF fields were measured in other studies. Most of these studies consistently showed detrimental health effects, and thus confirmed studies with long-term animals' MW exposure previously performed in Russia/The Soviet Union (18). This chapter represents an overview of recent studies on NT MW effects (SAR $\leq$ 2 W/kg) where EMF fields were measured.

4.2 ANIMAL *IN VIVO* STUDIES

4.2.1 Central Nervous System

Kesari et al. exposed 35-day old Wistar rats to MW from mobile phones for 2 h per day for a duration of 45 days, SAR being 0.9 W/Kg (19). A significant decrease in the levels of glutathione peroxidase and superoxide dismutase, and an increase in catalase activity were found in the exposed rats as compared to sham exposure. Moreover, protein kinase was significantly decreased in the hippocampus and whole brain of the exposed rats. Also, a significant decrease in the level of pineal melatonin and a significant increase in creatine kinase and caspase 3 were observed in the exposed group's whole brains as compared with the sham exposure. Finally, MW exposure significantly increased the level of reactive oxygen species (ROS). The authors concluded that a reduction or an increase in antioxidative enzyme activities, protein kinase C, melatonin, caspase 3, and creatine kinase are related to overproduction of ROS in animals under chronic exposure to mobile phone radiation.

Haghani et al. elucidated the possible effects of prenatal exposure of female Wistar rats to EMF from mobile phones (pulsed 900 MHz, SAR varying 0.5–0.9 W/kg, 6 h per day during gestation period) on the cerebellum of male and female offspring (20). Cerebellum-related behavioral dysfunctions were analyzed in offspring using motor learning and cerebellum-dependent functional tasks. Whole cell patch clamp recordings were used for electrophysiological evaluations. The results failed to show any behavioral abnormalities in rats chronically exposed to EMF from mobile phones. However, whole cell patch clamp recordings revealed decreased neuronal excitability of Purkinje cells in rats exposed to EMF. The changes were observed in after-hyperpolarization amplitude, spike frequency, half width, and first spike latency. The results showed that prenatal EMF exposure led to altered electrophysiological properties of Purkinje neurons. However, these changes might not be severe enough to alter the cerebellum-dependent functional tasks.

Ikinci et al. investigated changes in the spinal cords of Sprague-Dawley male rat pups exposed for 1 h daily between postnatal days 21 and 46 to the 900 MHz EMF (whole body SAR 0.01 W/kg) (21). At the end of exposure, the spinal cords in the upper thoracic region were collected for biochemical, light microscopic (LM), and transmission electron microscopic (TEM) examination. EMF exposure significantly increased malondialdehyde and glutathione levels as compared to control and sham exposed rats. LM revealed atrophy in the spinal cord, vacuolization, myelin thickening, and irregularities in the perikarya of the exposed rats. Marked loss of myelin sheath integrity and invagination into the axon and broad vacuoles in axoplasm was induced by EMF exposure as revealed by TEM. The authors concluded that biochemical alterations and pathological changes may occur in the spinal cords of male rats following chronic exposure to 900 MHz EMF.

Aslan et al. investigated possible pathological changes in the cerebellum of adolescent rats chronically exposed to 900 MHz EMF (13.4 V/m, the whole body SAR of 0.01 W/kg) 1 h daily for 25 days from postnatal days 21 through 46 (22). The cerebellums of animals were removed on postnatal day 47, then sectioned and stained with cresyl violet for histopathological and stereological analyses. Significantly fewer

Purkinje cells were found in the EMF exposed animals than in control and sham exposed rats. Histopathological evaluation revealed alteration of normal Purkinje cell arrangement and pathological changes including intense staining of neuron cytoplasm in the EMF exposed rats. The findings suggested that exposure to 900 MHz EMF for 1 h/day during adolescence can disrupt cerebellar morphology and reduce the number of Purkinje cells in the brain of adolescent rats.

Kerimoglu et al. exposed Sprague-Dawley male rats to MW (900 MHz, 8.4 V/m, 0.187 W/m2, whole body SAR 0.0067 W/kg, 1 h daily, days 21–59 throughout the adolescent period) and studied the 60-day old rat hippocampus (23). The left hemispheres were analyzed biochemically and the right hemispheres were subjected to stereological and histopathological evaluation. Histopathological examination revealed increased numbers of pyknotic neurons with black or dark blue cytoplasm in the brain of MW exposed rats. Fewer pyramidal neurons were found after MW exposure by stereological analysis. MW exposure increased malondialdehyde and glutathione levels, but decreased catalase levels in the brain. The data indicated that oxidative stress-related morphological damage and pyramidal neuron loss may be induced in the rat hippocampus following exposure to MW under given conditions throughout the adolescent period.

Deshmukh et al. investigated the effects of MW exposure at three different frequencies (900, 1800, and 2450 MHz, SAR being 5.953×10^{-4}, 5.835×10^{-4} and 6.672×10^{-4} W/kg, respectively) for 90 days on cognitive function, heat shock protein 70 (HSP70) level, and DNA damage in brain of Fischer rats (24). Cognitive functions were tested for using elevated plus maze and Morris water maze, HSP70 levels were estimated by enzyme-linked immunosorbent assay (ELISA), and DNA damage was assessed using alkaline comet assay. MW exposures at all frequencies led to decline in cognitive function and increased HSP70 level and DNA damage in the brain. The MW effects were significantly higher at 2450 MHz than at 900 MHz as measured with HSP70, tail length, the head and tail DNA content, the Olive tail moment, and the tail extent moment of the comets. The findings suggested that MW may lead to hazardous effects on the brain in dependence on frequency.

Gokcek-Sarac et al. studied effects of chronic exposure of young male albino Wistar rats to RF electromagnetic radiation (RF-EMR) at 900 and 2100 MHz (modulation frequency 217 Hz and pulse width 0.577 msec, 2 h/day, 5 days a week, for one week and ten weeks), on the hippocampal enzymes such as protein kinase A (PKA), Ca^{2+}/calmodulin-dependent protein kinase II alpha (CaMKIIalpha), cAMP response element-binding protein (CREB), and p44/42 mitogen-activated protein kinase (MAPK) from the N-methyl-D-aspartate receptor (NMDAR) related signaling pathways (25). The electric field strengths over the rat's head positioned 3.5 and 10 cm away from the antenna were 35.5 and 35.2 V/m for 900 and 2100 MHz RF-EMR, respectively. The average whole body SAR was 5.284 and 128 mW/kg for 900 and 2100 MHz, respectively. The average brain SAR was 0.66 and 0.27 W/kg for 900 and 2100 MHz, respectively. The hippocampal level/activity of selected enzymes was significantly higher after 10 week exposure as compared to 1-week exposures to RF-EMR at both 900 and 2100 MHz. Hippocampal level/activity of selected enzymes was significantly higher at 2100 MHz than at 900 MHz. The data indicated that chronic exposure of Wistar rats at different conditions had different effects on the protein expression of the hippocampus in dependence on duration of exposure.

Sharma et al. evaluated the effects of prolonged exposure of 2-week aged Swiss albino mice to MW (10 GHz, 0.25 mW/cm^2, 0.1790 W/kg, 2 h/day for 15 consecutive days) on developing mice brain (26). Various biochemical, behavioral, and histopathological parameters were analyzed in the exposed and sham exposed animals, which were autopsied either immediately after the completion of exposure or were allowed to attain 6 weeks of age for the follow-up study. Body weight showed significant changes immediately after exposure, whereas nonsignificant changes were observed in mice attaining 6 weeks of age. Brain weight, lipid peroxidation, glutathione, protein, catalase, and superoxide dismutase were found significantly altered in mice whole brain both immediately after exposure and in mice attaining 6 weeks of age. MW exposure affected spatial memory as measured using the Morris water maze test and histopathological parameters observed in the CA1 region of the hippocampus, cerebral cortex, and ansiform lobule of the cerebellum. The findings indicated that the brain of 2-week aged mice was sensitive to MW exposure as observed immediately after exposure and during follow-up study up to 6 weeks of age.

Tang et al. exposed male Sprague-Dawley rats to continuous wave EMF at 900 MHz, 1 mW/cm^2, SAR varying between 0.016 (whole body) and 2 W/kg (locally in the head), for 14 or 28 days, 3 h daily (27). The Morris water maze test was used to examine spatial memory performance. Morphological changes were investigated in the hippocampus and cortex, and the Evans Blue assay was used to assess blood brain barrier (BBB). Immunostaining was performed to identify heme oxygenase-1 (HO-1)-positive neurons and albumin extravasation detection. Western blot was used to determine HO-1 expression, expression of phosphorylated extracellular signal–regulated kinase (ERK) and upstream mediator mkp-1. EMF exposure did not affect the behavior of the rats at 14 days but impaired their performance at 28 days. BBB permeability increased 14 days after exposure to EMF and to a higher level after 28 days. Albumin uptake occurred more frequently in the cortex and hippocampal regions of brain in EMF exposed 28-d group than in the sham irradiated rats and EMF exposed 14-d group. Significant difference was found in HO-1 staining between the exposed rats and the sham exposed rats, as well as between the EMF 28-d group and the EMF 14-d group. Up-regulation of mkp-1 protein was observed at 28 days of exposure to EMF but not at 14 days. Dephosphorylation of ERK was detected in the rats at 28 days of exposure to EMF, and no difference between the nonexposed group and EMF 14-d group was observed. Taken together, the results demonstrated that chronic exposure to 900 MHz EMF for 28 days can significantly impair spatial memory and damage BBB permeability in rat by activating the mkp-1/ERK pathway.

Mugunthan et al. have investigated the effect of chronic exposure to radiations emitted from a 2G mobile phone (900–1800 MHz, SAR 1.6 W/kg, 48 minutes per day for a period of 30–180 days) in the hippocampus of mice (28). Random serial brain sections were analyzed for histomorphometric changes. The mean density of neurons in the hippocampus regions CA1, CA2 and dentate gyrus dorsal blade (DGDB) was significantly lower in the 2G exposed groups. However, the 2G exposed mice showed significantly higher density of neurons in CA3 and ventral blade/inferior limb (DGVB) regions. The mean nuclear diameter of neurons in the hippocampus region of CA1, CA2, CA3, DGDB, and DGVB showed lower nuclear diameter in 2G exposed mice. The authors concluded that chronic exposure to 900–1800 MHz frequency radiations emitted from 2G mobile phone could affect neuron density and decrease nuclear diameter in the hippocampus neurons of mice.

Finally, the emerging data have shown that chronic exposure to real signals from mobile communications under specific conditions can affect brain cells and important functions that may be related to various health effects including carcinogenesis.

4.2.2 Cognitive Functions

Zhao et al. analyzed the effects of chronic exposure of Wistar rats to MW (average power densities of 2.5, 5, and 10 mW/cm^2, SAR of 1.05, 2.1, and 4.2 W/kg, respectively, 6 min daily for 1 month) on hippocampal structure and function (29). Learning and memory abilities were assessed by the Morris water maze. High performance liquid chromatography was used to detect neurotransmitter concentrations in the hippocampus and hippocampal structures were subjected to histopathological analysis. MW exposure significantly decreased learning and memory activity as analyzed 7, 14, and 30 days in all three MW exposure groups. Neurotransmitter concentrations of four amino acids (glutamate, aspartic acid, glycine, and gamma-aminobutyric acid) in the hippocampus were increased in the 2.5 and 5 mW/cm^2 groups and decreased in the 10 mW/cm^2 group. There was evidence of neuronal degeneration and enlarged perivascular spaces in the hippocampus of exposed animals. Mitochondria became swollen and cristae were disordered after MW exposure. The rough endoplasmic reticulum exhibited sacculated distension and there was a decrease in the quantity of synaptic vesicles. These findings suggested that the hippocampus can be injured by long-term microwave exposure followed by impairment of cognitive function due to neurotransmitter disruption.

Given the suggested link between EMF exposure, iron overload in the brain, and neurodegenerative disorders including Parkinson's and Alzheimer's diseases, Maaroufi et al. investigated co-exposure to MW (900 MHz, SAR 0.05–0.18 W/kg, 1 h/daily) and iron overload (daily injection of 3 mg FeSO4 per kg body weight) during 21 consecutive days in Long-Evans rats (30). The co-exposed rats were tested in various spatial learning tasks (navigation task in the Morris water maze, working memory task in the radial arm maze, and object exploration task involving spatial and nonspatial processing). Biogenic monoamines and metabolites (dopamine, serotonin) and oxidative stress were measured. Rats exposed to MW were impaired in the object exploration task but not in the navigation and working memory tasks. They also showed alterations of monoamine content in several brain areas including the cerebellum and striatum, but mainly in the hippocampus. Rats that received combined treatment did not show greater behavioral and neurochemical deficits than MW-exposed rats. No oxidative stress was detected after treatments. These data indicated that MW affected the brain and cognitive processes but no synergistic effects were found between MW and iron overload in the brain.

Deshmukh et al. investigated the effects of chronic low-intensity MW exposure on cognitive function, heat shock protein 70 (HSP70), and DNA damage in rat brain (31). Male Fischer rats were exposed to MW for 180 days at 3 different mobile phone frequencies of 900, 1800, and 2450 MHz, SAR ranging 5.835×10^{-4}–6.672×10^{-4} W/kg. The rats were tested for cognitive function at the end of the exposure. The brain was analyzed for HSP70 by enzyme-linked immunotarget assay and DNA damage using alkaline comet assay. The results showed declined cognitive function, elevated HSP70 level, and DNA damage in the brain of MW-exposed animals. The results indicated that chronic low-intensity microwave exposure in the frequency range of 900–2450 MHz may cause hazardous effects on the brain.

Schneider and Stangassinger exposed male and female rats to EMF at a frequency of 900 MHz at GSM modulation or 1.966 GHz (Universal Mobile Telecommunications System [UMTS]) at 0.4 W/kg and analyzed memory performance of adult EMF-exposed and sham exposed female rats (at 6 months of age) and male rats (at 3 and 6 months of age) using a social discrimination procedure (32). The animals were exposed chronically for their entire lives to the far field linear polarized quasi-plane wave EMF. Differences in sniffing duration to the familiar and novel target rats were used to assess memory performance. EMF-exposed females exhibited no differences in sniffing duration compared with sham exposed controls. In contrast, the sniffing durations of EMF-exposed males at 3 months of age were significantly affected. At 6 months of age, GSM- but not UMTS-exposed male adults showed a memory performance deficit. This study showed that lifelong exposure to GSM EMF impairs social memory performance in adult male rats while lifelong exposure to UMTS EMF, with the same SAR, seems to display an age or exposure duration (3 months vs. 6 months) related adverse effect on the social memory retention.

Narayanan et al. investigated the effects of chronic EMF exposure from a mobile phone on spatial cognition and hippocampal architecture in prepubescent rats (33). Four weeks old male Wistar rats were exposed to EMF (GSM 900 MHz; SAR 1.15 W/kg with peak power density of 146.60 $\mu W/cm^2$ at 3 cm from mobile phone) for 1 h/day, 28 days. Spatial cognition was evaluated by Morris water maze test. Hippocampal morphology was studied in hippocampal sections by H&E staining, cresyl violet staining, and Golgi-Cox staining. CA3 pyramidal neuron morphology and surviving neuron count in CA3 region were studied using H&E and cresyl violet stained sections. Dendritic arborization pattern of CA3 pyramidal neuron was investigated by concentric circle method. Progressive learning abilities were found to be decreased in EMF exposed rats. Memory retention test performed 24 h after the last training revealed minor spatial memory deficit in the EMF-exposed group. However, EMF-exposed rats exhibited poor spatial memory retention when tested 48 h after the final trial. EMF exposure affected the viable cell count in the dorsal hippocampal CA3 region and the dendritic arborization pattern of both apical and basal dendritic trees. Structural changes found in the hippocampus of EMF-exposed rats could be one of the possible reasons for altered cognition.

Junior et al. investigated potential effects of mobile phone radiation on the central nervous system (CNS) using behavioral tests (open field and object recognition) in male Wistar rats (60 days old), which were exposed to EMR from a Global System for Mobile (GSM) cell phone (1.8 GHz, 2 V/m, 25-second long phone calls, every 2 minutes, for 3 days) (34). The exposed animals did not present anxiety patterns or working memory impairment, but stress behavior actions were observed upon exposure.

In some studies with chronic exposure to a specific RF signal generated by a signal generator (not by a mobile phone) neither neurodegenerative effects (35) nor effects on behavior and memory of exposed animals (36) were found.

In conclusion, most studies indicated that long-term chronic exposure to signals of mobile communications has a negative impact on cognition.

4.2.3 Immune Functions

Szmigielski reviewed studies on the impacts of weak RF/MW fields, including cell phone radiation, on various immune functions, both *in vitro* and *in vivo* (37). The bulk of available evidence clearly indicated that various shifts in the number and/or activity of immunocompetent cells are possible, while the results were inconsistent. In particular, a number of lymphocyte functions have been found to be either enhanced or weakened based on exposure to similar MW intensities although other important variables of experiments were different. The author concluded that, in general, short-term exposure to weak MW radiation may temporarily stimulate certain humoral or cellular immune functions, while chronic irradiation inhibits the same functions.

Ohtani et al. studied the effects of RF exposure (2.14 GHz wideband code division multiple-access (W-CDMA) signal, whole body SAR of 0.2 W/kg, for 20 h/day, 7 days/week) for a total of 9 weeks spanning in utero development, lactation, and the juvenile period on the immune system in Sprague-Dawley rats (38). Flow cytometry revealed no RF-induced changes in the numbers of CD4/CD8 T cells, activated T cells or regulatory T cells among peripheral blood cells, splenocytes, and thymocytes. Expression levels of 16 genes that regulate the immunological Th1/Th2 paradigm were analyzed using real time polymerase chain reaction (PCR) in the spleen and thymus. The Il5 gene was significantly upregulated in spleen and thymus, while Il4 and Il23a genes were significantly upregulated in thymus tissues only. ELISA showed no changes in serum IL-4 protein concentration. These data indicate no effects on immune-like T cell populations and T cell activation, while significant transcriptional effects of chronic RF exposure under given conditions were observed.

Kulaber et al. investigated changes in the thymic tissue of male Sprague-Dawley rats chronically exposed to MW (900 MHz, 8.86 V/m, 0.208 W/m2, 0.0067 W/kg) for 1 h every day between postnatal days 22 and 59 (39). On day 60, sections of thymus were assessed histologically and biochemically. MW exposure increased malondialdehyde (MDA) levels. Extravascular erythrocytes were observed in the medullary/corticomedullary regions in the sections of exposed rats. The findings indicated that MW exposure for 1 h/day on postnatal days 22–59 can increase tissue MDA and induce histopathological changes in the thymic tissue of male rats.

While the number of studies is still limited, available data indicate that chronic MW exposure may affect the immune system.

4.2.4 Sperm, Reproductive System, Fertility

Kesari and Behari chronically exposed Wistar rats to radiation from mobile phones (GSM 900 MHz, 0.9 W/kg, 2 h/day) for 45 days and analyzed the effects on sperm cells (40). EMF exposure significantly decreased the level of testosterone and increased caspase-3 activity, which is a marker of apoptosis. Distortions in sperm head and the mid-piece of sperm mitochondrial sheath were also observed by Transmission Electron Microscopy (TEM). A progeny from EMF-exposed rats showed a significant decrease in number and weight as compared with that of sham exposed animals.

Kumar et al. investigated the effect of 10 GHz chronic exposure (2 h per day for 45 days, power density 0.21 mW/cm^2, SAR 0.014 W/kg) on male Wistar rats' reproductive systems (41). Chromosomal aberrations (CA) and micronuclei were determined in blood samples of exposed and sham exposed animals. Spermatozoa were analyzed for Caspase-3, DNA damage, testosterone, and by electron microscopy. Scanning electron microscopy revealed shrinkage of the lumen of the seminiferous tubules. Apoptotic bodies and increased caspase 3 were found in exposed animals. A flow cytometry examination showed formation of micronuclei body in lymphocytes of the exposed group. While no CAs were detected, comet assay revealed DNA strand breaks. Testosterone level was found to be significantly decreased along with a shrinkage of testicular size. This study has shown that chronic exposure at 10 GHz, 0.21 mW/cm^2, and SAR of 0.014 W/kg has potentially deleterious effects on blood and fertility of exposed male Wistar rats.

Tas et al. investigated the effects of long-term (3 h per day, 7 d a week, for one year) mobile phone exposure at 900 MHz (point, 1 g and 10 g SAR levels of testis and prostate were 0.0623 W/kg, 0.0445 W/kg and 0.0373 W/kg, respectively) on reproductive organs of Wistar Albino male rats (42). Epididymal sperm concentration, progressive sperm motility, abnormal sperm rate, all genital organs weights, and testis histopathology were evaluated. No effect of RF exposure was observed on sperm motility and concentration. Although histological examination showed similarities in the seminiferous tubules diameters in exposed and sham exposed animals, RF exposure decreased tunica albuginea thickness and the Johnsen testicular biopsy score. The authors concluded that long-term exposure to 900 MHz RF radiation alters some reproductive parameters. Of note, at least some of the reported effects might be dismissed by applying the adjustment for multiple comparisons.

Qin et al. investigated whether chronic exposure to RF (1800 MHz, PD 205 μw/cm^2, SAR 0.0405 W/kg) for 2 h/day for 32 days at different zeitgeber time (ZT) points (ZT0, ZT4, ZT8, ZT12, ZT16, and ZT20) affects circadian rhythms of reproductive functional markers in adult male Sprague-Dawley rats (43). Testicular and epididymis tissues were collected and assessed for testosterone levels, daily sperm production and sperm motility, testis marker enzymes gamma-glutamyl transpeptidase (gamma-GT) and acid phosphatase (ACP), cytochrome P450 side-chain cleavage (p450cc) mRNA expression, and steroidogenic acute regulatory protein (StAR) mRNA expression. These measurements revealed pronounced circadian rhythms in sham exposed animals. RF exposure disrupted the circadian rhythms decreasing testosterone levels, lowering daily sperm production and sperm motility, down-regulating activity of gamma-glutamyl transpeptidase (gamma-GT) and ACP, and altering mRNA expression of cytochrome P450 and StAR. The most significant changes were observed in rats exposed to RF at ZT0. The findings indicated potential adverse effects of RF exposure on male reproductive functional markers in terms of daily overall levels and circadian rhythmicity.

The effect of prolonged MW exposure (2G, 900–1900 MHz, 48 minutes per day for a period up to 180 days) cell phone on rats' testis was evaluated (44). Body weight was found to be significantly reduced after 30, 60, and 120 days of exposure, mean testis weight was significantly reduced 30, 60, 90, 150, and 180 days of exposure, and the mean testis volume was significantly reduced in groups with 30, 60, and 90 days of exposure compared to sham exposed mice. In histological analysis, the mean density of seminiferous tubules was significantly lower in all exposure groups except for 30 days of exposure, the mean seminiferous tubule diameter was significantly reduced in all exposure group except for 60 days of exposure, and the numbers of Sertoli cells/tubule and Leydig cells was significantly reduced in all exposure groups compared to the sham exposure groups. For Johnson testicular biopsy score count and testosterone level, all exposure groups were pooled and a significantly reduced serum testosterone level and mild histological changes compared to sham exposed animals were found. The authors concluded that chronic exposure of mice to the 2G 900–1900 MHz mobile phone radiation might have detrimental effects on testes histology and function with possible consequences for fertility.

Kumar et al. chronically exposed male albino rats to EMF from a 3G cell phone (the frequency of the cell phone was fixed at 1910.5 MHz and kept in 'talk mode,' SAR varied from 0.28 to 0.0226 W/kg) for 60 days, two hours each day (6 days a week) and analyzed testicular functions (45). Significant decrease in sperm count, increase in the lipid peroxidation damage in sperm cells, reduction in seminiferous tubules and testicular weight, and DNA damage were revealed in rats following EMF exposure. The results demonstrated that exposure to the mobile phone radiation can negatively affect sperm functions via mechanisms that involve oxidative stress. The results suggest that mobile phone exposure adversely affects male fertility.

Liu et al. investigated whether chronic exposure of rats to MW (900 MHz, 0.66 ± 0.01 W/kg, 2 h/daily) for 50 days can trigger ROS, sperm cell apoptosis and affect semen morphology, concentration, and microstructure (46). The sperm count, morphology, apoptosis, ROS, and total antioxidant capacity (TAC), representing the sum of enzymatic and nonenzymatic antioxidants, were measured. Western blotting and reverse transcriptase PCR were used to determine the expression levels of apoptosis-related proteins and genes, including bcl-2, bax, cytochrome c, and capase-3. MW exposure increased ROS concentration and number of apoptotic sperm cells by 46.21% and 91.42%, respectively, while the TAC was decreased by 28.01%. MW exposure also significantly decreased the protein and mRNA expression of bcl-2 and increased that of bax, cytochrome c, and capase-3. The data indicated that MW exposure altered expression levels of apoptosis-related genes and triggered sperm apoptosis through induction of ROS and bcl-2, bax, cytochrome c, and caspase-3 signaling pathways.

Odaci and Ozyilmaz exposed Sprague-Dawley male rats to a 900 MHz EMF (whole body SAR 0.025 W/kg, 1 h daily, 30 days) and investigated EMF effects on the rat testicles (47). The levels of malondialdehyde, superoxide dismutase, catalase, and glutathione along with apoptotic index measured with terminal deoxynucleotidyl transferase dUTP nick end labeling (TUNEL) assay and histopathological damage scores were analyzed. EMF exposed rats exhibited vacuoles in seminiferous tubules basal membrane and edema in the intertubular space. Both seminiferous tubule diameters and germinal epithelium thickness were smaller, while apoptotic index was higher in the EMF exposed animals. The levels of malondialdehyde, superoxide dismutase, and catalase were increased in the EMF exposed rats as compared to the sham exposure group although glutathione was decreased. The authors concluded that chronic exposure to the mobile phone frequency of 900 MHz caused pathological alterations in rat testicular morphology and biochemistry.

Mugunthan et al. evaluated and compared effects of chronic exposure to 900–1800 MHz radiation emitted from 2G cell phone and 1900–2200 MHz from 3G cell phones on the testis of mice (48). Mice were intermittently exposed to 2G and 3G radiation, 48 minutes per day (2 min per each 30 min 8.00 a.m. – 8.00 p.m.) for a period of 30–180 days. The highest SAR value for this standard handset was 1.69 W/Kg (10 g). Measurements were performed at the end of 30, 60, 90, 120, 150, and 180 days of exposure. There was significant reduction of animal weight at first, second, and fourth months following chronic exposure to 2G and 3G cell phone radiation. The mean testis weight and volume of 2G and 3G radiation exposed mice were significantly reduced in the first three months. The comparison between 2G and 3G exposed groups showed no significant changes in mean body weight, mean testis weight, and mean testis volume. 2G and 3G chronic exposure decreased density of seminiferous tubules, mean seminiferous tubule diameter, and mean number of Sertoli and Leydig cells. Few changes were observed by microscopic analysis in the 2G and 3G exposed mice. Chronically exposed mice had significantly lower serum testosterone at the end of first, second, third, fourth, and sixth months of 2G and 3G exposures while no difference was observed between the 2G and 3G exposed groups. The authors concluded that chronic exposure to radiation from 2G and 3G cell phones could cause changes in the seminiferous epithelium, reduction of serum testosterone level, and reduction in the number of Sertoli cells and Leydig cells.

To conclude, most *in vivo* studies with animals indicated that NT MW induce detrimental effects in sperm, which can affect fertility and may occur through induction of ROS and ROS-dependent molecular pathways.

4.2.5 Other Tissues

Esmekaya et al. investigated whether chronic exposure to 900 MHz pulse-modulated RF fields (rectangular pulses with repetition frequency 217 Hz and pulse width 0.576 ms, the whole body average SAR 1.20 W/kg, 20 min/day for three weeks) induce oxidative damage in lung, heart, and liver tissues of Wistar albino rats (49). They assessed oxidative damage by investigating lipid peroxidation (malondialdehyde, MDA), nitric oxide (NOx), and glutathione (GSH) levels, which are the indicators of tissue toxicity. MDA and NOx levels were increased significantly in liver, lung, testis, and heart tissues of the exposed group compared to sham exposed animals. Conversely, GSH levels were significantly lower in exposed rat tissues. The authors concluded that pulse-modulated RF radiation causes oxidative injury in liver, lung, testis, and heart tissues mediated by lipid peroxidation, increased level of NOx, and suppression of antioxidant defense mechanism.

Tsybulin et al. elucidated the effects of MW emitted by a commercial model of GSM 900 MHz cell phone on embryo development in quails (*Coturnix coturnix japonica*) (50). Fresh fertilized eggs were irradiated during the first 38 h or 14 days of incubation by a cell phone in a connecting mode activated continuously through a computer system. Each connection attempt lasted about 45 s. Exposure during 38 h/14 days comprised of about 3000/26,900 calls. Maximum incident PD on the egg's surface was 0.2 $\mu W/cm^2$. The irradiation led to a significant increase in numbers of differentiated somites in 38-hour exposed embryos and to a significant increase in total survival of embryos from exposed eggs after 14 days exposure. The level of thiobarbituric acid (TBA) reactive substances was significantly higher in brains and livers of hatchlings from the exposed embryos. An especially conspicuous increase was detected in brains, where the TBA levels were higher by 3.5 fold in comparison with the unexposed samples. Consequently, it pointed to the increased lipid peroxidation of hatchling's tissues from exposed embryos, which is closely connected to levels of ROS. Thus, the observed effects of radiation from the commercial GSM 900 MHz cell phone on the developing quail embryos can be accounted for by the enhancement of metabolism provoked via peroxidation mechanisms due to radiation-induced ROS.

Ozorak et al. studied the effects of chronic exposures to EMF at 900 MHz, 1800 MHz, and 2.45 GHz (pulsed at 217 Hz, mean whole body SAR 0.18 $\pm$ 0.07 W/kg, 60 min/day, 5 days per week) on oxidative stress and trace element levels in the kidney and testis in rats growing from pregnancy to 6 weeks of age (51). EMF exposure decreased the level of lipid peroxidation in the kidney and testis and the copper, zinc, reduced glutathione (GSH), glutathione peroxidase (GSH-Px), and total antioxidant status (TAS) values in the kidney, while iron concentrations in the kidney as well as vitamin A and vitamin E concentrations in the testis increased at the 4th week of exposure. Iron, vitamin A, and beta carotene concentrations increased in the kidney of EMF exposed animals, while the GSH and TAS levels decreased after five weeks of exposure. Iron concentrations in the kidney and the extent of lipid peroxidation increased in the EMF groups in the kidney and testis after six weeks of exposure, while copper, TAS, and GSH concentrations decreased at this time. EMF exposure did not induce any changes in the kidney's concentrations of chromium, magnesium, and manganese. The authors concluded that chronic exposure to EMF caused oxidative damage by increasing the extent of lipid peroxidation and the iron level, while decreasing total antioxidant status, copper, and GSH values.

Eser et al. studied the histopathological and biochemical changes in the frontal cortex, brain stem, and cerebellum of Spraque-Dawley rats exposed to MW at 900, 1800, and 2450 MHz (average SAR 1.04 W/kg) 1 h daily for 2 months (52). MW exposures induced degenerative changes, shrunken cytoplasm, and extensively dark pyknotic nuclei in the frontal cortex and brain stem, which were more profound at 2400 MHz. The levels of Total Oxidative Capacity and Oxidative Stress Index were significantly increased in the frontal cortex, brain stem, and cerebellum of MW exposed animals. The frontal cortex was more affected at 900 MHz. MW exposures significantly increased the IL-1beta level in the brain stem, while exposure at 900 MHz was statistically significantly most efficient. MW exposures induced caspase-3 immunoreactivity in the frontal cortex and brain stem, although the frequency of 2450 MHz was most efficient. The data indicated that chronic MW exposure caused histopathological changes in the frontal cortex, brain stem, and cerebellum and impaired the oxidative stress and inflammatory cytokine system in dependence on frequency.

Tsybulin et al. assessed the effects of low intensity radiation from a GSM (Global System for Mobile communication) 900 MHz cellular phone on early embryogenesis in dependence on the duration of exposure (53). Embryos of Japanese Quails were exposed in ovo to GSM 900 MHz cellular phone radiation (890–915 MHz carrier frequency, nonmodulated by any voice signal while maintaining a pulse modulation which is equivalent to an amplitude modulation simultaneously by 217 Hz and harmonics, average power density 0.25 μW/cm^2, SAR 3 μW/kg) during the initial 38 h of brooding or alternatively during 158 h (120 h before brooding plus initial 38 h of brooding) interruptedly: 48 s on followed by 12 sec off intervals. A number of differentiated somites and DNA damage were assessed microscopically and by alkaline comet assay, respectively. Exposure significantly altered the number of differentiated somites. In embryos exposed during 38 h, the number of differentiated somites increased, while in embryos irradiated during 158 h, this number decreased. The lower duration of exposure led to a decrease in the level of DNA strand breaks in cells of 38-h embryos, while the higher duration of exposure significantly increased DNA damage as compared to the control. The authors concluded that effects of the GSM 900 MHz cellular phone radiation on early embryogenesis can be either stimulating or deleterious depending on the duration of exposure.

Ozgur et al. investigated effects of prenatal and/or postnatal chronic exposure to 1800 MHz RF radiation (pulsed with frequency of 217 Hz and a duty cycle of 1:8 (pulse width 0.576 ms), corresponding to the dominant modulation component of the GSM, 0.1 W output power) on the blood chemistry and lipid peroxidation levels of New Zealand female and male infant rabbits (54). Thirty-six females and 36 males were divided into four groups which were composed of nine infants each: (i) Group 1 was sham exposure; (ii) Group 2 was exposed to RF, 15 min daily for 7 days in the prenatal period (between 15th and 22nd days of the gestational period) (prenatal exposure group); (iii) Group 3 was exposed to RF 15 min/day (14 days for male, whereas 7 days for female) after they reached 1-month of age (postnatal exposure group); (iv) Group 4 was exposed to RF for 15 min daily during 7 days in the prenatal period (between 15th and 22nd days of the gestational period) and 15 min/day (14 days for male, whereas 7 days for female) after they reached 1-month of age (prenatal and postnatal exposure group). RF exposure affected serum lipid peroxidation level in both female and male rabbits and changed several biochemical parameters in blood (creatinine, uric acid, g-glutamyl transpeptidase (GGT), alanine transaminase (ALT), Albumin (ALB), and malondialdehyde (MDA) in males; urea, GGT, aspartate aminotransferase (AST), ALT, total protein (TP), MDA in females). Thus, the blood biochemistry of male and female infants was differently affected by RF exposure. The authors concluded that the whole body 1800 MHz GSM-like RF exposure may lead to oxidative stress and changes in some blood chemistry parameters.

Mugunthan et al. evaluated histological effects of chronic exposure to MW emitted from 2G (900–1900 MHz) cell phone on kidneys of mice (55). 21 days old mice were exposed to 2G MW, 48 minutes per day for a period up to 180 days. Animals were sacrificed at the end of 30, 60, 90, 120, 150, and 180 days of exposure and both kidneys were harvested and processed for histomorphometric study. MW exposure significantly reduced weight of kidney in mice exposed at the age of 21–51 days while kidney weight was significantly increased in the fifth month. In dependence on age and exposure time: (i) glomerulus showed dilated capillaries and increased urinary space; (ii) proximal convoluted tubule showed wider lumen with reduced cell size; (iii) brush border interrupted at places and vacuolated cytoplasm and pyknotic nuclei; and (iv) wider lumen with decreased cell size and marked basal striations were found in the distal convoluted tubule. The authors concluded that chronic exposure to radiation from 2G cell phone could cause microscopic changes in glomerulus, proximal, and distal convoluted tubules of the kidney.

Çiftçi et al. determined the effects of prenatal and postnatal exposure (2 h/day during the periods of pregnancy, 21 days, and lactation, 21 days) to Wi-Fi radiation (2.45 GHz, pulsed with 217 Hz, SAR 0.009 ± 0.002 W/kg per head) on tooth and surrounding tissue development as well as the element levels in growing Wistar albino rats (56). The offspring of these dams were also exposed to radiation up to decapitation. On the 7th, 14th, and 21st days after birth, EMR-exposed and sham exposed male offspring rats were decapitated and the jaws were taken for histological and immunohistochemical examination. Caspase-3 was used in the immunohistochemical examination for apoptotic activity. On the last day of the experiment, the rats' incisors were also analyzed. RF exposure induced no apoptotic activity. However, iron and strontium concentrations were increased in the Wi-Fi-exposed group, whereas boron, copper, and zinc concentrations were decreased. There were no statistically significant differences in calcium, cadmium, potassium, magnesium, sodium or phosphorus values between the groups. Histological and immunohistochemical examinations revealed no effects of exposure to 2.45 GHz radiation on the development of teeth and surrounding tissues. Given that Zn, B, and Cu can act as antioxidants by decreasing ROS while the increased Fe levels trigger $OH-$ formation, the authors concluded that the revealed alterations in the elemental composition of the teeth, especially affecting such oxidative stress-related elements as copper, zinc, and iron, suggest an imbalance in the oxidative stress condition in the teeth of growing rats exposed to Wi-Fi radiation. The authors noted that the animals were exposed to Wi-Fi radiation for a period which is equivalent to approximately 10 years in humans. Thus it is clear that the exposure period of this study is of too short a duration to draw conclusions as to the effects of Wi-Fi exposure over a lifetime.

Olgar et al. exposed Wistar male rats to 2.1 GHz EMF (217 Hz-pulse rate, SAR 0.83 W/kg, 2 h/day, 7 days/week, 10 weeks) and investigated nitric oxide (NO), contractility and beta-adrenergic (beta-AR) responsiveness of ventricular myocytes (57). Sarcomere shortening and Ca(2+) transients were recorded in isolated myocytes loaded with Fura2-AM and electrically stimulated at 1 Hz, while L-type Ca(2+) currents (I(CaL)) were measured using whole cell patch clamping at 36 ± 1°C. Cardiac NO levels were measured in tissue samples using a colorimetric assay kit. Fractional shortening and amplitude of the matched Ca(2+) transients were not changed in the EMF exposed rats. Although the basal I(CaL) density in myocytes was similar between exposed and sham exposed groups, the isoproterenol-induced (10(−6) M) I(CaL) response was reduced in rats exposed to EMF. Moreover, EMF exposure led to a significant increase in nitric oxide levels in the rat heart. The authors concluded that long-term exposure to 2.1 GHz EMF decreases beta-AR responsiveness of ventricular myocytes through NO signaling.

Cao et al. studied whether circadian rhythms of the plasma antioxidants (Mel, GSH-Px, and superoxide dismutase [SOD]) are affected by chronic exposure of male Sprague Dawley rats to the 1.8 GHz RF (201.7 $\mu W/cm^2$ power density, 0.05653 W/kg SAR) (58). The animals were exposed to RF for 2 h/day at six specific times during the 24 h light-dark cycle (3, 7, 11, 15, 19 and 23 h Greenwich Mean Time (GMT), respectively) for 32 consecutive days. The concentrations of three antioxidants

(Mel, GSH-Px and SOD) were determined in blood samples. RF exposure shifted circadian rhythms in the synthesis of Mel and antioxidant enzymes, GSH-Px, and SOD. The Mel, GSH-Px, and SOD levels were significantly decreased when RF exposure was given at 23 and 3 h GMT. The overall results indicate that there may be adverse effects of RF exposure on antioxidant function, in terms of both the daily antioxidative levels, as well as the circadian rhythmicity.

Zhu et al. exposed adult male Institute for Cancer Research (ICR) mice to MW (continuous wave 900 MHz, 1.6 mW/cm^2, whole body average SAR 0.731 W/kg) for 4 hour/day for 15 days (59). At the end of exposure, each mouse was caged with 3 mature virgin female mice for mating. After 7 days, each male mouse was transferred to a fresh cage and mated with a second batch of 3 females. This process was repeated for a total of 4 consecutive weeks. All females were subjected to examination on the 18th day of gestation and presumptive mating. The overall observations during the 4 weeks of mating indicated that the unexposed female mice mated to MW-exposed male mice showed no significant differences in the percentage of pregnancies, total implants, live implants, and dead implants when compared with those mated with sham exposed mice. In contrast, female mice mated with GR-exposed males showed a consistent pattern of significant differences in the above indices in each and all 4 weeks of mating. These data indicated an absence of dominant lethal mutations upon exposure of the germ cells of male mice to MW under given conditions.

Kuybulu et al. investigated oxidative stress and apoptosis in kidney tissues of male Wistar rats, which were chronically exposed to MW (2.45 GHz, pulsed with 217 Hz, whole body SAR of 0.143 W/kg, 60 min/day) in pre- and postnatal periods (60). Exposure during the prenatal period increased renal tissue malondialdehyde (MDA) and total oxidant (TOS) levels and decreased total antioxidant (TAS) and superoxide dismutase (SOD) levels. Spot urine N-acetyl-beta-D-glucosaminidase (NAG)/creatinine ratio was significantly higher in animals exposed in both pre- and postnatal periods. Tubular injury was detected in most of the specimens in postnatally exposed animals. Immunohistochemical analysis showed low-intensity staining with Bax in cortex and high-intensity staining with Bcl-2 in cortical and medullar areas of prenatally exposed rats. Bcl2/Bax ratios of medullar and cortical area were higher in prenatally exposed rats than in sham exposed animals. These findings indicated that chronic MW exposure during pre- and postnatal periods may cause kidney injury.

In conclusion, available data encourage evaluation of risks for a wide spectrum of diseases before any new type of mobile communications is set up.

4.2.6 Carcinogenesis

In 2011, the International Agency for Research on Cancer (IARC) Working Group reviewed more than 40 studies in which the carcinogenicity of RF-EMF was assessed in rodents; among these studies were seven two-year oncogenicity bioassays (4,61). All these studies explored very few RF signals including the frequency of 2450 MHz and some frequencies within the frequency range of emissions from cell phones. An increased total number of malignant tumors were identified in RF-exposed animals in one of the seven chronic bioassays in animals exposed to RF-EMF for two years. Increased cancer incidences in exposed animals were noted in two of twelve studies with tumor-prone animals and in one of eighteen studies using initiation-promotion protocols. However, four of six cocarcinogenesis studies provided evidence of increased cancer incidences after exposure to RF. Overall, the IARC Working Group concluded in 2011 that there is limited evidence in experimental animals for the carcinogenicity of RF-EMF (61).

One cocarcinogenesis lifetime study with mice suggested tumor-promoting effects of UMTS signals (62). Lerchl et al. have recently performed a replication of this study using higher numbers of animals per group and including two additional exposure levels (0 (sham), 0.04, 0.4, and 2 W/kg SAR) (63). This study confirmed and extended the originally published observations of tumor-promoting effects of life-long RF-EMF exposure. Numbers of tumors of the lungs and livers in RF-exposed animals were significantly higher than in sham exposed controls. In addition, lymphomas were also found to be significantly elevated by exposure. The same tumor-promoting effects were seen at nonthermal exposure levels (0.04, and 0.4 W/kg SAR), thus well below exposure limits for the users of mobile phones. The authors concluded that these findings may help explain the repeatedly reported increased incidences of brain tumors in heavy users of mobile phones.

A report has recently been released from The National Toxicology Program (NTP) under the National Institutes of Health (NIH) in USA on the largest ever animal 2-year study on cell phone RF radiation and cancer (64). Rats were exposed to either GSM- or code-division multiple access (CDMA)-moduleated signals at 900 MHz beginning in utero (SAR 0, 1.5, 3, 6 W/kg, 9 h per day, 10 min on/off, 7 days per week). An increased incidence of glioma in the brain and malignant schwannoma in the heart was found in rats at all SAR values and both types of signal. This effect was statistically significant in males only. A statistically significant SAR-dependent trend for GSM and CDMA exposures in males was found. Comet assay showed a statistically significant increased trend and SAR-dependent increase of DNA damage in the frontal cortex of males. Acoustic neuroma or vestibular schwannoma is a similar type of tumor as the one found in the heart, although it is benign. Thus, this animal study supported human epidemiological findings on chronic exposure to RF radiation and brain tumor risk (5,65,66). The strength of the NTP study is in its: (i) long term exposure covering *in utero* period and comparable with life span, (ii) usage of GSM/CDMA modulations and intermittent exposure that is close to exposure from mobile phones in real life, and (iii) large animal group providing high statistical power. The limitation of this study is in using only one GSM and one CDMA frequency, 900 and 1900 MHz, respectively, from multiple frequency channels used in mobile communication. The previously reviewed data showed frequency dependent effects of nonthermal RF (8). In particular, our studies showed that the mobile phone frequency channels vary in their efficiency to affect human cells (67–69). In particular, the frequency of 915 MHz was shown to affect the blood brain barrier and inhibit DNA repair in rats and human cells, respectively. The frequency of 905 MHz was much less effective in experiments with human cells. Thus, some of mobile phone frequency channels may be more or less detrimental. The usage of only two frequencies from GSM/CDMA mobile communication in the NTP study might underestimate carcinogenic effects from everyday exposures to mobile phone RF at various frequency channels. The finding that increased cancer risks was revealed in RF-exposed males only is not a limitation of this study. According to IARC, "‘the probability that tumors will occur may depend on the species, sex, strain, genetic background, and age of the animal, and on the dose, route, timing, and duration of the exposure. Evidence of an increased incidence of neoplasms with increasing levels of exposure strengthens the inference of a causal association between the exposure and the development of neoplasms." p. 22 (4).

4.3 HUMAN STUDIES WITH VOLUNTEERS AND EPIDEMIOLOGICAL STUDIES

4.3.1 Sperm, Reproductive System, and Fertility

Recent review included meta-analysis of 11 studies on human males of reproductive age (70). Based on this meta-analysis, mobile phone use was associated with deterioration in semen quality. The traits adversely affected were sperm concentration, sperm morphology, sperm motility, sperm viability, proportion of nonprogressive motile sperm, and slow progressive motile sperm. Direct exposure of spermatozoa to mobile phone radiation in *in vitro* studies also significantly deteriorated the sperm quality by reducing straight line velocity, fast progressive motility, hypo-osmotic swelling (HOS) test score, major axis, minor axis, total sperm motility, perimeter, area, average path velocity, curvilinear velocity, motile spermatozoa, and acrosome reacted spermatozoa. The strength of evidence for the different outcomes varied from very low to very high. The analysis shows that mobile phone use is possibly associated with a number of deleterious effects on human spermatozoa.

Al-Ali et al. evaluated association of cell phone usage with erectile function (EF) in men (71). 20 men complaining of erectile dysfunction (ED) for at least six months (Group A), and 10 healthy men with no complaints of ED (Group B) were evaluated. Anamnesis, basic laboratory investigations, and clinical examinations were performed. All men completed the German version of the Sexual Health Inventory for Men (SHIM) for evaluation of the International Index of Erectile Function (IIEF), as well as another questionnaire designed for assessing cell phone usage habits. There was no significant difference between both groups enrolled regarding age, weight, height, and total testosterone. The SHIM scores of Group A were significantly lower than that of Group B. While total time spent talking on the cell phone per week was not significantly higher in Group A over B, men with ED were found to carry their 'switched on' cell phones for a significantly longer time than those without ED. The data indicated that the total time of chronic exposure to EMF of the cell phone might be more important than the relatively short duration of intense exposure during making cellular phone calls.

El-Helaly and Mansour studied the effects of cell phones usage on the quality of human semen from 262 male attending an andrology clinic for infertility evaluation (72). The study analyzed cell phone use, duration of daily use in minutes, and how the participants kept or handled their cell phones in relation to their bodies. Semen quality parameters of the participants did not differ significantly between cell phone users and cell phone nonusers. Also, semen quality parameters did not differ significantly according to daily use of cell phone in minutes or in years. Those who kept their cell phones in their trouser pockets had lower sperm motility compared to those who kept their cell phone in their waist pouch, shirt pocket or in hands, but the diffidence was not statistically significant. This study failed to find any significant reduction of semen quality parameters in association with cell phone use.

Zilberlicht et al. investigated an association between characteristics of cell phone usage and semen quality in 106 men who underwent a first-time semen analysis as a part of infertility workup (73).Talking for ≥1 h/day and during device charging were statistically significantly associated with higher rates of abnormal semen concentration. Among men who reported holding their phones ≤50 cm from the groin, a nonsignificantly higher rate of abnormal sperm concentration was found (47.1% versus 11.1%). Multivariate analysis revealed that talking while charging the device and smoking were risk factors for abnormal sperm concentration. These findings suggested that certain aspects of cell phone usage may bear adverse effects on sperm concentration.

While not universal, available studies indicate that prolonged usage of mobile phone may affect human sperm and fertility.

4.3.2 Hearing

Few studies have recently evaluated the effects of chronic MW exposure on hearing (74–77). While these studies did not usually find any effects of using mobile phone up to 5 years on hearing, the latency of waves in auditory brainstem responses (ABR) was significantly prolonged in subjects using mobile phones for 10 years for a maximum of 30 min/day as compared to the control group in one study (76). The authors concluded that long term exposure to mobile phones may affect conduction in the peripheral portion of the auditory pathway. No endpoints relevant for carcinogenicity were evaluated in these studies and the number of participants enrolled to these studies was rather limited suggesting further investigations with a larger group.

4.3.3 Type 2 Diabetes Mellitus

Meo et al. studied the association of exposure to RF EMF generated by mobile phone base stations for 6 h daily, five days in a week, with glycated hemoglobin (HbA1c), which is commonly used as a marker of hyperglycemia and an independent and reliable marker for diabetes mellitus, and occurrence of type 2 diabetes mellitus (78). For this study, 159 male students aged 12–17 years were recruited from two different elementary schools (school-1 and school-2). Mobile phone base stations were about 200 m away from each school. RF EMF was measured inside both schools; 9.601 nW/cm^2 in school 1 and 1.909 nW/cm^2 in school 2. HbA1c was measured in blood samples collected from the students. The mean HbA1c for the students who were exposed to higher RF EMF was significantly higher than the mean HbA1c for the students who were exposed to lower RF EMF. Moreover, students who were exposed to higher RF EMF had a significantly higher risk of type 2 diabetes mellitus relative to their counterparts who were exposed to lower RF-EMF. These findings indicated that chronic exposure to RF-EMF of 9.601 nW/cm^2 is associated with elevated levels of HbA1c and risk of type 2 diabetes mellitus.

4.4 ACADEMIC PERFORMANCE, SLEEPINESS, MENTAL HEALTH, AND SUBJECTIVE WELL-BEING

Lepp et al. investigated the relationships between total cell phone use and texting on Satisfaction with Life (SWL), Academic Performance (GPA), and anxiety in college students (79). Both cell phone use and texting were negatively related to GPA and positively related to anxiety while GPA was positively related to SWL and anxiety was negatively related to SWL. These findings indicate that increased use may negatively impact academic performance, mental health, and subjective well-being or happiness.

Byun et al. evaluated the association between mobile phone use and symptoms of Attention Deficit Hyperactivity Disorder (ADHD) considering the modifying effect of lead exposure (80). A total of 2422 children at 27 elementary schools in 10 Korean cities were examined and followed up 2 years later. Parents filled in a questionnaire including the Korean version of the ADHD rating scale and questions about mobile phone use, as well as socio-demographic factors. The ADHD symptom risk for mobile phone use was estimated at two time points using logistic regression and combined over 2 years using the generalized estimating equation model with repeatedly measured variables of mobile phone use, blood lead, and ADHD symptoms, adjusted for covariates. Voice call use variables (number of outgoing calls per day, average time spent per voice call, and cumulative time spent for voice calls) showed increased risks for ADHD symptoms according to increasing mobile phone exposure. The ADHD symptom risk associated with mobile phone use for voice calls, but the association was limited to children exposed to relatively high lead after adjustment for several covariates. The authors concluded that simultaneous exposure to lead and RF from mobile phone use was associated with increased ADHD symptom risk.

Redmayne et al. evaluated associations between self-reported use of wireless telephone and internet technology and well-being of New Zealand adolescents (81). The participants completed questionnaires in class about their mobile phone and cordless phone use, their self-reported well-being, and possible confounders. Parental questionnaires provided data on whether they had WiFi at home and cordless phone ownership and model. The 373 enrolled participants were reported to use analogue and digital cordless phones, the latter utilizing DECT, DECT6, Wideband Digital Enhanced Cordless Telecommunication (WDECT), Digital Signal Standard (DSS), and frequency hopping spread spectrum (FHSS) modulation systems. They were categorized in four groups: (A) nonusers of cordless phone, (B) analogue phone, (C) DECT and DECT6 phones, and (D) the remainder. The frequency ranges were (1) 30–40 and 900 MHz, (2) 1.8 and 1.9 GHz, (3) 2.4 GHz, and (4) 5.8 GHz. Use of mobile phone and cordless phone $\geq$3 times weekly was associated with increased risk of headaches. Several cordless phone frequencies bands were statistically significantly related to tinnitus, feeling down/depressed, and sleepiness at school. This study revealed more statistically significant associations (36%) of mobile phone use and well-being than could be expected by chance (5%), with several of these associations being dependent on dose (number and duration of calls). The data also suggested apparent significance of some frequency bands or systems used by cordless phones.

Nathan et al. investigated an association between mobile phone use, especially at night, and sleepiness in a group of 191 US teenagers using a questionnaire containing an Epworth Sleepiness Scale (ESS) modified for teens and questions about qualitative and quantitative use of the mobile phone (82). Multivariate regression analysis indicated that ESS score was significantly associated with being female, feeling a need to be accessible by mobile phone all of the time, and a past attempt to reduce mobile phone use. The number of daily texts or phone calls was not directly associated with ESS. The relationship between daytime sleepiness and mobile phone use was not directly related to the number of daily texts or phone calls, but may be related to the temporal pattern of mobile phone use.

Zheng et al. studied the association between mobile phone (MP) use and inattention in 7102 students in 4 middle schools (83). The mean age was 15.26 ± 1.77 years. Participants owned mobile phones at the time of the survey and had been using a mobile phone for a mean of 3.50 ± 2.48 years. Participants spent 57.36 ± 71.96 minutes on entertainment and 8.64 ± 15.48 minutes on making calls daily. Inattention was assessed as defined for the Attention Deficit component of Attention deficit/Hyperactivity disorder (ADHD) by the Diagnostic and Statistical Manual of Mental. After adjustment for confounders, inattention in adolescents was significantly associated with MP ownership, the time spent on entertainment on mobile phone per day, the position of the MP during the day, and the mode of the mobile phone at night. The strongest association between inattention and the time spent on the mobile phone was among students who spent $\geq$60 minutes per day playing on their mobile phone. This data indicated association between mobile phone use and inattention in Chinese adolescents. The authors advised that decreasing mobile phone usage to $\leq$60 minutes per day may help adolescents to stay focused and centered.

In their cross-sectional study, Zheng et al. investigated associations between mobile phone use and well-being among 746 children in the two primary schools in Chongqing, China (84). The average age of the participants in the survey was 10.6 ± 0.6 years and the average year of mobile phone usage was 1.3 ± 1.5 years. Fatigue was significantly associated with the years of mobile phone usage and the daily duration of mobile phone calls. Headache was significantly associated with the daily duration of mobile phone calls. However, only the association between fatigue and mobile phone usage remained statistically significant after adjusting for confounders. There was no significant association between MP use and other physical symptoms (dizziness, sleeping problems, feeling low, heart beating fast) in children. This study indicated that there was a consistent significant association between mobile phone use and fatigue in children.

Huss et al. evaluated association of chronic exposure to RF-EMF with reported quality of sleep in 2361 Amsterdam born children, aged 7 years (85). When children were about five years old, school and residential exposure to RF-EMF from base stations was assessed with a geospatial model (NISMap) and from indoor sources (cordless phone/WiFi) using parental self-reports. Parents also reported their children's use of mobile or cordless phones. When children were seven years old, sleep quality was evaluated with the Child Sleep Habits Questionnaire (CSHQ) filled in by parents. Of eight CSHQ subscales, sleep onset delay, sleep duration, night wakening, parasomnias, and daytime sleepiness were evaluated with logistic or negative binomial regression models, adjusting for child's age and sex and indicators of socio-economic position of the parents. The remaining three subscales (bedtime resistance, sleep anxiety, sleep disordered breathing) were evaluated as unrelated outcomes (negative control). Sleep onset delay, night wakening, parasomnias, and daytime sleepiness were not associated with residential exposure to RF-EMF from base stations. Sleep duration scores were associated with RF-EMF levels from base stations. Higher mobile phone use was associated with less favorable sleep duration, night wakenings, and parasomnias, and also with bedtime resistance. Cordless phone use was not related to any of the sleeping scores. Based on inconsistent findings for different RF sources, which otherwise are well expected based on studies and mechanisms reviewed previously (2,3,8), the authors suggested that the revealed sleep disorders may also be potentially caused by other factors that are related to mobile phone usage such as the displacement of sleep by media use, physiological arousal when using media in the evenings or bright (blue) light from screens suppressing melatonin.

Schoeni et al. investigated association of memory performance in adolescents with the dose of RF exposure from mobile communication devices in their longitudinal epidemiological cohort study with 439 adolescents (86). Verbal and figural memory tasks at baseline and after one year were completed using a standardized, computerized cognitive test battery. Use of wireless devices was inquired by questionnaire and operator recorded mobile phone use data was obtained for a subgroup of 234 adolescents. Exposure from cordless phone base stations, WLAN access points, and other people's mobile phones were estimated by linear regression models calibrated on the personal measurement data available from 95 study participants. RF-EMF dose measures considering various factors affecting RF-EMF exposure were computed for the brain and the whole body. A substantial correlation was found between self-reported mobile phone call duration and brain dose of the whole sample. In linear exposure-response models, an interquartile increase in cumulative operator recorded mobile phone call duration was associated with a decrease in figural memory performance score by 0.15 (95% CI: 0.33, 0.03) units. For cumulative RF-EMF brain and whole body dose, corresponding decreases in figural memory scores were 0.26 (95% CI: 0.42, 0.10) and 0.40 (95% CI: 0.79, 0.01), respectively. Compared to the low exposure group (below median), significant decreases were observed in the high exposure group for brain dose (−1.16; 95% CI: −1.99, −0.34) and whole body dose (−0.86; 95% CI: −1.67, −0.05) of the whole sample and for the brain dose of the sample with operator data (−1.62; 95% CI: −2.63, −0.61). Stratified analyses according to the preferred side of mobile phone use revealed for the analyses of the figural memory test in the whole sample a stronger effect estimate for the brain dose of right side mobile phone users compared to the group of left side and no preference side users (change per interquartile range: −0.52 (95% CI: −0.82, −0.22) vs. 0.27 (95% CI: −0.35, 0.89)). For the verbal memory test, the pattern tended to be reversed with somewhat stronger effect estimates for the left side users and those without a side preference compared to the right side users. Of note, during figural memory processes, encoding elicits bilateral prefrontal activity and retrieval increases the activity in bilateral or right-sided temporal regions and in bilateral prefrontal regions. In contrary, during verbal encoding increases in prefrontal and temporal brain activity in the left hemisphere can be seen. Stronger overall effects observed for figural memory processes predominantly involving the right hemisphere compared to the verbal memory tasks mostly involving the left hemisphere were compatible with the fact that 81.2% of the study participants reported mainly used mobile phones on the right side, but only 18.8% on the left side or with no laterality preference. No exposure-response associations were observed for sending text messages and duration of gaming, which produced tiny RF-EMF emissions. Finally, the data indicated that negative effects on memory performance over one year were associated with cumulative duration of wireless phone use and more strongly with RF-EMF dose. Within various dose measures, stronger associations were observed for brain than for whole body dose. The laterality analyses indicated stronger associations for right side users for the figural memory task whereas the reverse pattern was seen for the verbal task.

In conclusion, several studies provided evidence that that long-term chronic exposure to signals of mobile communications may affect cognitive functions.

4.5 PRENATAL EXPOSURE TO MOBILE PHONE

Studies examining prenatal exposure to mobile phone use and its effect on child neurodevelopment showed different results depending on the child's developmental stages. Adverse effects have been reported in later ages at 7 years (87,88), and 11 years (89). However, no effects were reported for earlier ages, at 14 months (90), at 6 and 18 months (91), at 3 years (92) and 5 years (93). All these studies were based on retrospective assessment of cell phone use. Birks et al. have recently assessed this association in a multi-national analysis, using data from three cohorts with prospective data on prenatal cell phone use, together with previously published data from two cohorts with retrospectively collected cell phone use data (94). They used individual participant data from 83,884 mother-child pairs in the five cohorts from Denmark (1996–2002), Korea (2006–2011), the Netherlands (2003–2004), Norway (2004–2008), and Spain (2003–2008). Cell phone use was categorized into none, low, medium, and high based on frequency of calls during pregnancy reported by the mothers. Child behavioral problems were classified in the borderline/clinical and clinical ranges using validated cut-offs in children aged 5–7 years. Overall, 38.8% of mothers, mostly from the Danish cohort, reported no cell phone use during pregnancy and these mothers were less likely to have a child with overall behavioral, hyperactivity/inattention or emotional problems. The trend of increased risk of child behavioral problems through the maternal cell phone use categories was observed for hyperactivity/inattention problems (OR for problems in the clinical range: 1.11, 95% CI 1.01, 1.22; 1.28, 95% CI 1.12, 1.48, among children of medium and high users, respectively). This association was fairly consistent across cohorts and between cohorts with retrospectively and prospectively collected cell phone use data. The authors concluded that maternal cell phone use during pregnancy may be associated with an increased risk for behavioral problems, particularly hyperactivity/inattention problems, in the offspring.

Tan et al. assessed the association between maternal lifestyle factors and risk of threatened miscarriage in their recent case-control study in the largest maternity hospital in Singapore, with over 12,000 deliveries a year (95). Cases were 154 women with threatened miscarriage in the 5th to 10th weeks of gestation; controls were 264 women without threatened miscarriage. Lifestyle variables were: current and past cigarette smoking, current second-hand cigarette smoke exposure, computer and mobile phone use, perceived stress, past contraceptive use, past menstrual regularity, and consumption of fish oils, caffeine, and alcohol. A positive association of threatened miscarriage with second-hand smoke exposure, computer usage (>4 hours/day), caffeine consumption and mobile phone usage (>1 hour/day) was found using multivariate analysis. Mobile phone use for 1–2 hours/day had an odds ratio (OR) of 2.94 (95% CI 1.32–6.53) and use for >2 hours/day had an OR of 6.32 (95% CI 2.71–14.75) as compared to <1 hour/day. Thus, longer duration of mobile phone use was associated with higher risk. The data suggested that prolonged mobile phone use correlated with threatened miscarriage and a dose-response relationship was observed.

Mahmoudabadi et al. investigated possible association between chronic exposure to electromagnetic fields of cell phones and spontaneous abortion (96). In this case-control study, 292 women who had an unexplained spontaneous abortion at <14 weeks gestation and 308 pregnant women >14 weeks gestation were enrolled. The data about socioeconomic and obstetric characteristics, medical and reproductive history, lifestyles, and use of cell phones during pregnancy were collected. The data on cell usage included the average calling time per day, the location of the cell phones when not in use, use of hands-free equipment, use of phones for other applications, the phone SAR reported by the manufacturer, and the effective SAR determined as average duration of calling time per day x SAR. This last parameter estimated the per day dose of RF exposure from a phone. All the data pertaining to mobile phones were different between the two groups except the use of hands-free devices. Logistic regression analysis revealed a significant association between the effective SAR (per day RF dose) with the risk of spontaneous abortions after adjustment for maternal age, paternal age, history of abortions, and family relationships. These findings suggested that use of mobile phones can be related to the early spontaneous abortions.

To conclude, the available data encourage warnings against prenatal usage of mobile communication.

4.6 CARCINOGENESIS AND MOBILE PHONE USE

Several epidemiological studies had examined the association between cell phone use and tumors in the parotid glands. These studies provided contradictory results. de Siqueira et al. evaluated the available literature to determine their statistical significance using meta-analysis (97). Only three studies satisfied the criteria to be included in the meta-analysis. Using these independent samples representing 5087 subjects from retrospective case-control studies, cell phone use was revealed to be associated with greater odds (1.28, 95%-confidence interval 1.09–1.51) to develop salivary gland tumor.

West et al. reported a case series of four young women aged from 21 to 39 with multifocal invasive breast cancer that raises the concern of a possible association with exposure to electromagnetic fields from cellular phones (98). All patients regularly carried their smartphones directly against their breasts in their brassieres for up to 10 hours a day, for several years, and developed tumors in areas of their breasts immediately underlying the phones. While breast cancer occurring in women under the age of 40 is uncommon in the absence of family history or genetic predisposition such as mutated BRCA1 and BRCA2, all patients had no family history of breast cancer, tested negative for BRCA1 and BRCA2, and had no other known breast cancer risks. Their breast imaging has shown clustering of multiple tumor foci in the breast directly under the area of phone contact. Pathology of all four cases revealed striking similarity; all tumors were hormone-positive, low-intermediate grade, having an extensive intraductal component, and all tumors have near identical morphology. The findings supported the notion that prolonged direct cellular phone contact may be associated with the development of breast carcinoma.

de Vocht analyzed the 1985–2014 incidence of selected brain cancer subtypes in England and compared to counterfactual 'synthetic control' time series were (99). More specifically, two specific hypotheses are addressed: (1) trends in histologically-defined brain cancers that have previously been linked to mobile phone exposure; malignant glioma and glioblastoma multiforme (Grade IV astrocytoma) or GBM4, and (2) malignant neoplasms of the temporal and parietal lobes, which receive the highest exposures, and for which the temporal lobe has especially been highlighted as an important location of interest. Annual 1985–2014 incidence of malignant glioma, glioblastoma multiforme, and malignant neoplasms of the temporal and parietal lobes in England were modeled based on population-level covariates using Bayesian structural time series models assuming 5, 10, and 15 year minimal latency periods. Post-latency counterfactual 'synthetic England' time series were nowcast based on covariate trends. The impact of mobile phone use was inferred from differences between measured and modelled time series. There was no evidence of an increase in malignant glioma, glioblastoma multiforme or malignant neoplasms of the parietal lobe not predicted in the 'synthetic England' time series. Malignant neoplasms of the temporal lobe, however, have increased faster than expected. A latency period of 10 years reflected the earliest latency period when this was measurable and related to mobile phone penetration rates, and indicated an additional increase of 35% (95% Credible Interval 9%:59%) during 2005–2014; corresponding to an additional 188 (95% CI 48–324) cases annually. The author concluded that a causal factor, of which mobile phone use (and possibly other wireless equipment) is in agreement with the hypothesized temporal association, is related to an increased risk of developing malignant neoplasms in the temporal lobe.

Few recent meta-analyses of available case-control studies have consistently shown that long term mobile phone use is associated with statistically significant increased risks of brain tumors while no such association is seen with shorter usage (5,6,66,100). The impact of study quality and source of finding has also been estimated.

Bortkiewicz et al. conducted a systematic review and meta-analysis of multiple works on the association between the use of mobile phones and brain cancer (66). The inclusion criteria were: original papers, case-control studies, published after the end of March 2014, measures of association (point estimates as odds ratio and confidence interval of the effect measured), and data on individual exposure. Twenty-four studies (26,846 cases, 50,013 controls) were included in the meta-analysis. A significantly higher risk of an intracranial tumors (all types) was noted for the time from the first regular mobile phone use over 10 years (odds ratio (OR) = 1.25, 95%

confidence interval (CI): 1.04–1.52), and for the ipsilateral location (OR = 1.29, 95% CI: 1.06–1.57). The results indicated that long-term use of mobile phones increased risk of intracranial tumors, especially in the case of ipsilateral exposure.

Prasad et al. investigated whether the methodological quality of studies and source of funding can explain the variation in results for increased brain tumor risks accumulated in epidemiologic studies (6). Twenty-two case-control studies were included for systematic review. Meta-analysis of 14 case-control studies showed practically no increase in risk of brain tumor (OR 1.03 (95% CI 0.92–1.14)). However, for mobile phone use of 10 years or longer (or >1640 h), the overall result of the meta-analysis showed a significant 1.33 times increase in risk. The summary estimate of government funded as well as phone industry funded studies showed 1.07 times increase in odds, although it was not significant. The mixed funded studies did not show any increase in risk of brain tumor. Relationship between source of funding and log OR for each study was not statistically significant ($p < 0.32$, 95% CI 0.036–0.010). Meta-regression analysis indicated that the increased risk was significantly associated with methodological study quality ($p < 0.019$, 95% CI 0.009–0.09). Studies with higher quality showed a trend toward high risk of brain tumor, while lower quality showed a trend toward lower risk/protection. This data provided evidence linking mobile phone use and risk of brain tumors especially in long-term users while lower quality studies underestimated this risk.

Garlberg and Hardell used Bradford Hill's viewpoints from 1965 on association or causation for assessment of glioma risk and use of mobile or cordless phones (65). All nine viewpoints were evaluated based on epidemiology and laboratory studies. (1) Strength: meta-analysis of case-control studies gave odds ratio (OR) = 1.90, 95% confidence interval (CI) = 1.31–2.76 with highest cumulative exposure. (2) Consistency: the risk increased with latency, meta-analysis gave in the 10+ years' latency group OR = 1.62, 95% CI = 1.20–2.19. (3) Specificity: increased risk for glioma was in the temporal lobe. Using meningioma cases as a comparison group still increased the risk. (4) Temporality: highest risk was in the 20+ years' latency group, OR = 2.01, 95% CI = 1.41–2.88, for wireless phones. (5) Biological gradient: cumulative use of wireless phones increased the risk. (6) Plausibility: animal studies showed an increased incidence of glioma and malignant schwannoma in rats exposed to RF radiation. There is increased production of ROS from RF radiation. (7) Coherence: there is a change in the natural history of glioma and increasing incidence. (8) Experiment: antioxidants reduced ROS production from RF radiation. (9) Analogy: there is an increased risk in subjects exposed to extremely low-frequency electromagnetic fields (see also present report. V.). The authors concluded that RF radiation should be regarded as a human carcinogen causing glioma.

A growth in brain cancer incidence including most exposed temporary lobe was described by the cancer registers of some countries (101,102). However, comparison of these data with increased cancer risks from mobile telephony should be done with caution due to reported incompleteness of cancer registers in different countries, which may mask increased cancer incidence (101,103,104).

4.7 DISCUSSION

4.7.1 Chronic Exposures to NT MW and Safety Guidelines

The effects of exposure to NT MW depend on many biological and physical parameters including exposure duration (2,3,8). This dependence is a key reason for variability in the NT MW effects reported in different studies. However, many studies have consistently shown that significant biological and health effects are observed under prolonged durations of exposure (7,105). This chapter reviewed recent studies on health effects of chronic exposure to NT MW.

Available studies show that chronic exposure to NT MW may result in various health effects affecting the central nervous system, memory, leaning, reproductive system, fertility, and immune functions. Chronic exposure to NT MW from mobile communication at $\geq$10 years correlated with increased cancer risk. Overall, there is strong evidence that chronic exposure to NT MW from mobile communication adversely affects health. As far as the ICNIRP safety guidelines, which were adopted by many countries, are based on acute thermal MW effects only, they do not save the population from the adverse effects from chronic exposure to NT MW. Moreover, the SAR concept, which is only relevant to thermal effects and acute exposures, is not useful for protection against adverse effects from chronic exposures to NT MW. Thus, all available data strongly suggest that power density along with duration of exposure should be applied for safety limits (7,106).

Russia was the first country in the world to develop the safety standards for RF/MW exposure, which were based on a 30-year research performed in several Soviet institutions. In these studies, different types of animals (mice, rats, rabbits, guinea pigs) were chronically exposed to NT MW at different PD, frequencies, and modulations. According to 40 Soviet studies selected by the Russian National Committee of Non-Ionizing Radiation Protection (RCNIRP) based on standard quality criteria, the unfavorable bioeffects were observed in animals under chronic MW exposures (18). The studied endpoints included histological analysis of tissues, central nervous system, arterial pressure, blood and hormonal studies, immune system, metabolism and enzymatic activity, reproductive system, teratogenic, and genetic effects. RCNIRP concluded that: (1) data on chronic MW exposure should be considered during development of guidelines; (2) application of SAR concept at nonthermal PD less than 100 $\mu W/cm^2$ is questionable; (3) the role of other parameters such as modulation and duration of exposure should be taken into account; (4) development of safety guidelines would greatly benefit from the knowledge of the biophysical mechanisms for the NT MW effects. Based on multiple data on chronic exposure to NT MW, Soviet/Russian safety standards limited exposure by duration and power density PD while the SAR concept was not applied (10).

Significant progress has recently been reached in understanding the biophysical mechanisms for the NT MW bioeffects (2). Emerging evidence suggests that these nonthermal effects occur due to oxidative stress, induced intracellular signaling cascades, transmembrane processes, conformational changes, changes in gene/protein expression, cellular metabolism, transmembrane signal transduction, and cell cycle progression (3).

4.8 COMBINED ASSESSMENT OF NONTHERMAL AND THERMAL EFFECTS UPON CHRONIC EXPOSURES TO MOBILE PHONE

This chapter considered the effects of chronic exposure to nonthermal MW (less than or equal to 2 W/kg) only. However, the French government agency L'Agence Nationales des Fréquences (ANFR) reported that despite non-thermal SAR values less than 2 W/kg are commonly indicated in the manuals from mobile phone, most of them significantly exceed these values if used in contact with head (https://data.anfr.fr/explore/dataset/das-telephonie-mobile/?disjunctive.marque&disjunctive.modele). The ANFR tested hundreds of mobile phones for SAR when the phones operated at maximum power. If phones were measured at the distance of 15 mm from the body, the SAR complied with the ICNIRP guidelines of 2 W/kg. When the same phones were measured at 5 mm from the body, most, but not all phones complied. On the other hand, many phones had SAR levels above the ICNIRP guidelines in contact with the body. These new data complicate assessment of risks from chronic exposures to mobile phone suggesting consideration of the combined nonthermal and thermal effects.

4.8.1 New Technologies, 5G

New mobile communication technologies are implemented every 5–10 years without any test for potential health risks under chronic exposures. As soon as the laboratory and epidemiological studies have collected data on potential health risks of currently used technologies (e.g. brain tumor risks associated with 1G, 2G, and 3G mobile communication), these signals are replaced by newer ones. However, given the dependence of MW effects on multiple parameters, generally established dependence of health effects on duration of chronic exposure, and latency time $\geq$10 years, the obtained data on current and past technologies are almost useless for prediction of health risks for newer developed mobile communication signals. At the moment, 5G communications, which use extremely high frequency MW or millimeter waves (MMW, wavelength 1–10 mm), is planned to be introduced in many countries. It follows from multiple studies that MMW can affect biological systems and human health, both positively and negatively, under specific conditions of exposure at very low intensities below the ICNIRP guidelines (107–109). Various biological and health effects have been described, which commonly depend on multiple physical and physiological parameters. In particular, MMW inhibited repair of DNA damage induced by ionizing radiation under specific conditions of exposure (109). On other hand, MMW exposure at individually selected frequencies has been used in ex-USSR countries for treatment of various diseases since the 1980s. For example, Sit'ko et al. described the frequency of 56.46 GHz, which was found during an ordinary search for therapeutic frequencies based on sensorial reactions of a patient with duodenal ulcer (110). A negative sensation (defined as spastic contraction of musculus quadricepts femoris) was repeatedly observed under applying MMW at this frequency. This sensory reaction allowed tracking the stomach meridian by using a static magnet at 4 mT. Exposure at the frequency of 56.46 GHz worsened the health condition of the patient. Thus, this exposure was aborted and the patient received treatment at the resonance therapeutic frequency found by typical positive sensations reviewed by Kositsky et al. (https://www.salzburg.gv.at/gesundheit_/Documents/2001_kositsky_et_al._-_ussr_review-2.pdf). After successfully healing the duodenal ulcer at the MMW resonance therapeutic frequency, the negative response of the patient to the frequency of 56.46 GHz disappeared.

To what extent the 5G technology, the Internet of Things, will affect the biota and human health is definitely not known. However, based on the possible fundamental role of MMW in regulation of homeostasis (111,112) and almost complete absence of MMW in the atmosphere due to effective absorption suggesting lack of adaptation to this type of radiation, the health effects of chronic exposures to MMW may be more significant than for any other frequency range.

4.9 CONCLUSION

Chronic exposure to nonthermal microwaves (NT MW) may result in various health effects affecting the central nervous system, fertility, immune functions, and causing/promoting cancer. Taken together, available studies indicate that response to NT MW depends on PD and duration exposure (7). The SAR based ICNIRP safety standards, which have been widely adopted for protection against acute thermal effects of MW, are insufficient to protect the public from chronic exposures to NT MW from mobile communication. New safety standards should commonly be adopted based on data from multiple studies on chronic exposures and mechanisms for nonthermal MW effects (106). It should be anticipated that definite parts of human population, such as children, pregnant women, and hypersensitive persons, which constitute about 1%–10% of the general population in economically developed counties (113), could be especially vulnerable to chronic NT MW exposures. In general, new signals of mobile communication should be tested with chronic exposures before being put into practice.

ACKNOWLEDGMENTS

Financial support from the National Scholarship Program of the Slovak Republic, the Russian Foundation for Basic Research, the Slovak Research and Development Agency (APVV-15-0250), and the VEGA Grant Agency (2/0109/15) of the Slovak Republic are gratefully acknowledged.

REFERENCES

1. Morgan LL, Miller AB, Sasco A, Davis DL. Mobile phone radiation causes brain tumors and should be classified as a probable human carcinogen (2A) (Review). *Int J Oncol* 2015;46:1865–71.
2. Belyaev I. Biophysical mechanisms for nonthermal microwave effects. In: Markov M, editor. *Electromagnetic Fields in Biology and Medicine.* Boca Raton, London, New York: CRC Press; 2015. pp. 49–68.

3. Belyaev I. Electromagnetic field effects on cells and cancer risks from mobile communication. In: Rosch PJ, editor. *Bioelectromagnetic and Subtle Energy Medicine*. Volume Second Edition. Boca Raton, London, New York: CRC Press; 2015. pp. 517–539.
4. IARC. *IARC Monographs on the Evaluation of Carcinogenic Risks to Humans. Non-Ionizing Radiation, Part 2: Radiofrequency Electromagnetic Fields*. Volume 102. Lyon, France: IARC Press; 2013. pp. 1–406, http://monographs.iarc.fr/ENG/Monographs/vol102/mono102.pdf
5. Yang M, Guo W, Yang C, Tang J, Huang Q, Feng S, Jiang A, Xu X, Jiang G. Mobile phone use and glioma risk: A systematic review and meta-analysis. *PLoS One* 2017;12:e0175136.
6. Prasad M, Kathuria P, Nair P, Kumar A, Prasad K. Mobile phone use and risk of brain tumours: A systematic review of association between study quality, source of funding, and research outcomes. *Neurol Sci* 2017;38:797–810.
7. Belyaev I. 9 duration of exposure and dose in assessing nonthermal biological effects of microwaves. In: Markov M, editor. *Dosimetry in Bioelectromagnetics*. Boca Raton, London, New York: CRC Press; 2017. pp. 171–184.
8. Belyaev IY. Dependence of non-thermal biological effects of microwaves on physical and biological variables: Implications for reproducibility and safety standards. *European Journal of Oncology - Library* 2010;5:187–218.
9. ICNIRP. ICNIRP Guidelines. Guidelines for limiting exposure to time-varying electric, magnetic, and electromagnetic fields (up to 300 GHz). *Health Phys* 1998;74:494–522.
10. SanPiN. *[Radiofrequency Electromagnetic Radiation (RF EMR) Under Occupational and Living Conditions]*. Moscow: Minzdrav; 1996.
11. Jokela K, Puranen L, Sihvonen AP. Assessment of the magnetic field exposure due to the battery current of digital mobile phones. *Health Phys* 2004;86:56–66.
12. Perentos N, Iskra S, McKenzie R, Cosic I. Characterization of pulsed ELF magnetic fields generated by GSM mobile phone handsets. *World Congress on Medical Physics and Biomedical Engineering 2006, Vol 14, Pts 1-6* 2007;14:2706–2709.
13. Cook CM, Saucier DM, Thomas AW, Prato FS. Exposure to ELF magnetic and ELF-modulated radiofrequency fields: The time course of physiological and cognitive effects observed in recent studies (2001–2005). *Bioelectromagnetics* 2006;27:613–27.
14. Heath B, Jenvey S, Cosic I. Investigation of analogue and digital mobile phone low frequency radiation spectrum characteristics. *Proceedings of the 2nd International Conference on Bioelectromagnetism* 1998:83–84.
15. Linde T, Mild KH. Measurement of low frequency magnetic fields from digital cellular telephones. *Bioelectromagnetics* 1997;18:184–6.
16. Ilvonen S, Sihvonen AP, Karkkainen K, Sarvas J. Numerical assessment of induced ELF currents in the human head due to the battery current of a digital mobile phone. *Bioelectromagnetics* 2005;26:648–56.
17. IARC. IARC (International Agency for Research on Cancer) monographs on the evaluation of carcinogenic risks to humans. In: *Non-Ionizing Radiation, Part I: Static and Extremely Low Frequency (ELF) Electric and Magnetic Fields*. Volume 80. Lyon, France: IARC Press; 2002. p. 429.
18. Grigoriev YG, Stepanov VS, Nikitina VN, Rubtcova NB, Shafirkin AV, Vasin AL. *ISTC Report. Biological Effects of Radiofrequency Electromagnetic Fields and the Radiation Guidelines*. Results of Experiments Performed in Russia/Soviet Union. Moscow: Institute of Biophysics, Ministry of Health, Russian Federation; 2003.
19. Kesari KK, Kumar S, Behari J. 900-MHz microwave radiation promotes oxidation in rat brain. *Electromagn Biol Med* 2011;30:219–234.
20. Haghani M, Shabani M, Moazzami K. Maternal mobile phone exposure adversely affects the electrophysiological properties of Purkinje neurons in rat offspring. *Neuroscience* 2013;250:588–98.

21. Ikinci A, Mercantepe T, Unal D, Erol HS, Sahin A, Aslan A, Bas O et al. Morphological and antioxidant impairments in the spinal cord of male offspring rats following exposure to a continuous 900MHz electromagnetic field during early and mid-adolescence. *J Chem Neuroanat* 2016;75:99–104.
22. Aslan A, Ikinci A, Bas O, Sonmez OF, Kaya H, Odaci E. Long-term exposure to a continuous 900 MHz electromagnetic field disrupts cerebellar morphology in young adult male rats. *Biotech Histochem* 2017;16:1–7.
23. Kerimoglu G, Hanci H, Bas O, Aslan A, Erol HS, Turgut A, Kaya H, Cankaya S, Sonmez OF, Odaci E. Pernicious effects of long-term, continuous 900-MHz electromagnetic field throughout adolescence on hippocampus morphology, biochemistry and pyramidal neuron numbers in 60-day-old Sprague Dawley male rats. *J Chem Neuroanat* 2016;77:169–175.
24. Deshmukh PS, Megha K, Nasare N, Banerjee BD, Ahmed RS, Abegaonkar MP, Tripathi AK, Mediratta PK. Effect of low level subchronic microwave radiation on rat brain. *Biomed Environ Sci* 2016;29:858–867.
25. Gokcek-Sarac C, Er H, Kencebay Manas C, Kantar Gok D, Ozen S, Derin N. Effects of acute and chronic exposure to both 900 and 2100 MHz electromagnetic radiation on glutamate receptor signaling pathway. *Int J Radiat Biol* 2017;1:1–29.
26. Sharma A, Kesari KK, Saxena VK, Sisodia R. Ten gigahertz microwave radiation impairs spatial memory, enzymes activity, and histopathology of developing mice brain. *Mol Cell Biochem* 2017;435:1–13.
27. Tang J, Zhang Y, Yang L, Chen Q, Tan L, Zuo S, Feng H, Chen Z, Zhu G. Exposure to 900 MHz electromagnetic fields activates the mkp-1/ERK pathway and causes blood-brain barrier damage and cognitive impairment in rats. *Brain Res* 2015;15:019.
28. Mugunthan N, Shanmugasamy K, Anbalagan J, Rajanarayanan S, Meenachi S. Effects of long term exposure of 900–1800 MHz radiation emitted from 2G mobile phone on mice hippocampus- A histomorphometric study. *J Clin Diagn Res* 2016;10:AF01–6.
29. Zhao L, Peng RY, Wang SM, Wang LF, Gao YB, Dong J, Li X, Su ZT. Relationship between cognition function and hippocampus structure after long-term microwave exposure. *Biomed Environ Sci* 2012;25:182–188.
30. Maaroufi K, Had-Aissouni L, Melon C, Sakly M, Abdelmelek H, Poucet B, Save E. Spatial learning, monoamines and oxidative stress in rats exposed to 900 MHz electromagnetic field in combination with iron overload. *Behav Brain Res* 2014;258:80–89.
31. Deshmukh PS, Nasare N, Megha K, Banerjee BD, Ahmed RS, Singh D, Abegaonkar MP, Tripathi AK, Mediratta PK. Cognitive impairment and neurogenotoxic effects in rats exposed to low-intensity microwave radiation. *Int J Toxicol* 2015;34:284–90.
32. Schneider J, Stangassinger M. Nonthermal effects of lifelong high-frequency electromagnetic field exposure on social memory performance in rats. *Behav Neurosci* 2014;128:633–637.
33. Narayanan SN, Kumar RS, Karun KM, Nayak SB, Bhat PG. Possible cause for altered spatial cognition of prepubescent rats exposed to chronic radiofrequency electromagnetic radiation. *Metab Brain Dis* 2015;30:1193–206.
34. Junior LC, Guimaraes Eda S, Musso CM, Stabler CT, Garcia RM, Mourao-Junior CA, Andreazzi AE. Behavior and memory evaluation of Wistar rats exposed to 1.8 GHz radiofrequency electromagnetic radiation. *Neurol Res* 2014;36:800–3.
35. Kumlin T, Iivonen H, Miettinen P, Juvonen A, van Groen T, Puranen L, Pitkäaho R, Juutilainen J, Tanila H. Mobile phone radiation and the developing brain: Behavioral and morphological effects in juvenile rats. *Radiat Res* 2007;168:471–479.
36. Klose M, Grote K, Spathmann O, Streckert J, Clemens M, Hansen VW, Lerchl A. Effects of early-onset radiofrequency electromagnetic field exposure (GSM 900 MHz) on behavior and memory in rats. *Radiat Res* 2014;182:435–447.
37. Szmigielski S. Reaction of the immune system to low-level RF/MW exposures. *Sci Total Environ* 2013;454–455:393–400.

38. Ohtani S, Ushiyama A, Maeda M, Ogasawara Y, Wang J, Kunugita N, Ishii K. The effects of radio-frequency electromagnetic fields on T cell function during development. *J Radiat Res* 2015;56:467–74.
39. Kulaber A, Kerimoglu G, Ersoz S, Colakoglu S, Odaci E. Alterations of thymic morphology and antioxidant biomarkers in 60-day-old male rats following exposure to a continuous 900 MHz electromagnetic field during adolescence. *Biotech Histochem* 2017;9:1–7.
40. Kesari KK, Behari J. Evidence for mobile phone radiation exposure effects on reproductive pattern of male rats: Role of ROS. *Electromagn Biol Med* 2012;31:213–222.
41. Kumar S, Behari J, Sisodia R. Influence of electromagnetic fields on reproductive system of male rats. *Int J Radiat Biol* 2013;89:147–54.
42. Tas M, Dasdag S, Akdag MZ, Cirit U, Yegin K, Seker U, Ozmen MF, Eren LB. Long-term effects of 900 MHz radiofrequency radiation emitted from mobile phone on testicular tissue and epididymal semen quality. *Electromagn Biol Med* 2014;33:216–22.
43. Qin F, Zhang J, Cao H, Guo W, Chen L, Shen O, Sun J et al. Circadian alterations of reproductive functional markers in male rats exposed to 1800 MHz radiofrequency field. *Chronobiol Int* 2014;31:123–33.
44. Mugunthan N, Anbalagan J, Meenachi S. Effects of long term exposure to a 2G cell phone radiation (900–1900 MHz) on mouse testis. *Int J Sci Res* 2014;3:523–529.
45. Kumar S, Nirala JP, Behari J, Paulraj R. Effect of electromagnetic irradiation produced by 3G mobile phone on male rat reproductive system in a simulated scenario. *Indian J Exp Biol* 2014;52:890–7.
46. Liu Q, Si T, Xu X, Liang F, Wang L, Pan S. Electromagnetic radiation at 900 MHz induces sperm apoptosis through bcl-2, bax and caspase-3 signaling pathways in rats. *Reprod Health* 2015;12:65.
47. Odaci E, Ozyilmaz C. Exposure to a 900 MHz electromagnetic field for 1 hour a day over 30 days does change the histopathology and biochemistry of the rat testis. *Int J Radiat Biol* 2015;91:547–54.
48. Mugunthan N, Anbalagan J, Shanmuga Samy A, Rajanarayanan S, Meenachi S. Effects of chronic exposure to 2G and 3G cell phone radiation on mice testis – A randomized controlled trial. *Int J Curr Res Rev* 2015;7:36–47.
49. Esmekaya MA, Ozer C, Seyhan N. 900 MHz pulse-modulated radiofrequency radiation induces oxidative stress on heart, lung, testis and liver tissues. *Gen Physiol Biophys* 2011;30:84–9.
50. Tsybulin O, Sidorik E, Kyrylenko S, Henshel D, Yakymenko I. GSM 900 MHz microwave radiation affects embryo development of Japanese quails. *Electromagn Biol Med* 2012;31:75–86.
51. Ozorak A, Naziroglu M, Celik O, Yuksel M, Ozcelik D, Ozkaya MO, Cetin H, Kahya MC, Kose SA. Wi-Fi (2.45 GHz)- and mobile phone (900 and 1800 MHz)-induced risks on oxidative stress and elements in kidney and testis of rats during pregnancy and the development of offspring. *Biol Trace Elem Res* 2013;156:221–9.
52. Eser O, Songur A, Aktas C, Karavelioglu E, Caglar V, Aylak F, Ozguner F, Kanter M. The effect of electromagnetic radiation on the rat brain: An experimental study. *Turk Neurosurg* 2013;23:707–15.
53. Tsybulin O, Sidorik E, Brieieva O, Buchynska L, Kyrylenko S, Henshel D, Yakymenko I. GSM 900 MHz cellular phone radiation can either stimulate or depress early embryogenesis in Japanese quails depending on the duration of exposure. *Int J Radiat Biol* 2013;89:756–63.
54. Ozgur E, Kismali G, Guler G, Akcay A, Ozkurt G, Sel T, Seyhan N. Effects of prenatal and postnatal exposure to GSM-like radiofrequency on blood chemistry and oxidative stress in infant rabbits, an experimental study. *Cell Biochem Biophys* 2013;67:743–51.
55. Mugunthan N, Anbalagan J, Meenachi S, Shanmuga Samy A. Exposure of mice to 900–1900 Mhz radiations from cell phone resulting in microscopic changes in the kidney. *Int J Curr Res Rev* 2014;6:44–49.

56. Çiftçi ZZ, Kırzıoğlu Z, Nazıroğlu M, Özmen Ö. Effects of prenatal and postnatal exposure of Wi-Fi on development of teeth and changes in teeth element concentration in rats: Wi-Fi (2.45 GHz) and teeth element concentrations. *Biol Trace Elem Res* 2014;163(1–2):193–201.
57. Olgar Y, Hidisoglu E, Celen MC, Yamasan BE, Yargicoglu P, Ozdemir S. 2.1 GHz electromagnetic field does not change contractility and intracellular Ca2+ transients but decreases beta-adrenergic responsiveness through nitric oxide signaling in rat ventricular myocytes. *Int J Radiat Biol* 2015;91:851–7.
58. Cao H, Qin F, Liu X, Wang J, Cao Y, Tong J, Zhao H. Circadian rhythmicity of antioxidant markers in rats exposed to 1.8 GHz radiofrequency fields. *Int J Environ Res Public Health* 2015;12:2071–87.
59. Zhu S, Zhang J, Liu C, He Q, Vijayalaxmi, Prihoda TJ, Tong J, Cao Y. Dominant lethal mutation test in male mice exposed to 900 MHz radiofrequency fields. *Mutat Res Genet Toxicol Environ Mutagen* 2015;792:53–7.
60. Kuybulu AE, Oktem F, Ciris IM, Sutcu R, Ormeci AR, Comlekci S, Uz E. Effects of long-term pre- and post-natal exposure to 2.45 GHz wireless devices on developing male rat kidney. *Ren Fail* 2016;38:571–80.
61. Baan R, Grosse Y, Lauby-Secretan B, El Ghissassi F, Bouvard V, Benbrahim-Tallaa L, Guha N et al. Carcinogenicity of radiofrequency electromagnetic fields. *Lancet Oncology* 2011;12:624–626.
62. Tillmann T, Ernst H, Streckert J, Zhou Y, Taugner F, Hansen V, Dasenbrock C. Indication of cocarcinogenic potential of chronic UMTS-modulated radiofrequency exposure in an ethylnitrosourea mouse model. *Int J Radiat Biol* 2010;86:529–41.
63. Lerchl A, Klose M, Grote K, Wilhelm AF, Spathmann O, Fiedler T, Streckert J, Hansen V, Clemens M. Tumor promotion by exposure to radiofrequency electromagnetic fields below exposure limits for humans. *Biochem Biophys Res Commun* 2015;459:585–90.
64. Wyde M, Cesta M, Blystone C, Elmore S, Foster P, Hooth M, Kissling G et al. Report of Partial findings from the National Toxicology Program Carcinogenesis Studies of Cell Phone Radiofrequency Radiation in Hsd: Sprague Dawley® SD rats (Whole Body Exposure). bioRxiv 2016.
65. Carlberg M, Hardell L. Evaluation of mobile phone and cordless phone use and glioma risk using the bradford hill viewpoints from 1965 on association or causation. *Biomed Res Int* 2017;2017:9218486.
66. Bortkiewicz A, Gadzicka E, Szymczak W. Mobile phone use and risk for intracranial tumors and salivary gland tumors: A meta-analysis. *Int J Occup Med Environ Health* 2017;30:27–43.
67. Markova E, Malmgren LO, Belyaev IY. Microwaves from mobile phones inhibit 53BP1 focus formation in human stem cells more strongly than in differentiated cells: Possible mechanistic link to cancer risk. *Environ Health Perspect* 2010;118:394–9.
68. Belyaev IY, Markova E, Hillert L, Malmgren LO, Persson BR. Microwaves from UMTS/GSM mobile phones induce long-lasting inhibition of 53BP1/gamma-H2AX DNA repair foci in human lymphocytes. *Bioelectromagnetics* 2009;30:129–41.
69. Markova E, Hillert L, Malmgren L, Persson BR, Belyaev IY. Microwaves from GSM mobile telephones Affect 53BP1 and gamma-H2AX Foci in human lymphocytes from hypersensitive and healthy persons. *Environ Health Perspect* 2005;113:1172–1177.
70. Dama MS, Bhat MN. Mobile phones affect multiple sperm quality traits: A meta-analysis. *F1000Res* 2013;2:40.
71. Al-Ali BM, Patzak J, Fischereder K, Pummer K, Shamloul R. Cell phone usage and erectile function. *Cent European J Urol* 2013;66:75–7.
72. El-Helaly M, Mansour M. Cell phone usage and semen quality, hospital based study. *SJAMS* 2014;2:1978–1982.

73. Zilberlicht A, Wiener-Megnazi Z, Sheinfeld Y, Grach B, Lahav-Baratz S, Dirnfeld M. Habits of cell phone usage and sperm quality - Does it warrant attention? *Reprod Biomed Online* 2015;31:421–426.
74. Gupta N, Goyal D, Sharma R, Arora KS. Effect of prolonged use of mobile phone on brainstem auditory evoked potentials. *J Clin Diagn Res* 2015;9:CC07–9.
75. Bhagat S, Varshney S, Bist SS, Goel D, Mishra S, Jha VK. Effects on auditory function of chronic exposure to electromagnetic fields from mobile phones. *Ear Nose Throat J* 2016;95:E18–22.
76. Khullar S, Sood A, Sood S. Auditory brainstem responses and EMFs generated by mobile phones. *Indian J Otolaryngol Head Neck Surg* 2013;65:645–9.
77. Mohan M, Khaliq F, Panwar A, Vaney N. Does chronic exposure to mobile phones affect cognition? *Funct Neurol* 2016;31:47–51.
78. Meo SA, Alsubaie Y, Almubarak Z, Almutawa H, AlQasem Y, Hasanato RM. Association of exposure to radio-frequency electromagnetic field radiation (RF-EMFR) generated by mobile phone base stations with glycated hemoglobin (HbA1c) and risk of type 2 diabetes mellitus. *Int J Environ Res Public Health* 2015;12:14519–28.
79. Lepp A, Barkley JE, Karpinski AC. The relationship between cell phone use, academic performance, anxiety, and Satisfaction with Life in college students. *Comput Hum Behav* 2014;31:343–350.
80. Byun YH, Ha M, Kwon HJ, Hong YC, Leem JH, Sakong J, Kim SY et al. Mobile phone use, blood lead levels, and attention deficit hyperactivity symptoms in children: a longitudinal study. *PLoS One* 2013;8:e59742.
81. Redmayne M, Smith E, Abramson MJ. The relationship between adolescents' well-being and their wireless phone use: A cross-sectional study. *Environ Health* 2013;12:90.
82. Nathan N, Zeitzer J. A survey study of the association between mobile phone use and daytime sleepiness in California high school students. *BMC Public Health* 2013;13:840.
83. Zheng F, Gao P, He M, Li M, Wang C, Zeng Q, Zhou Z, Yu Z, Zhang L. Association between mobile phone use and inattention in 7102 Chinese adolescents: a population-based cross-sectional study. *BMC Public Health* 2014;14:1022.
84. Zheng F, Gao P, He M, Li M, Tan J, Chen D, Zhou Z, Yu Z, Zhang L. Association between mobile phone use and self-reported well-being in children: A questionnaire-based cross-sectional study in Chongqing, China. *BMJ Open* 2015;5:e007302.
85. Huss A, van Eijsden M, Guxens M, Beekhuizen J, van Strien R, Kromhout H, Vrijkotte T, Vermeulen R. Environmental radiofrequency electromagnetic fields exposure at home, mobile and cordless phone use, and sleep problems in 7-year-old children. *PLoS One* 2015;10:e0139869.
86. Schoeni A, Roser K, Röösli M. Memory performance, wireless communication and exposure to radiofrequency electromagnetic fields: A prospective cohort study in adolescents. *Environ Int* 2015;85:343–351.
87. Divan HA, Kheifets L, Obel C, Olsen J. Prenatal and postnatal exposure to cell phone use and behavioral problems in children. *Epidemiology* 2008;19:523–529.
88. Divan HA, Kheifets L, Obel C, Olsen J. Cell phone use and behavioural problems in young children. *J Epidemiol Community Health* 2012;66:524–529.
89. Sudan M, Olsen J, Arah OA, Obel C, Kheifets L. Prospective cohort analysis of cellphone use and emotional and behavioural difficulties in children. *J Epidemiol Community Health* 2016;70:1207–1213.
90. Vrijheid M, Martinez D, Forns J, Guxens M, Julvez J, Ferrer M, Sunyer J. Prenatal exposure to cell phone use and neurodevelopment at 14 months. *Epidemiology* 2010;21:259–62.
91. Divan HA, Kheifets L, Olsen J. Prenatal cell phone use and developmental milestone delays among infants. *Scand J Work Environ Health* 2011;37:341–348.

92. Choi KH, Ha M, Ha EH, Park H, Kim Y, Hong YC, Lee AK et al. Neurodevelopment for the first three years following prenatal mobile phone use, radio frequency radiation and lead exposure. *Environ Res* 2017;156:810–817.
93. Guxens M, van Eijsden M, Vermeulen R, Loomans E, Vrijkotte TGM, Komhout H, van Strien RT, Huss A. Maternal cell phone and cordless phone use during pregnancy and behaviour problems in 5-year-old children. *J Epidemiol Community Health* 2013;67:432–438.
94. Birks L, Guxens M, Papadopoulou E, Alexander J, Ballester F, Estarlich M, Gallastegi M et al. Maternal cell phone use during pregnancy and child behavioral problems in five birth cohorts. *Environ Int* 2017;104:122–131.
95. Tan TC, Neo GH, Malhotra R, Allen JC, Lie D, Østbye T. Lifestyle risk factors associated with threatened miscarriage: A case-control study. *J Fertil In Vitro IVF Worldw Reprod Med Genet Stem Cell Biol* 2014;02:100123.
96. Mahmoudabadi FS, Ziaei S, Firoozabadi M, Kazemnejad A. Use of mobile phone during pregnancy and the risk of spontaneous abortion. *J Environ Health Sci Eng* 2015;13:34.
97. de Siqueira EC, de Souza FT, Gomez RS, Gomes CC, de Souza RP. Does cell phone use increase the chances of parotid gland tumor development? A systematic review and meta-analysis. *J Oral Pathol Med* 2016;9:12531.
98. West JG, Kapoor NS, Liao SY, Chen JW, Bailey L, Nagourney RA. Multifocal breast cancer in young women with prolonged contact between their breasts and their cellular phones. *Case Rep Med* 2013.
99. de Vocht F. Inferring the 1985–2014 impact of mobile phone use on selected brain cancer subtypes using Bayesian structural time series and synthetic controls. *Environ Int* 2016;97:100–107.
100. Wang Y, Guo X. Meta-analysis of association between mobile phone use and glioma risk. *J Cancer Res Ther* 2016;12:C298–C300.
101. Hardell L, Carlberg M. Mobile phones, cordless phones and rates of brain tumors in different age groups in the Swedish National Inpatient Register and the Swedish Cancer Register during 1998–2015. *PLoS One* 2017;12:e0185461.
102. Hardell L, Carlberg M, Hansson Mild K. Use of mobile phones and cordless phones is associated with increased risk for glioma and acoustic neuroma. *Pathophysiology* 2013;20:85–110.
103. Meguerditchian AN, Stewart A, Roistacher J, Watroba N, Cropp M, Edge SB. Claims data linked to hospital registry data enhance evaluation of the quality of care of breast cancer. *J Surg Oncol* 2010;101:593–9.
104. German RR, Fink AK, Heron M, Stewart SL, Johnson CJ, Finch JL, Yin D. The accuracy of cancer mortality statistics based on death certificates in the United States. *Cancer Epidemiol* 2011;35:126–31.
105. Cucurachi S, Tamis WL, Vijver MG, Peijnenburg WJ, Bolte JF, de Snoo GR. A review of the ecological effects of radiofrequency electromagnetic fields (RF-EMF). *Environ Int* 2013;51:116–40.
106. Belyaev I, Dean A, Eger H, Hubmann G, Jandrisovits R, Kern M, Kundi M et al. EUROPAEM EMF Guideline 2016 for the prevention, diagnosis and treatment of EMF-related health problems and illnesses. *Rev Environ Health* 2016;31:363–97.
107. Rojavin MA, Ziskin MC. Medical application of millimetre waves. *QJM* 1998;91:57–66.
108. Pakhomov AG, Murphy MB. Comprehensive review of the research on biological effects of pulsed radiofrequency radiation in Russia and the former Soviet Union. In: Lin JC, editor. *Advances in Electromagnetic Fields in Living System*. Volume 3. New York: Kluwer Academic/Plenum Publishers; 2000. pp. 265–290.
109. Belyaev IY, Shcheglov VS, Alipov ED, Ushalov VD. Nonthermal effects of extremely high-frequency microwaves on chromatin conformation in cells *in vitro* - Dependence on physical, physiological, and genetic factors. *IEEE Trans Microw Theory Tech* 2000;48:2172–2179.

110. Sitko SP, Andreev EA, Dobronravova IS. The whole as a result of self-organization. *J Biol Phys* 1988;16:71–73.
111. Frohlich H. Long-range coherence and energy storage in biological systems. *Int J Quantum Chem* 1968;2:641–652.
112. Frohlich H. The biological effects of microwaves and related questions. In: Marton L, Marton C, editors. *Advances in Electronics and Electron Physics*. Volume 53. New York: Academic Press; 1980. pp. 85–152.
113. Belpomme D, Campagnac C, Irigaray P. Reliable disease biomarkers characterizing and identifying electrohypersensitivity and multiple chemical sensitivity as two etiopathogenic aspects of a unique pathological disorder. *Rev Environ Health* 2015;30:251–271.

5 Can Electromagnetic Field Exposure Caused by Mobile Communication Systems in a Public Environment Be Counted as Dominant?

Jolanta Karpowicz, Dina Šimunić, and Krzysztof Gryz

CONTENTS

5.1 INTRODUCTION

Various types of applications of the electromagnetic field (EMF) are used to improve the quality of life, as well as for industrial and medical purposes. The core of mobile (in other words wireless) communication technologies used for various purposes consists of the transfer of information via wireless links involving the emission and reception of EMF in the radio frequency band (RF), also called radio frequency electromagnetic radiation. All users of such systems, as well as the entire population, are nowadays exposed to the radio frequency electromagnetic field (RF-EMF) emitted by mobile terminals (such as mobile phone handsets, wireless internet access – tablets, laptops, routers, etc.) and their base stations which ensure the transmission of information between them. However, it needs to be pointed out that the same frequency bands – that is, RF-EMF from the frequency band (0.1–6000) MHz (in other words, frequencies from 100 kHz to 6 GHz), are also used by other technologies, such as radio and television broadcasting, cordless phones, wireless internet links, for example, in offices or schools, microwave heating, anti-theft systems, radio frequency identification (RFID) systems, security cameras, baby monitors, Bluetooth devices, ZigBee devices, other industrial, scientific or medical devices, and so on.

Considering the variety of mobile communication technologies, it may be extremely difficult to identify dominant sources of RF-EMF affecting a particular workplace or space accessible to the general public (such as offices, schools, libraries, public transport facilities, shopping infrastructure, open spaces in the city – where both workers and members of the general public, including children, may spend many hours a day). On the other hand – when considering protection measures to reduce electromagnetic exposure in the RF band or considering possible health adverse effects from such exposure – the difficult but core question is about the exposure components and which of them are dominant in order to address the conclusions and any safety actions to the proper (the real dominant) source of environmental hazard. Identifying the dominant sources of RF-EMF exposure is especially difficult because of dynamic changes in wireless communication technologies over the years, which have caused the continuous reorganisation of both the frequency pattern of emitted RF-EMF and the location and technical parameters of active (emitting) components of specific systems.

5.1.1 Physical Properties of RF-EMF

The time-varying nonionizing EMF from extremely low frequency radiation (including power frequency 50/60 Hz), through the intermediate frequency, radio frequency and microwaves are discussed here. The boundary frequency at which ionization appears can be taken as 30×10^6 GHz (in other notation – photons of 12.5 eV energy).

Systematic research and applications of electromagnetic energy were strongly triggered by the work of James Clerk Maxwell, who, in 1864, presented equations summarising all known laws on electricity and magnetism. Maxwell's equations remain the basics of all systems operating with EMF, including wireless systems, as well as interactions between human beings and EMF. Minkowski's form of the set of Maxwell's equations, describing electromagnetic energy by electric and magnetic field vector quantities, consists of four vector fields: E(r,*t*), H(r,*t*), D(r,*t*) and B(r,*t*):

$$\nabla \times \mathrm{E}(\mathrm{r},t) = -\frac{\partial}{\partial t}\mathrm{B}(\mathrm{r},t) \tag{5.1}$$

$$\nabla \times \mathrm{H}(\mathrm{r},t) = \mathrm{J}(\mathrm{r},t) + \frac{\partial}{\partial t}\mathrm{D}(\mathrm{r},t) \tag{5.2}$$

$$\nabla \cdot D(r,t) = \rho(r,t) \tag{5.3}$$

$$\nabla \cdot B(r,t) = 0 \tag{5.4}$$

where E and H are electric field strength and magnetic field strength, respectively; D and B are electric flux density and magnetic flux density, respectively; J is current density, and ρ is electric charge density.

The term EMF formally covers the complete set of field vectors (E, H, D, B), space- (r) and time-dependent (*t*). The SI units of the E and H fields are Volt per metre (V/m) and Ampere per metre (A/m), respectively; the D unit is Ampere-second per metre squared (As/m^2), known as a Coulomb per metre squared (C/m^2), and the B unit is Volt-second per metre squared (Vs/m^2) called a Tesla (T).

The distribution of EMF around any source depends mostly on frequency and distance and the dimensions and geometrical pattern of the radiating structure (usually called an antenna), as well as objects present in the vicinity. In the area closest to the antenna, a reactive near field is formed. The reactive near field develops first into a reactive-radiative near field, and then into a radiative near field (known as a Fresnel zone). As shown in Figure 5.1, at a certain distance from the source, the electromagnetic wave transitions and propagates in the far or radiation field (known as the Frauenhofer zone).

Table 5.1 shows the scheme of four main EMF types developed at various distances from the emitting antenna located in a free space. When discussing safety issues concerning the use of mobile communication systems, the highest attention is drawn to the close proximity of EMF sources (the case of exposure from mobile terminals) or the far distance (the case of exposure from the base station), (Zradziński, 2015b). The reactive near field appears near an antenna without the propagation (or radiation) of electromagnetic energy in a certain direction, because the electric field changes to a magnetic field and vice versa within the time period of the time-changing signal. Wave impedance in the near field differs considerably from wave impedance of the far field (which is established as being approximately 377 V/A),

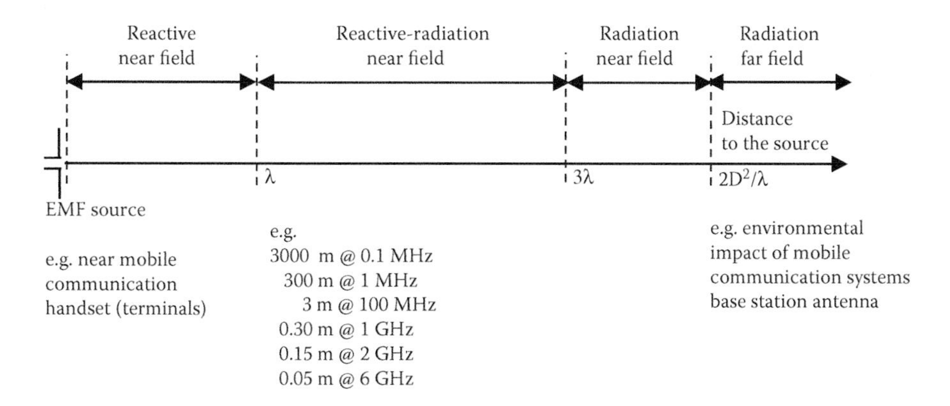

FIGURE 5.1 Simplified scheme of the field distribution around EMF antenna in the free space.

TABLE 5.1
Simplified Characteristics of Near and Far Field in the Vicinity of Antenna in the Free Space

	Near Field			Far Field
	Reactive	**Reactive-Radiation**	**Radiation**	**Radiation**
Inner border	0	λ	3λ	$2D^2/\lambda$
Outer border	λ	3λ	$2D^2/\lambda$	$\propto$
Power density, S	$S \neq \|E\| \cdot \|H\|$	$S \neq \|E\| \cdot \|H\|$	$S \neq \|E\| \cdot \|H\|$ or $S = \|E\|^2/\eta_0$	$S = \|E\| \cdot \|H\| = \|E\|^2/\eta_0$
Wave impedance	different from η_0		in certain points/equals η_0	in the whole space equals η_0

Notes: λ – wavelength of EMF, D – dimension of antenna, $\eta_0 = 377$ V/A – free-space wave impedance

and does not actually exist as a concept of the radiating field. The **radiation far field** begins on the outer border of the Fresnel zone and propagates to infinity. The electric and the magnetic field vectors are time-synchronised in the spatial quadrature and are rectangular to the propagation direction of electromagnetic energy. The presence of objects reflecting EMF energy influences the EMF, even at large geometrical distances to antennas. This basically means that the far field parameters of EMF may not exist in a particular location in the real environment, even at a significant distance from the EMF source. So, in case of an assessment of EMF affecting the human body, both components – the E and H fields – need attention (Hansson Mild et al., 2009, ICNIRP, 1998, Karpowicz and Gryz, 2007).

5.1.2 Biophysical Interaction between RF-EMF and the Human Body

The physical interaction between EMF and human beings can be described via the direct and indirect effects (ICNIRP, 1998). The direct effects are a result of direct interaction of the EMF with the body, and may also be caused by environmental EMF. Indirect effects initially involve EMF interactions with another exposed object present in the vicinity of humans, and may result from physical contact between a person and an exposed object, such as a metallic structure present in the EMF, and as result of exposure being at a different electric potential where the contact results in what is known as contact current. It is highly complex to estimate the value of EMF induced inside the human body (by measurements or numerical calculations) while under exposure from certain EMF sources, and especially when more than one EMF source is present in the near environment (Hansson Mild et al., 2009, Zradziński, 2013, 2015a,b). One of the main reasons for this is that EMF distribution around an emitting device and coupling with the exposed person heavily depends mainly on the environment around the antenna, the antenna structure and polarisation, the EMF frequency and modulation type, and the distance between the EMF source and the human body.

The established mechanisms of human biophysical interaction with EMF include: synapse activity alteration by cell membrane polarisation (phosphenes), peripheral and central nervous systems excitation by cell membrane depolarisation, muscle cell (skeletal) excitation by membrane depolarisation, electroporation, resistive (joule) heating, audio effects by thermoelastic expansion (Frey effect), and magnetohydrodynamic effects (IARC, 2002, IARC, 2013, ICNIRP, 1998, Reilly, 1998). In the case of EMF at the frequencies used by mobile communication systems, the most relevant mechanism of biophysical interaction is the heating effect, which may cause a thermal effect in tissues (tissue heating or even serious burns caused by the absorbed electromagnetic energy in the whole body or in the localised area only). It happens when thermoregulation mechanisms of the body are not efficient enough to dissipate the heat deposed in tissues by EMF exposure. EMF exposures at levels that may be found in the environment accessible by the public are too weak to cause significant thermal effects in the whole body, and usually not even localised effects in any part of the body – evaluated in any 10 g of tissues, as defined by international guidelines (ICNIRP, 1998). However, it needs to be noted that with regard to any possible adverse health effects of EMF exposure, the scientific debate considers that nonthermal mechanisms of interaction (i.e., not related to the temperature rise in a body) may exist, especially when other environmental cofactors have an influence on the body (SCENIHR, 2009, 2015). EMF at levels of normal environmental exposure is not perceived by the human senses.

5.1.3 Health and Safety Hazards from Environmental RF-EMF Exposure

The health consequences of various interactions of EMF with the human body are not yet established, because the scientific background for an assessment considering such complex exposures is not sufficient – still nonsystematic and limited. It is based mainly on studies on the health impact from RF-EMF emitted by mobile phone systems, and limited studies on the health of workers from RTV broadcasting centres.

So far, the results of investigations are inconclusive – they still include a lot of uncertainty, but have not ruled out the possibility of adverse health effects from chronic exposure, especially to high levels (e.g., the development of tumours or malfunctions of the cardiovascular, nervous, and immunological systems are under consideration). For example, the results of epidemiological investigations linked the heavy use of mobile phone handsets with the more frequently diagnosed cancers in the head (Ahlbom et al., 2009, Bortkiewicz et al., 2017, Hardell et al., 2008, 2016, IARC, 2013, ICNIRP, 2009, INTERPHONE Study Group, 2010, Szmigielski, 2013). Such evidence was taken into consideration when the International Agency for Research on Cancer (IARC), affiliated to World Health Organisation (WHO), classified RF-EMF as an environmental factor that is possibly carcinogenic to humans – recognised as 2B classification (classification summarised as: a causal association is considered credible, but bias or confounding cannot be ruled out with reasonable confidence, and based mainly on risks associated with wireless phone use), (IARC, 2011, 2013). Other observations suggest, for example, that chronic, long-term (over years) RF-EMF exposure may also be a risk factor for cardiovascular diseases (Bortkiewicz et al., 2012, Israel et al., 2013, Vangelova et al., 2006, Vesselinova, 2013). A specific environmental factor in that area is the long-term exposure to low-level complex RF-EMF from wireless communication systems – terminals and base stations. Thanks to the intensive development of wireless communication technologies with a growing number of various new types of communication devices, RF-EMF exposure has varied significantly over the years, and scientific knowledge on the health results of such exposure (especially chronic), and how far it may affect health when it is extended over years is still limited and needs to be continuously updated. This is why the topic of safe exposure conditions to EMF is still high in the focus of the general public and even medical doctors (healthychildren.org, 2015, Berg-Beckhoff et al., 2014).

A better understanding of the RF-EMF exposure pattern of subjects involved in studies is a key element for more systematic investigations. Further studies to improve the monitoring of complex RF-EMF exposure and to identify exposure profiles in the context of possible adverse health effects due to chronic exposure are covered, among other things, by recommendations from the Scientific Committee on Emerging and Newly Identified Health Risks (SCENIHR, 2009, 2015). Those studies need also to provide tools for identifying the dominant sources of RF-EMF affecting a particular workplace or a space accessible to the general public. The use of frequency-selective (recognising the types of sources emitting recorded components of exposure by EMF frequency), personal, pocket-sized exposure meters (known as personal exposimeters) and designed for autonomous long-terms, over hours or days, recordings of the variability of RF-EMF levels in real time, allow for more detailed investigations of the profiles of individual RF-EMF exposure – in comparison to classic measurement techniques, which involve broadband measurements (covering the total exposure only) of electric or magnetic field strengths in selected locations (i.e., spot EMF measurements). By exposimetric measurements, it is possible to record correlations between selected parameters of RF-EMF exposure and to identify the relative exposure contributions from various sources – covering the variability of exposure levels over the time of recording caused by a person's movement or changes in the operation of RF-EMF sources (Gryz et al., 2014a,b,c, Gryz and Karpowicz 2015, Karpowicz et al., 2017, Neubauer et al., 2010, Röösli et al., 2010).

On the other hand, the cumulative scientific background on the health impact of RF-EMF is raising public concern over EMF health hazards – both at the level of individuals and at a political level (e.g., European Parliament resolutions) – which indicates the need to take action to prevent any adverse health effects of EMF exposure among the population (European Council, 1999, European Parliament, 2009, European Directive, 2013, healthychildren.org, 2015, IARC, 2013, SCENIHR, 2015, Precautionary Policies and Health Protection 2001, WHO, 1993). It presents a challenge to public health experts to properly identify the most important problems related to EMF, to understand their nature, and to select the most efficient tools in order to eliminate health hazards. This problem may also be supported by the results of exposimetric studies. Further discussion on the state of the art in RF-EMF environmental exposures – sources and exposure profiles – presents what outcome of technical studies may support epidemiologists and decision makers in further decisions and actions on this environmental issue.

5.2 SOURCES OF PUBLIC RF-EMF EXPOSURE

The novel wireless communications technologies grow every day and have changed over years. The oldest systems still functioning are radio and television broadcasting, though these too have recently undergone a change from analogue to digital technology.

FM broadcasting refers to radio broadcasting still using old-fashioned analogue frequency modulation (FM). The frequency band used is the very high frequency (VHF) band (87.5–108 MHz). FM radio waves propagate only to the visual horizon, which is also the radio horizon (usually 40–60 km) (ITU, 2001).

The term **"analogue television"** covers the television technology using analogue signals for transmitting video and audio, meaning that the rapid variations of amplitude, frequency or phase correspond to the brightness, colours, and sound on the transmitted program. Analogue signals propagate or are propagated in the VHF low-band or VHF band I (48–88 MHz), the VHF high-band or VHF band III (174–216 MHz), and ultra-high frequency (UHF) band (470–806 MHz). The analogue television receiver reconstructs the signal from the time-varying signal with timing and synchronisation information.

"Digital TV" uses VHF band III with 7 MHz bandwidth and UHF band with 8 MHz bandwidth (ITU-R, 2016).

Global System for Mobile Communications (GSM) is a European standard developed for 2G networks as a digital, circuit-switched network for duplex voice telephony in 1991, which in later phases was expanded to include data communications (General Packet Radio Services (GPRS) and Enhanced Data rates for GSM Evolution (EDGE), and bearing the name 2.5G) to become a global standard with a market share of over 90% in 2014 (3GPP, 2016).

GSM is based on the following network subsystems: base stations, network and switching, an optional GPRS part, and an operations support system. GSM is designed to be a cellular network with various cell sizes: from the largest (umbrella – covering the whole city and overcoming shadowed regions), through macro (covering up to 35 km distance), micro, and pico to the smallest (femto – with very limited indoor coverage) cells. Most 2G GSM networks operate in the 900 MHz (for the mobile-to-base: 890–915 MHz (uplink, UL); for the base-to-mobile: 935–960 MHz (downlink, DL)) and 1800 MHz bands (1710.2–1784.8 MHz (UL) and 1805.2–1879.8 MHz (DL)), but these networks in some countries may operate in the 450 MHz bands (e.g., 450.6–457.6 MHz (UL) and 460.6–467.6 MHz (DL)). GSM is based on Time Division Multiple Access (TDMA) technology, with time slots independent of the operating frequency. Thus, there are eight full-rate or sixteen half-rate speech channels per radio frequency, which are combined into a TDMA frame. In the same time slot, half-rate channels use alternate frames with the channel data rate for all eight channels of 270.833 kbit/s, and the frame duration of 4.615 ms. The transmission handset power is limited to a maximum of 2 W in GSM900 and 1 W in GSM1800.

Universal Mobile Telecommunications System (UMTS) is the 3G mobile telecommunications technology, supporting conventional cellular voice, text, and multimedia messaging services. Due to the much higher speeds in comparison to GSM, UMTS supported a great expansion of internet access technology, including video calling, e-mail, and web browsing. The UMTS complete network system consists of a radio access network, the same 2G core network, and a user authentication part. UMTS is a technology based on Code Division Multiple Access (CDMA), in a combination with a frequency-division duplexing method. It uses a pair of 5 MHz wide channels. The used frequency bands are 1885–2025 MHz (UL) and 2110–2200 MHz (DL). The UMTS2100 is the most widely deployed UMTS band. The average transfer speed is ~3.6 Mbits/s. In the ideal case, with implemented Evolved High Speed Packet Access (HSPA+) technology, the maximum theoretical data transfer rate is 42 Mbit/s. However, users can expect a transfer rate of up to 384 kbit/s for UMTS and 7.2 Mbit/s (later to 21 Mbit/s) for an HSPA downlink connection. If these values are compared to a single GSM circuit switched data channel with 9.6 kbit/s, it is a significant improvement in technology. The maximum transmission UMTS handset power is 2 W (ETSI TS125101, 2011).

Long Term Evolution (LTE) project (ETSI TS 136101, 2011) was launched to ensure user demand for higher data rates and quality of service, to improve the packet switch optimised system, to further decrease the roundtrip time and user costs, and to avoid the unnecessary fragmentation of technologies related to the frequency spectrum. The newly developed system (called the Evolved Packet System (EPS)) is purely Internet Protocol-based for both real time services and data communications services. It enables speeds of up to 100 Mbit/s for downlink and 50 Mbit/s for uplink, using another air interface technology with Orthogonal Frequency-Division Multiple Access (OFDMA) and higher order modulation of Quadrature Amplitude Modulation (QAM), actually up to 64 QAM, as well as even larger bandwidths (up to 20 MHz). In the downlink with spatial multiplexing, the highest rate can be up to 300 Mbit/s. The downlink and uplink technologies are different in relation to power radiation. The downlink uses OFDMA, which is a multicarrier technology, depicted in Figure 5.2.

The available bandwidth is subdivided into a multitude of mutual orthogonal narrowband subcarriers, which can be shared among multiple users. On the other hand, this means that the power consumption is increased for the sender due to the high peak-to-average power ratio. It also means that the required power amplifiers are quite expensive because of the high requirements on linearity. The fixed part of the network can perform it without problem, but the handsets could be very expensive, even prohibitively so. Therefore, a different frequency access was chosen for the connection of the user to the network recognised as Frequency Division Multiple Access (FDMA), used in the mode of: Single

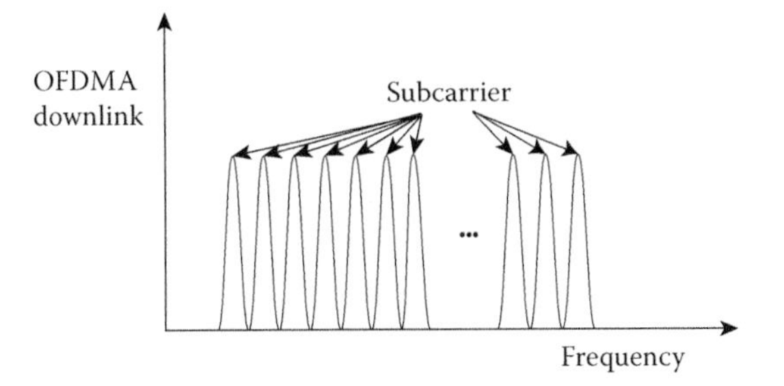

FIGURE 5.2 Subdivision of band into a multitude of mutual orthogonal narrowband subcarriers (OFDMA).

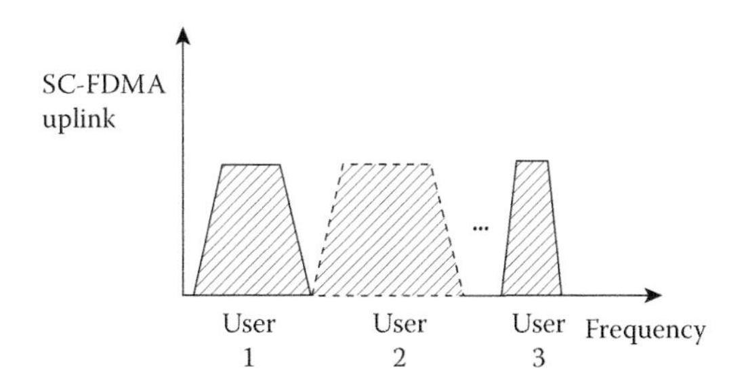

FIGURE 5.3 SC-FDMA signal with single carrier characteristics.

Carrier – Frequency Division Multiple Access (SC-FDMA). As shown in Figure 5.3, the SC-FDMA has a signal with single carrier characteristics, and thus with a low peak-to-average power ratio. LTE uses a frequency range from 700–2700 MHz (i.e., 0.7–2.7 GHz). The available bandwidths are also flexible, starting with 1.4 MHz up to 20 MHz. LTE supports time-division duplex technology (TDD) in eight frequency bands, and frequency-division duplex (FDD) in 15 frequency bands. The transmitter handset power is 0.2 W.

The third generation (3G) standard (UMTS) and the fourth generation (4G) standard (LTE), which followed the 2G standard, were meant to be developed to become global standards.

Digital Enhanced Cordless Telecommunications (or, as before, Digital European Cordless Telecommunications, **DECT**), was developed in Europe for supporting cordless telephone systems (ETSI, 2005). DECT is usually used as a single-cell cordless phone to an analog telephone line, or as a Private Branch Exchange (PBX) for small offices and home systems. However, DECT can be used also for various purposes (e.g., for connection of different kinds of sensors, such as baby monitors).

Technical operation of DECT is designed as an FDMA / TDMA system. The frequency band used for the DECT system (e.g., in Europe: 1880–1900 MHz) is divided up into 10 frequency channels, and an additional 24 time slots per every frame of 10 ms are used. On the top of this, DECT applies TDD technology, which uses different time slots for transmission and reception in the same frequency channel. This is why it is possible for DECT to provide 12 duplex speech channels in each frame and 120 carriers, where each of them can support 32 kbit/s. The maximum power for both the base stations and portable unit is 250 mW. This means that the portable unit usually radiates up to 10 mW during the call, since it is using only one out of 24 time slots.

Wireless Fidelity (Wi-Fi) is a technology for Wireless Local Area Networking (WLAN) where the system operation is based on Institute of Electrical and Electronics Engineers (IEEE) standard number 802.11 (ISO/IEC/IEEE 8802–11, 2012, IEEE Std 802.11-2016, 2016). Wi-Fi most commonly uses the Industrial, Scientific, and Medical (ISM) radio bands: 2.4 GHz (central frequencies: 2.412–2.484 GHz) and 5.7 GHz (central frequencies: 5.745–5.825 GHz). The transmitted power in the European Union is limited to 0.1 W, and in the US to 1 W. In the past, the so-called "WiFi 2G" and "WiFi 5G" (meaning that it is not a mobile 5G) was divided relative to frequency and the kind of technology (IEEE 802.11–2007, 2007). The very new generation combines the two technologies in the best manner, which means that the dual-band wireless technology is applied (IEEE 802.11ac, 2013). This newest generation is compatible with all the older devices at 2.4 GHz, but still has the advantages of the bandwidth rated up to 450 Mbit/s in the 2.4 GHz band and up to 1300 Mbit/s in the 5 GHz band.

The **Radio Frequency Identification (RFID)** system is widely used for the automatic identification of objects, animals, and people and for various tasks in the world of the **Internet of Things** (IoT).

The RFID system consists of readers or interrogators and tags. A reader or interrogator is a piece of equipment that will activate an adjacent tag and read its data. RFID tags can be read-only with an already assigned number which is used as a key for the database, read/write with information written by the system user, or once-write/multi-read with information written by the user. Basic RFID tags are made of three parts: an antenna to transmit/receive the data; an integrated circuit for storing and processing data; and a direct current (DC) power collector from the incident reader signal. RFID tags can be passive (without a battery), active (battery-powered) or battery-assisted passive. From the side of human exposure to EMF, as well as of interference with other devices, the highest RF power is generated by the RFID system with passive tags due to them having the highest transmitted power level (ETSI, 2014).

RFID systems operate in different frequency bands. In the low-frequency (LF) band (125–134.2 kHz and 140–148.5 kHz), LF-RFID tags can be used globally without a licence, and in the high-frequency (HF) band (ISM band – 13.56 MHz), HF-RFID tags can be used the same way. In the UHF band (865–928 MHz), UHF-RFID tags cannot be used globally uniformly, but they are defined for every country, depending on the country's regulations. In Europe, RFID operation is restricted to the band 865–868 MHz in such a way that readers are required to monitor a channel before transmitting (Listen Before Talk, (LBT-RFID)); this requirement has led to some restrictions on performance. In North America, UHF can be used unlicensed for 902–928 MHz (±1 MHz from the 915 MHz centre frequency), but restrictions exist for transmission power. The UHF band also includes 433 MHz and ISM band 2.45 GHz. RFID systems may use also the super-high frequency (SHF) band (ISM 5.8 GHz and UWB 3.1–10 GHz).

RFID in the band 865–868 MHz provides fifteen channels, three of 100 mW, ten of up to 2 W, and two of up to 500 mW. The current plan provides for an LBT-RFID system so that only one device in a radio space can occupy a channel at a time. If the interrogators transmit 2 W in a high density RFID environment, a maximum of 10 interrogators can operate simultaneously. In the case of more than 10 interrogators transmitting at the same time, they have to share time on the same channels. It can happen that at busy sites, all ten of the high power channels are occupied for extended periods of time.

5.3 CURRENT MEASUREMENT TECHNIQUES INVOLVED IN THE PUBLIC RF-EMF EXPOSURE EVALUATION

The measurement techniques used for the public RF-EMF exposure control are nowadays usually continuously and automatically carried out in the studied frequency range. For the case of RF sources, the frequency range should cover all frequencies of all the sources in the considered area (van Deventer et al., 2006). In recent years, the frequency band between 80 MHz and 3 GHz was used. However, this is no longer sufficient, given that WiFi at 5 GHz band and 5G networks are coming to the market more and more in various versions.

The measurements of RF-EMF components emitted by base stations or broadcasting antennas (the case of whole body EMF exposure) are usually taken in the far distance to antennas, where far field EMF may be expected and power density may be converted from the measurements of only one component of EMF. However, as mentioned, for the human body exposure evaluation, there are significant limitations to such an approach. Therefore, it is not justified to use W/m^2 or mW/cm^2 notations in any presentation of the results of measurements of E-field strength, which are an acceptable equivalent to V/m notation when assessing real 'far-field' exposure only. Additionally, in measurements of RF-EMF emitted by mobile communications terminals (the case of localised EMF exposure), it is important to take into account the fact that exposure is in the near field area and the direct coupling between a human body and the EMF source needs evaluation for both purposes – an evaluation of the hazards caused by exposure, as well as the direct coupling between the measurement devices and the human body (Gryz et al., 2014a,b,c, Gryz and Karpowicz, 2015, Hansson Mild et al., 2009, Karpowicz et al., 2010, Karpowicz and Šimunić, 2009).

The usual measurement equipment is a device consisting of a measurement probe (broadband and/or narrowband in the frequency response), a frequency selective measuring instrument (monitor), measurement automation, and housing to protect the instrument from mechanical and atmospheric damage (Šimunić, 2001). This measurement device should be calibrated as a complete system in the reference EMF of a well-known level, spatial distribution, frequency, and modulation – at the measurement frequencies. The total measurement uncertainty depends on various factors that may be related to the probe and the measurement device (type of measuring instrument, type of measurement probe, calibration, isotropy, linearity, noise, mismatch, influence of temperature and humidity), related to the environment (perturbation and influence of the body) and related to post-processing (time- and spatial averaging). In general, the total measurement uncertainty needs to be counted at least 20% in environmental RF-EMF measurements.

This is most widely used measurement technique involving broadband measurements of electric and magnetic fields in the environment, but does not provide data for consideration regarding the contribution to total RF-EMF exposure caused by particular sources emitting EMF. The use of body-worn, personal, RF-EMF frequency-selective exposure meters (known as exposimeters, or more precisely electric field (E-field) exposimeters) is a suitable, still-developing investigation method that may assist the analysis of RF-EMF exposure with respect to the significance of particular sources. The main goal for the design of such devices was to establish a relationship between an individual person's exposure parameters and their activities when the contribution of various sources is assessed, excluding the personal use of mobile phone handsets which cause localised exposure to the palm and head (through classical phone use) and which have to be assessed by SAR values (Electromagnetic-Fields-A-Hazard-to-Your-Health.aspx, Gajsek et al., 2013, Joseph et al., 2010, Neubauer et al., 2010, Röösli et al., 2010). However, these devices may also be used to examine the parameters of RF-EMF exposure in selected locations, including variability over many hours of monitoring.

The environmental investigations discussed in this article have been performed in the RF-EMF from the frequency band 27 MHz–6 GHz, with the use of spectrum analysers and exposimeters. The used frequency-selective exposimeters of electric field (E-field) – EME SPY series (from Satimo, France) – are portable, pocket-sized (not exceeding 500 g), battery-powered, RF-EMF data loggers of the root-mean-square (RMS) value of E-field strength in the frequency range from 88 MHz to 2500 (5850) MHz. Each predefined frequency band of the exposimeters corresponds to the most common RF-EMF applications currently in use in the public environment (Table 5.2), which help identify dominant components of exposure and evaluate the relative levels of exposure from various sources. The measurement results also cover the total RMS value of E-field exposure – representing the value almost equal to broadband measurement results covering each frequency component. Some examples of RF-EMF components of exposure that are not covered by the mentioned exposimetric measurements are: citizens band radio (CB radio) (27 MHz), amplitude modulation radio (AM radio) (100–300 kHz), short-wave radio (several MHz), analogue radiophones (approximately 150 MHz), radio links (operating at frequencies exceeding 6 GHz, for example, approximately 18 GHz, 60 GHz), and almost any pulsed signal (because of the relatively slow sampling rate of exposimeters). The data logger of exposimeters is equipped with a nonvolatile internal memory to store samples of measurement results and actual real time recording with a programmable sampling rate of which the fastest is several seconds. The exposimeters are able to operate autonomously without charging for up to many days (dependent on the sampling

TABLE 5.2
Predefined Measurement Frequency Bands of Frequency-Selective Exposimeters used in Environmental Investigations on RF-EMF Exposures from Various Mobile Communication Systems

Label	Frequency Band, MHz	The use of Frequency Bands
FM	88–108	FM radio broadcasting
TV3	174–233	TV VHF band broadcasting
Tetra (I, II, III)	380–400 410–430 450–470	Mobile communications system for closed groups
TV4&5	470–830 (470–770)	TV UHF band broadcasting
LTE 800	791–821 and 832–862	LTE network (UL and DL bands)
GSM 900 (GSM + UMTS 900)	880–915 and 925–960	Digital cellular network (UL and DL bands)
DCS 1800 (GSM 1800)	1710–1785 and 1805–1880	Digital cellular network (UL and DL bands)
DECT	1880–1900	Digital enhanced cordless tele-communications of short distance
UMTS 2100	1920–1980 and 2110–2170	Digital cellular network (UL and DL bands)
WLAN/ WiFi 2G	2400–2500 (2400–2483)	Wireless local area network, e.g., access to internet
LTE 2600	2500–2570 and 2620–2690	LTE network (UL and DL bands)
WiFi 5G	5150–5850	Internet access

rate and the quality of batteries). Investigations involving the use of exposimeters in various environments (ongoing in the authors' research activities since 2011) have included a systematic study on the relationship between the results of exposimetric investigations and unperturbed RF-EMF, the metrological properties of frequency-selective exposimeters, and RF-EMF exposure profiles in various environments (Gryz et al., 2012, Gryz et al., 2014a,b,c, Gryz and Karpowicz, 2015). It must also be pointed out that misinterpretations may result from focusing only on the maximum recorded value, which may come from any irregular function of the exposimeter, influence from the EMF source, reflecting objects or the human body. Because of that, a more stable parameter characterising the upper level of RF-EMF exposure is advised as the measurement outcome – that is, the use of particular percentiles from recorded values – the most frequently used are 75th or 95th percentiles of the recorded data set (Gryz et al., 2014a,b,c, Gryz and Karpowicz, 2015, Neubauer et al. 2010).

5.4 EXAMPLES OF RF-EMF EXPOSURE SCENARIOS WITH RESPECT TO VARIOUS COMPONENTS OF DAILY EXPOSURE OF INDIVIDUALS

Frequency-selective exposimeters (with predefined frequency measurement ranges, dedicated to investigating RF-EMF from typical wireless telecommunication systems) were used to evaluate the stationary and mobile components of RF-EMF exposure in the public accessible environment where various mobile communication systems were being used. The main aim of the work was to analyse the pattern of RF-EMF exposure in the context of identified mobile services available in particular locations and the results of more precise frequency analysis of frequency composition of RF-EMF (Figures 5.4 and 5.5).

Examples of the results of studies discussed further were selected to draw attention to the exposure conditions in which exposure components from mobile phone systems may be not dominant in the total exposure in a particular location or of a particular

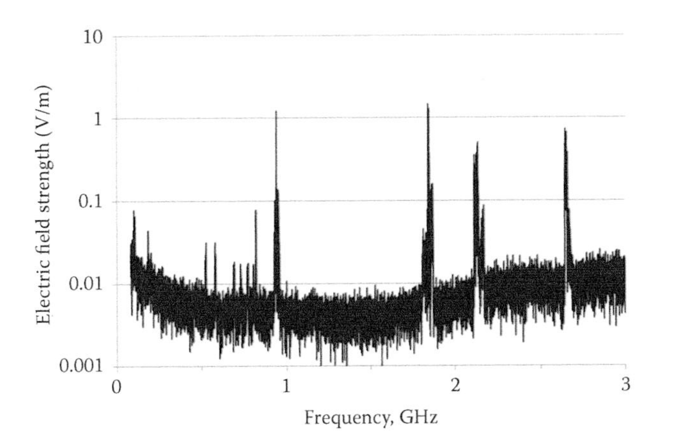

FIGURE 5.4 Electric field strength versus frequency, recorded by RF-EMF spectrum analyser in the 0.08–3 GHz frequency band.

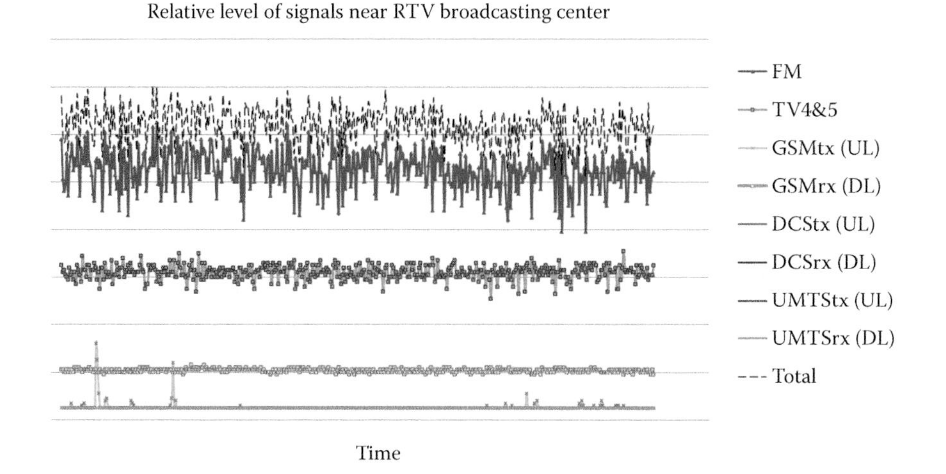

FIGURE 5.5 Electric field strength versus time, recorded by RF-EMF exposimeter near the radio-television broadcasting center located in the rural area.

person. The variability of the level of RF-EMF exposure was analysed by calculating the statistical parameters of registered over time exposimetric profiles: minimum, maximum, and median values, and the range between the 5–95th percentiles – from profiles registered in each frequency range as well as the total level of exposure (Gryz et al., 2014a,b,c, Gryz and Karpowicz, 2015).

A well-known situation where mobile phone RF-EMF signals may be less significant than other components of RF exposure is the environmental influence from nearby radio-television high power (long distance) broadcasting centres that may be located in a rural area or in a city centre. The first example is RF-EMF exposure recorded near an RTV broadcasting tower located in a rural area where the following frequencies of emitters have been identified by spectrum analyser: FM radio (88–107.5 MHz); TV3 and TV4&5 (223–794 MHz); mobile phone base stations (915–960 MHz, and 1820–1870 MHz). All the EMF emitters were located at a height of 50–90 m from the ground. In this kind of environment, the dominant component in the recorded RF-EMF exposure was the contribution from the FM radio (Figure 5.6). Other sources of EMF were much lower or negligible because the RTV tower was located far from other radiation sources and far from users of mobile communication services.

A similar profile of RF-EMF exposure is expected in the vicinity of RTV broadcasting centres located inside a city. Examples of the results of investigations of RF-EMF exposure covering the locations in a city with a downtown broadcasting centre were collected from measurements in an urban area with ~2 million habitants. In this kind of location, exposure with a dominant FM radio component may be found – an example of measurements on the 15th floor of an apartment building located downtown near to the broadcasting centre is shown in Figure 5.7. A small difference to the previous example consists of weaker TV signals, because digital emissions were already introduced to the broadcasting centre under consideration. In both cases, there is almost no uplink signal, because no users of mobile communication systems were

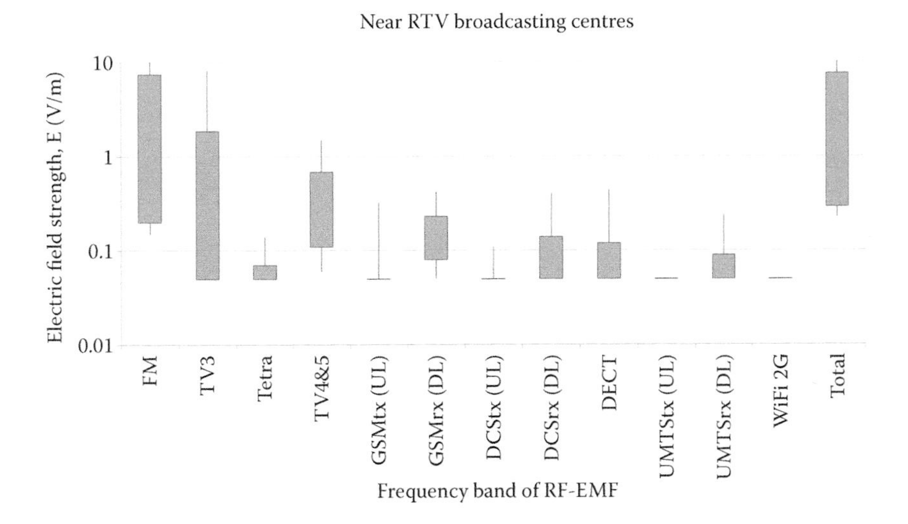

FIGURE 5.6 The components of RF-EMF exposure recorded near the RTV broadcasting centre located in rural area (outdoor measurements); whiskers: min–max, bars: 5%–95%.

present near the measurement location (except for the personnel taking measurements and the inhabitants of the apartment). Almost the entire RF-EMF exposure comes in such situations from external sources not controlled by individuals. The opposite situation is found in rural areas located far from broadcasting installations and mobile networks base stations – where almost all the RF-EMF exposure is under the control

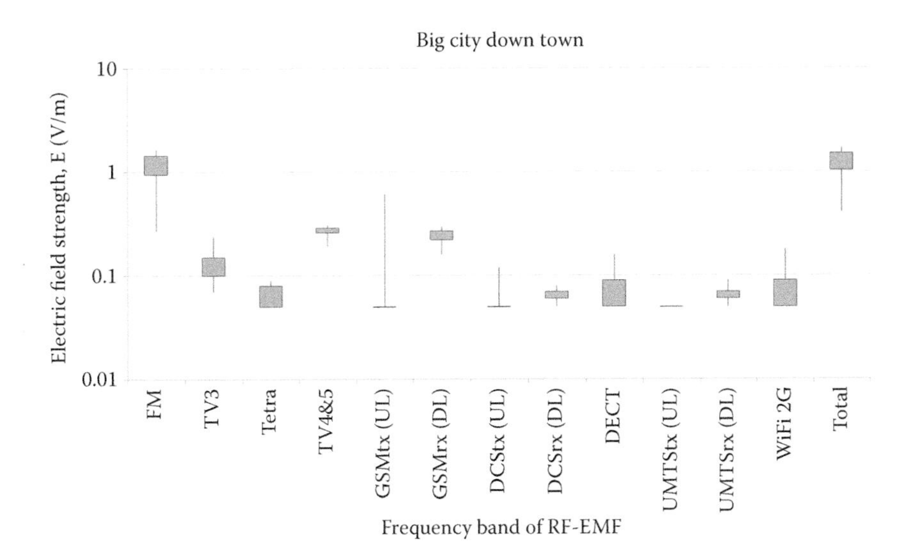

FIGURE 5.7 The components of RF-EMF exposure recorded near the RTV broadcasting centre located in downtown of the city (indoor measurements); whiskers: min–max, bars: 5%–95%.

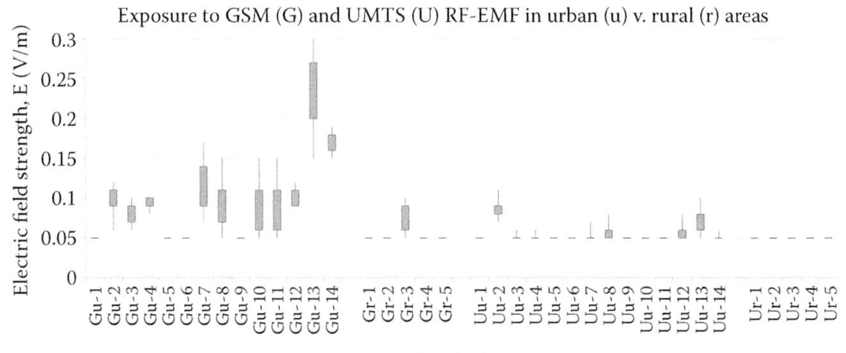

FIGURE 5.8 The components of RF-EMF exposure from base station to terminals, recorded in urban and rural areas, far from the RTV broadcasting centre and mobile networks base stations (indoor measurements) – the comparison of results derived from 19 exposimetric profiles – recording in GSM-DL (G) and UMTS-DL (U) range, in urban (u) and rural (r) areas; whiskers: min-max, bars: 5%–95%.

of individuals who may decide to use an RF-EMF emitter or not (such as mobile phone handsets, WiFi emitters, routers, etc.), (Figure 5.8).

The RF-EMF exposure profile changes where it concerns locations where other, especially many, users of mobile communication services are present. The example of such locations may be in city centres, where the influence of many emitters – RTV broadcasting antennas, mobile networks base stations antennas, mobile phone handsets of many users, wireless Internet access users, and so on – can reasonably be expected. Examples of such complex exposure situations are summarised in Figure 5.9, which covers samplings split into subsets recorded during: (a) rides on a public bus; (b) walks along various locations in the city centre; and (c) participation in the meeting with approximately 70 users of various wireless communication tools. The investigations cover a set of locations that represents the variability of typical exposure conditions in the urban area (during a daily commute to/from home/hotel/school/office/job/shopping/etc.), as well as the frequent situation of being in a large room with many users of mobile communication tools, such as public library, museums, waiting halls, shopping galleries, and so on. When both LTE and Wi-Fi systems are available in a particular location, where many users of mobile phones, laptops, and tablets are simultaneously connected to the internet and using voice communications, the RF-EMF exposure level may double or triple (Karpowicz et al., 2017).

Special attention is needed with respect to the proper interpretation of frequency selective measurements in parallel multi-channel measurements (such as in the presented examples of exposimetric measurements). The results of recording of a particular frequency band may come from various other sources using the same frequency band (an example of such a situation is recording RF-EMF emitted by a kitchen microwave oven at 2450 MHz frequency, which may be recorded to the frequency bands labelled as WiFi) (Lopez-Iturri et al., 2015). However, it may also happen that a recorded signal is from a mobile phone network, but partly appears

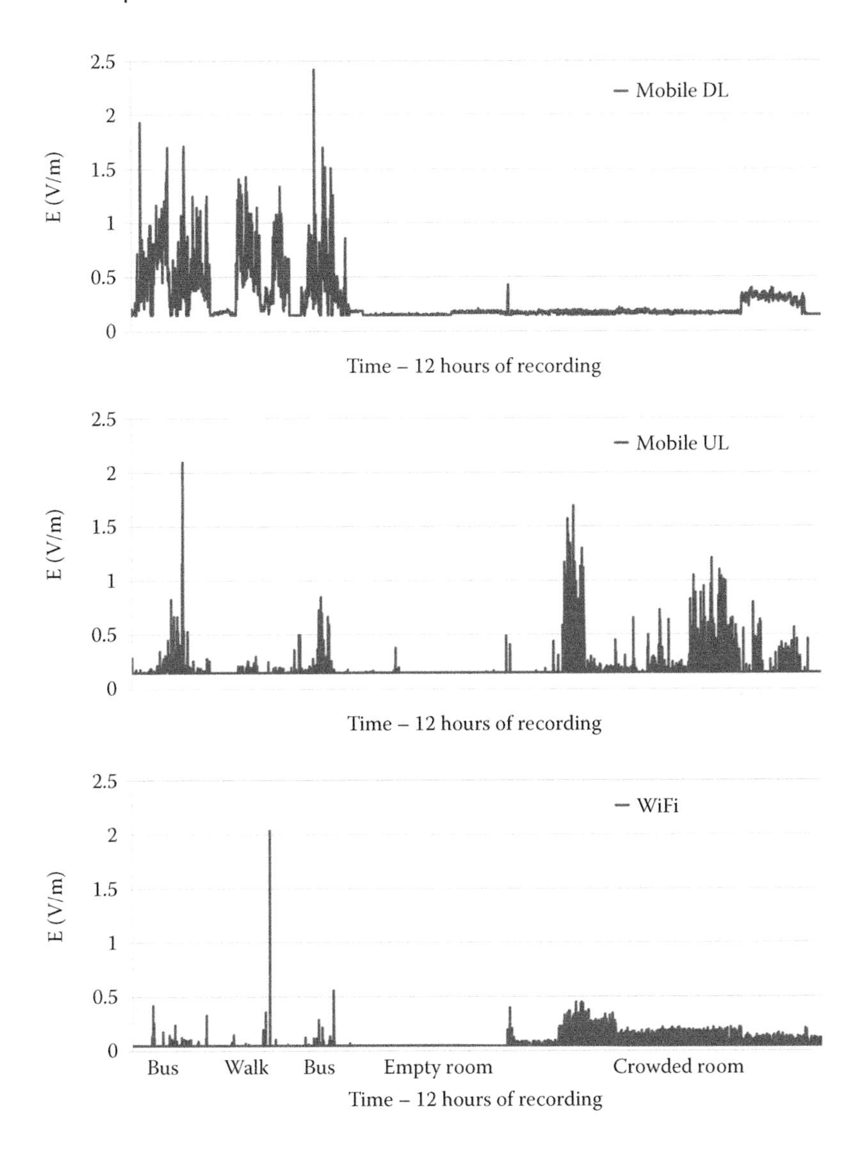

FIGURE 5.9 Logged data on E-field exposures in various locations (12 hours), stationary and mobile components recorded in the public bus, open area of the city center, public bus, and in the large meeting room – first empty and than crowded: WiFi, Mobile DL (GSM, DCS and UMTS downlink channels), Mobile UL (GSM, DCS and UMTS downlink channels).

in the frequency bands labelled in a different way, such as recordings to a DECT-frequency band – during indoor and outdoor measurements as well (see Figures 5.6 and 5.7). In both cases, such recordings were the result of what is known as crosstalk, where the signals in fact come to the DECT band of exposimeter from neighbouring DCS and UMTS bands (as shown in details by Gryz et al., 2012).

In the case of locations where a DECT phone is one of the RF-EMF sources, the recorded DECT component of exposure is usually much more significant and exists during the use of the DECT phone, as well as when it is not in use (e.g., during the night in an empty office). It happens because a DECT phone usually consists of two sources of RF-EMF – a base station which is permanently active, and a cordless handset which is active only during phone calls (Figure 5.10). This is significant also in that cross-talks may cause the DECT signal recording partly to neighbouring frequency bands (e.g., the recordings in the DSC frequency band shown in Figure 5.10 comes from a DECT phone).

RF-EMF exposure inside the underground metro infrastructure (tubes and stations) has been identified as an example of an environment where some specific parameters of the exposure profile are expected, such as: relatively short distances between base stations' (BTS) antenna locations (in the walls or ceilings of underground stations) and

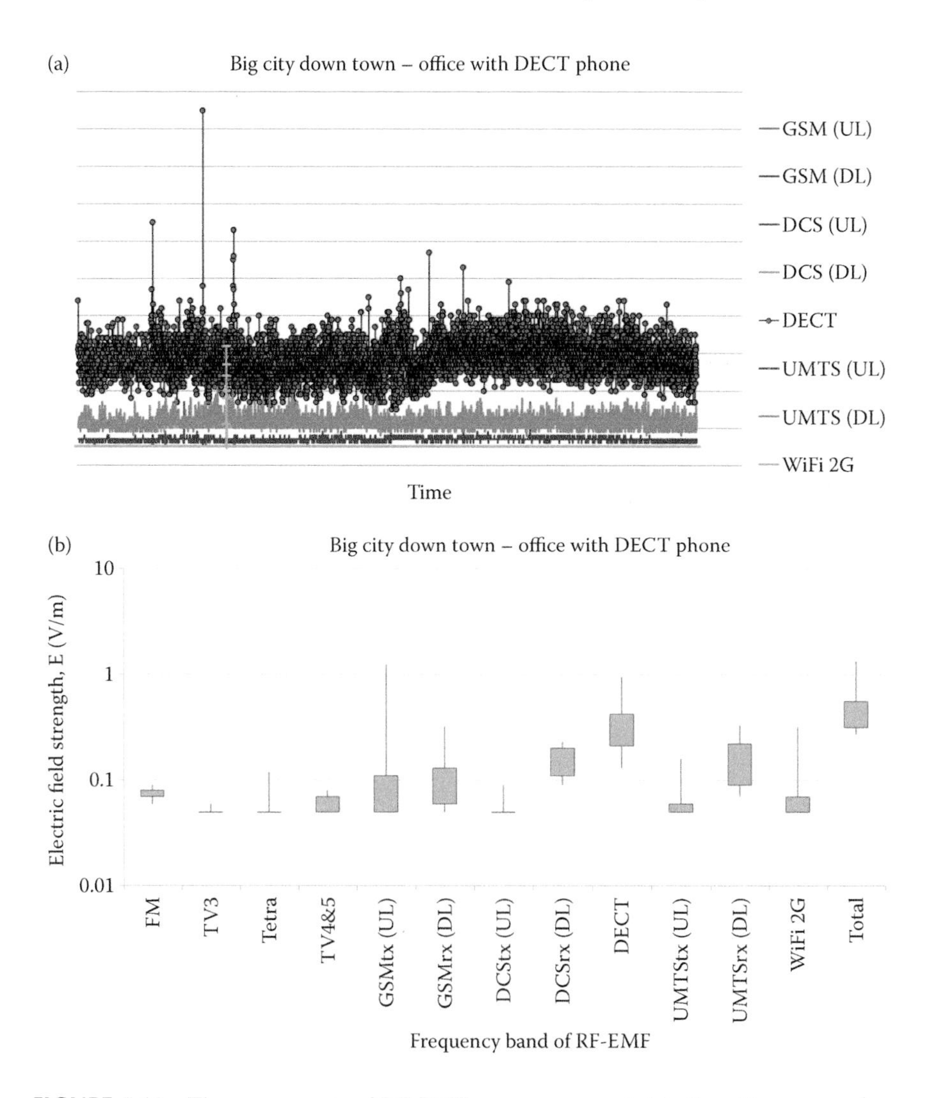

FIGURE 5.10 The components of RF-EMF exposure recorded in the office room where DECT cordless phone is used (indoor measurements); whiskers: min–max, bars: 5%–95%.

humans present on platforms, a crowd of mobile handset users on the platforms and in metro cars, and also a waveguide-like structure of a tube for RF-EMF propagation. Additionally, external to the metro infrastructure, the RF-EMF signals may be reduced in comparison to the locations on the ground because of shielding effects from the ground above the tube (Figures 5.11 and 5.12). Similar relations between RF-EMF exposure components are also expected in other locations, such as traffic or railway tunnels, aeroplanes, underground parking areas or sport halls (Aguirre et al., 2014, 2015, de Miguel-Bilbao et al., 2015, Gryz and Karpowicz, 2015, Hardell et al., 2016).

As a result of such exposure conditions, a significant component of RF-EMF exposure registered inside underground metro infrastructure came from mobile phone

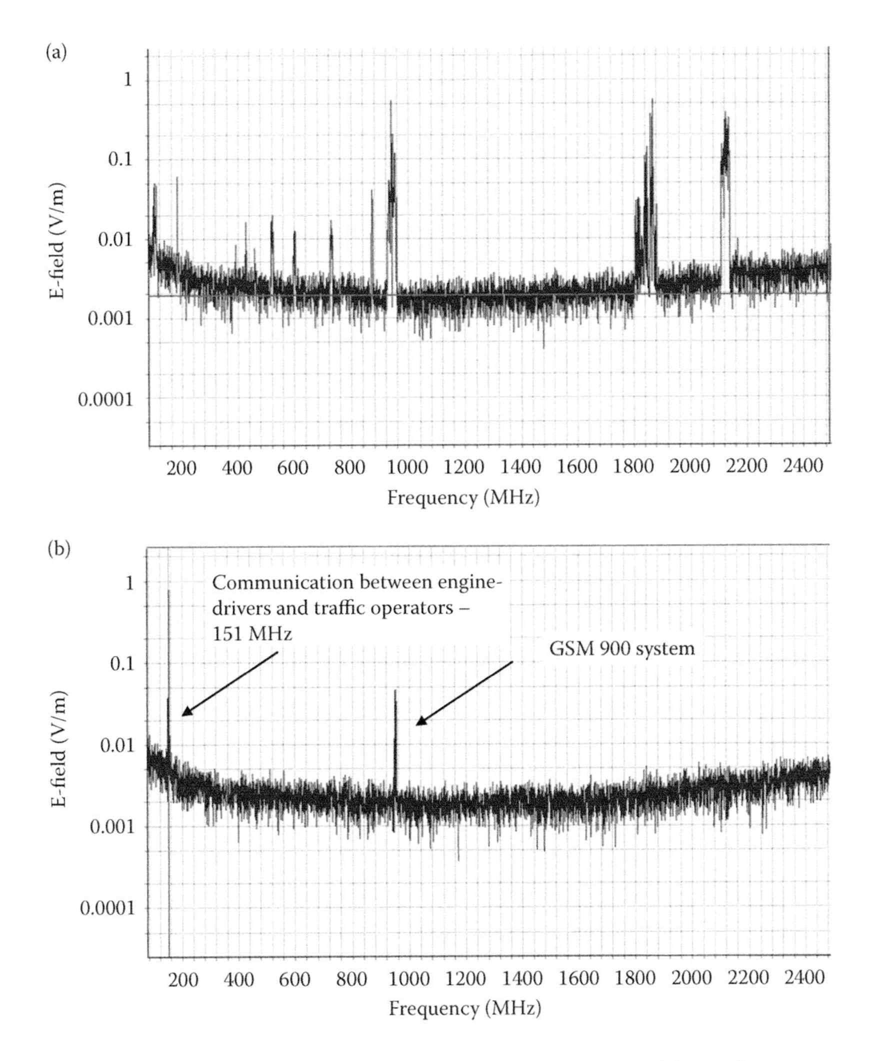

FIGURE 5.11 An example of the RF-EMF spectrum recorded in: (a) in the down town – at the ground (Warszawa – location of the RF-EMF exposimetric profile shown at Figure 5.7); (b) and the same day in the underground metro infrastructure.

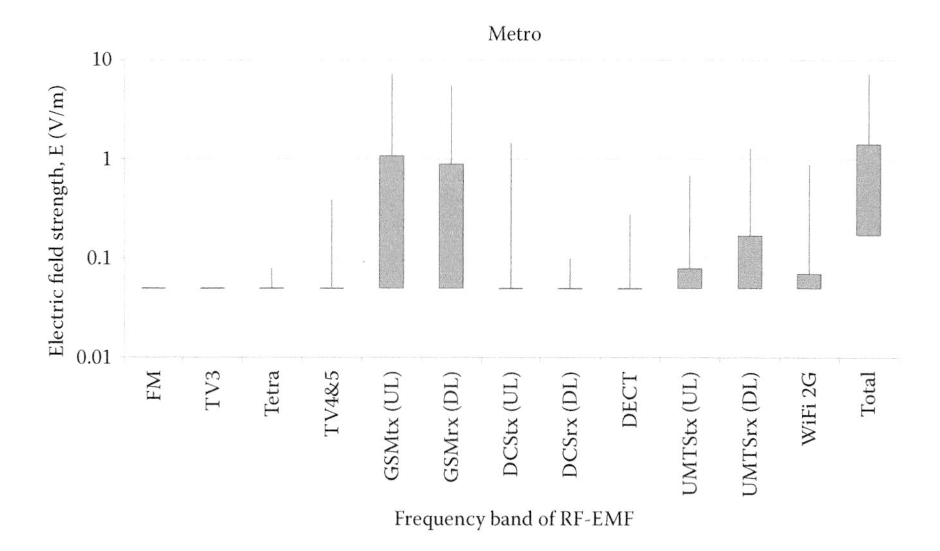

FIGURE 5.12 An example of RF-EMF exposimetric profiles recorded at locations covered by Figure 5.11b.

terminals of users who were present near the volunteer performing the exposimetric measurements (UL signals) – exposure inside the metro needs to be considered as a composition of "far-field" (from BTS) and 'near-field' (from mobile phone and Internet terminals) components (Hansson Mild et al., 2009, Karpowicz and Gryz, 2007). Similar conditions may be found in other public transportation facilities (such as buses, trams, trains, aeroplanes), and also in crowded locations like meeting rooms, shopping centres, libraries, and city centres visited by many habitants or tourists.

5.5 DISCUSSION AND CONCLUSIONS

The level of exposure to RF-EMF recorded in the discussed investigations performed in environments accessible to the public is usually significantly lower than the general public exposure limits provided by international guidelines and legislation established in various countries (4–61 V/m) (Council Recommendation, 1999, Gryz et al., 2014a, Stam, 2011). It is worth noting that, when approaching RF emitting antennas, especially BTS of mobile networks or RTV broadcasting, over a short distance the level of RF-EMF increases and may even significantly exceed the mentioned limits. However, the investigations show that in locations where many users of mobile communication tools are present in a crowded space, the components of RF-EMF exposure caused by their activities (which significantly vary over time) may together exceed components from the stationary emitters of RF-EMF (such as mobile networks base stations and RTV broadcasting antennas). Furthermore, other studies showed that local hot spots of exposure may also be created in such locations as a result of the multipath propagation of RF-EMF. Together, this is significant in the context of the safety of the vulnerable population, such as individuals with medical implants and users of telemedicine body worn sensors, because it may cause local hot spot overexposure with respect to the limit of radio frequency exposure, which may influence the function of electronic devices. In order to avoid medical device malfunction, it is usually recommended to maintain a distance from the transmitting terminals (handsets) greater than 1 m. At such distances, medical device malfunction is extremely rare because exposure is kept below the level of 3 V/m – recommended by the International Electrotechnical Commission (IEC) standard regarding electromedical devices (standard IEC60601-1-2) (International Electrotechnical 2007, Pantchenko et al., 2011, de Miguel Bilbao et al., 2015). The discussed situations determining RF-EMF exposure components also need attention when any protection measures with respect to RF-EMF exposure is considered in order to ensure that they are properly addressed to the dominant components of exposure.

It is also important to keep in mind that the rapidly developing mobile communication services are including continuously higher frequencies – AM and FM radio transmissions initially operated at kHz and MHz frequencies and analogue radiophones and cellular phones started from frequencies 27–450 MHz, whereas today's digital cellular phones use frequencies up to 2.2 GHz and wireless internet access explores frequencies up to almost 6 GHz, where the next generation of cellular phones is also going to be. Even much higher frequencies are explored by radio links, almost up to 100 GHz.

Electromagnetic Quantities and Corresponding SI Units

Symbol	Quantity	Unit
H	Magnetic field strength	ampere per metre (A/m)
B	Magnetic flux density	tesla (T)
E	Electric field strength	volt per metre (V/m)
U	Voltage	volt (V)
I	Current	ampere (A)
σ	Conductivity	siemens per metre (S/m)
λ	Wavelength	meter (m)
ε	Permittivity	farad per metre (F/m)
f	Frequency	hertz (Hz)
t	Time	second (s)
SAR	Specific energy absorption rate	watt per kilogram (W/kg)

Submultiple and Multiple Units Applicable in the Environmental EMF Discussion

Prefix to Unit	Symbol	Submultiple or Multiple Meaning	
nano	n	$\times 10^{-9}$	($\times$0.000 000 001)
micro	μ (micro)	$\times 10^{-6}$	($\times$0.000 001)
milli	m	$\times 10^{-3}$	($\times$0.001)
—	—	$\times 10^{0}$	($\times$1)
kilo	k	$\times 10^{3}$	($\times$1000)
mega	M	$\times 10^{6}$	($\times$1000 000)
giga	G	$\times 10^{9}$	($\times$1000 000 000)

ABBREVIATIONS

AIMD	Active Implantable Medical Devices
Bluetooth	an Anglicised version of the Scandinavian Blåtand/Blåtann (Old Norse blátǫnn), the epithet of the tenth-century king Harald Bluetooth who united dissonant Danish tribes into a single kingdom and, according to legend, also introduced Christianity; Bluetooth radio is a wireless standard that enables various network topologies, including point-to-point broadcast and mesh.
AM	Amplitude Modulation
AM radio	Amplitude Modulation Radio
BTS	Base Transceiver Station
CB	Citizen's Band
CB radio	Citizens Band radio
CDMA	Code Division Multiple Access
CENELEC	European Committee for Electrotechnical Standardization
CW	Continuous Wave
DC	Direct Current
DECT	Digital Enhanced Cordless Telecommunications (or, as before, Digital European Cordless Telecommunications)
DL	Downlink
EC	European Commission
EDGE	Enhanced Data rates for GSM Evolution
EMC	Electromagnetic compatibility
EMF	Electromagnetic Field
EP	European Parliament
EPS	Evolved Packet System
ETSI	European Telecommunications Standards Institute
EU	European Union
FDD	Frequency-Division Duplex
FDMA	Frequency Division Multiple Access
FM	Frequency Modulation
GPRS	General Packet Radio Services
GSM	Global System for Mobile Communications
HF	High Frequency
HF-RFID	RFID in High Frequency band
HSPA+	Evolved High Speed Packet Access
ISM radio bands	Industrial, Scientific, and Medical radio bands
IARC	International Agency for Research on Cancer
ICNIRP	International Commission on Non-Ionizing Radiation Protection
IEC	International Electrotechnical Commission
IEEE	Institute of Electrical and Electronics Engineers
ITU	International Telecommunication Union
IoT	Internet of Things
IQR	Interquartile Range
LBT-RFOD	Listen Before Talk RFID

LF	Low Frequency
LF-RFID	RFID in Low Frequency band
LTE	Long Term Evolution
MW	Microwave
OFDMA	Orthogonal Frequency-Division Multiple Access
QAM	Quadrature Amplitude Modulation
PBX	Private Branch Exchange
PM	Pulsed-Modulation
RF	Radio frequency
RF-EMF	Radio frequency Electromagnetic Field
RFID	Radio frequency Identification
RMS	Root-Mean-Square
RTV	Radio Television – public broadcasting
SC-FDMA	Single Carrier – Frequency Division Multiple Access
SHF	Super-High Frequency
TDMA	Time Division Multiple Access
TDD	Time-Division Duplex
VHF	Very High Frequency
UHF	Ultra High Frequency
UHF-RFID	RFID in Ultra High Frequency band
UL	Uplink
UMTS	Universal Mobile Telecommunications System
WHO	World Health Organisation
WiFi	Wireless Fidelity
WLAN	Wireless Local Area Network
ZigBee	high-level communication protocols used to create personal area networks with small, low-power digital radios, such as for home automation, medical device data collection, and other low-power low-bandwidth needs, designed for small scale projects which need wireless connection – the name refers to the waggle dance of honey bees after their return to the beehive

ACKNOWLEDGMENTS

This article has been based on the results of research tasks carried out within the scope of the National Programme "Improvement of safety and working conditions" partly supported by the Ministry of Science and Higher Education/National Centre for Research and Development (within the scope of research and development), and by the Ministry of Family, Labour and Social Policy (within the scope of state services) in Poland (1.G.12, II.N.19, II.B.07). The Central Institute for Labour Protection – National Research Institute is the Programme's main co-ordinator.

Prof.Dr.sc. Dina Šimunić wishes to acknowledge the support of the project "Information and communication technology for generic and energy-efficient communication solutions with application in e-/m-health (ICTGEN)" co-financed by the "European Union from the European Regional Development Fund."

The authors thank Dr. Patryk Zradziński and Mr. Wiesław Leszko from Laboratory of Electromagnetic Hazards of Central Institute for Labour Protection (CIOP-PIB), Warszawa, Poland, for their support in collecting exposimetric measurements which were summarised in the article.

REFERENCES

3GPP 2016. GSM/EDGE Physical layer on the radio path; General description.

Aguirre E, Arpón J, Azpilicueta L, López P, de Miguel S, Ramos V, Falcone F. 2014. Estimation of Electromagnetic Dosimetric Values from Non-Ionizing Radiofrequency Fields in an Indoor Commercial Airplane Environment. *Electromagn. Biol. and Med.*, 33(4), 252–263.

Aguirre E, Iturri López P, Azpilicueta L, de Miguel-Bilbao S, Ramos V, Garate U, Falcone F. 2015. Analysis of estimation of electromagnetic dosimetric values from non-ionizing radiofrequency fields in conventional road vehicle environments. *Electromagn. Biol. and Med.*, 34, 19–28.

Ahlbom A et al. 2009. ICNIRP (International Commission on Non-Ionizing Radiation Protection) Standing Committee on Epidemiology. Epidemiology evidence on mobile phones and tumor risk: a review. *Epidemiology*. 20(5), 639–652.

Berg-Beckhoff G, Breckenkamp J, Veldt Larsen P, Kowall B. 2014. General Practitioners' Knowledge and Concern about Electromagnetic Fields. *Int J Environ Res Public Health*, 11(12):12969–12982.

Bortkiewicz A, Gadzicka E, Szymczak W. 2017. Mobile phone use and risk for intracranial tumors and salivary gland tumors – A meta-analysis. *Int J Occup Med Environ Health* 30(1):27–43, doi: https://doi.org/10.13075/ijomeh.1896.00802.

Bortkiewicz A, Gadzicka E, Szynczak W, Zmyślony M. 2012. Heart rate variability (HRV) analysis in radio and TV broadcasting stations workers. *Int. J. of Occupational Medicine and Environmental Health*, 25(4):446–455.

Council of the European Union (EU). 1999. Recommendation of 12 July 1999 on the limitation of exposure of the general public to electromagnetic fields (0 Hz to 300 GHz), 1999/519/EC. *Official Journal of the European Communities*, L 199; 59–70.

de Miguel-Bilbao S, Aguirre E, Lopez-Iturri P, Azpilicueta L, Roldán J, Falcone F, Ramos V. 2015. Evaluation of Electromagnetic Interference and Exposure Assessment from s-Health Solutions Based on Wi-Fi Devices. *BioMed Research International*, 2015(2015), Article ID 784362, 9 pages. Doi: 10.1155/2015/784362.

Electromagnetic-Fields-A-Hazard-to-Your-Health.aspx. Adapted from Pediatric Environmental Health, 3rd Edition.

ETSI TR101178. 2005. Digital Enhanced Cordless Telecommunications (DECT): A high level guide to the DECT standardization.

ETSI TS136101. 2011. LTE; Evolved Universal Terrestrial Radio Access (E-UTRA); User Equipment (UE) radio transmission and reception.

ETSI TS125101. 2011. Universal Mobile Telecommunications System (UMTS); User Equipment radio transmission and reception (FDD).

ETSI TR102436. 2014. Electromagnetic compatibility and Radio spectrum Matters (ERM); Short range devices intended for operation in the bands 865 MHz to 868 MHz and 915 MHz to 921 MHz; Guidelines for the installation and commissioning of Radio Frequency Identification (RFID) at UHF.

European Parliament resolution of 2 April 2009 on health concerns associated with electromagnetic fields (2008/2211(INI)) http://www.europarl.europa.eu/sides/getDoc.do?pubRef=-//EP//NONSGML+TA+P6-TA-2009-0216+0+DOC+PDF+V0//EN.

European Parliament (EP) and the Council. 2013. Directive 2013/35/EU of the European Parliament and of the Council of 26 June 2013 on the minimum health and safety requirements regarding the exposure of workers to the risks arising from physical agents (electromagnetic fields) (20th individual Directive within the meaning of Article 16(1) of Directive 89/391/EEC), Official Journal of the European Union, 29.6.2013, L 179/1–21.

Gajsek P, Ravazzani P, Wiart J, Grellier J, Samaras T, Thuróczy G. 2013. Electromagnetic field exposure assessment in Europe radiofrequency fields (10 MHz - 6 GHz). *Journal of Exposure Science and Environmental Epidemiology*, doi: 10.1038/jes.2013.40.

Gryz K, Karpowicz J, Leszko W. 2012. Exposimeters of radiofrequency electromagnetic radiation – an overview of functional and technical parameters. *Bezpiecz Pr.* 2:12–15. [in Polish].

Gryz K, Karpowicz J, Leszko W, Zradziński P. 2014a. Evaluation of exposure to electromagnetic radiofrequency radiation in the indoor workplace accessible to the public by the use of frequency-selective exposimeters. *International Journal of Occupational Medicine and Environmental Health*, 27(6):1043–1054.

Gryz K, Karpowicz J, Leszko W, Zradziński P. 2014c. The frequency-selective evaluation of radiofrequency electromagnetic radiation in the public accessible indoor environment. *Proceedings of EMC Europe 2014*, September 1-14, Gothenburg, Sweden.

Gryz K, Karpowicz J. 2015. Radiofrequency electromagnetic radiation exposure inside the metro tube infrastructure in Warszawa. *Electromagnetic Biology and Medicine*, 34(3), 265–273.

Gryz K, Zradziński P, Karpowicz J. 2014b. The role of the location of personal exposimeters on the human body in their use for assessing exposure to electromagnetic field in the radiofrequency range 98-2450 MHz and compliance analysis – evaluation by virtual measurements. *BioMed Research International*, 2015(2015), Article ID 272460, 12 pages. Doi: 10.1155/2015/272460.

Hansson Mild K, Alanko T, Decat G, Falsaperla R, Gryz K, Hietanen M, Karpowicz J, Rossi P, Sandström M. 2009. Exposure of Workers to Electromagnetic Fields. A Review of Open Questions on Exposure Assessment Techniques. *International Journal of Occupational Safety and Ergonomics (JOSE)*, 15(1):3–33.

Hardell L et al. 2008. Meta-analysis of long-term mobile phone use and the association with brain tumours. *International Journal of Oncology*. 32(5).

Hardell L, Koppel T, Carlberg M, Ahonen M, Hedendahl L. 2016. Radiofrequency radiation at Stockholm Central Railway Station in Sweden and some medical aspects on public exposure to RF fields. *International Journal of Oncology* 49:1315–1324.

healthychildren.org (21.11.2015) American Academy of Pediatrics. Internet page: https://www.healthychildren.org/English/safety-prevention/all-around/Pages/.

IARC (International Agency for Research on Cancer). 2002. Non-ionizing radiation, part 1: Static and Extremely Low-Frequency (ELF) Electric and Magnetic Fields, Lyon, France, The WHO/IARC, IARC Monographs Volume 80.

IARC (International Agency for Research on Cancer). 2011. *Classifies Radiofrequency Electromagnetic Fields As Possibly Carcinogenic To Humans*. Lyon, France, May 31, 2011, The World Health Organization (WHO)/International Agency for Research on Cancer (IARC), Press Release No 208.

IARC (International Agency for Research on Cancer). 2013. Non-ionizing radiation, part 2: Radiofrequency electromagnetic fields, Lyon, France, The WHO/IARC, IARC Monographs Volume 102.

IEEE 802.11-2007. 2007. IEEE Standard for Information technology-Telecommunications and information exchange between systems. *Local and metropolitan area networks-Specific requirements- Part 11: Wireless LAN Medium Access Control and Physical Layer Specifications.*

IEEE 802.11ac-2013. 2013. IEEE Standard for Information technology-Telecommunications and information exchange between systems. *Local and metropolitan area networks-Specific requirements- Part 11: Wireless LAN Medium Access Control and Physical*

Layer Specifications; Amendment 4: Enhancements for Very High Throughput for Operation in Bands below 6 GHz.

IEEE Std 802.11-2016. 2016. IEEE Standard for Information technology – Telecommunications and information exchange between systems. *Local and metropolitan area networks-Specific requirements-Part 11:Wireless LAN Medium Access Control and Physical Layer Specifications.*

ICNIRP (International Commission on Non-Ionizing Radiation Protection). 2009. Exposure to high frequency electromagnetic fields, biological effects and health consequences (100 kHz–300 GHz). Review of the scientific evidence on dosimetry, biological effects, epidemiological observations, and health consequences concerning exposure to high frequency electromagnetic fields (100 kHz to 300 GHz). 16.

ICNIRP (International Commission on Non-ionizing Radiation Protection). 1998. Guidelines for Limiting Exposure to Time-Varying Electric, Magnetic, and Electromagnetic Fields (up to 300 GHz). *Health Physics*, 4(74):494–522.

International Electrothecnical Commission (IEC) Standard IEC 60601-1-2 Electromedical devices. 2007.

INTERPHONE Study Group. 2010. Brain tumour risk in relation to mobile telephone use: results of the INTERPHONE international case-control study. *International Journal of Epidemiology*, 39, 675–694, doi: 10.1093/ije/ dyqO79.

ITU-R BS.450-3 Transmission standards for FM sound broadcasting at VHF, 2001.

ISO/IEC/IEEE 8802-11. 2012. Information technology – Telecommunications and information exchange between systems. *Local and metropolitan area networks-Specific requirements-Part 11: Wireless LAN Medium Access Control and Physical Layer Specifications.*

Israel M, Zaryabova V, Ivanova M. 2013. Electromagnetic field occupational exposure: Non-thermal vs. thermal effects. *Electromagnetic Biology and Medicine*. 32(2), ITU. International Telecommunication Union (2001) Transmission standards for FM sound broadcasting at VHF". ITU Rec. BS.450. International Telecommunications Union. 4–5.

ITU-R. International Telecommunication Union. 2016. Handbook on Digital Terrestrial Television Broadcasting Networks and Systems Implementation, ITU.

Joseph W, Frei P, Röösli M, Thuroczy G, Gajsek P, Trcek T, Bolte J, Vermeeren G, Mohler E, Juhasz P, Finta V, Martens L. 2010. Comparison of Personal Radio Frequency Electromagnetic Field Exposure in Different Urban Areas Across Europe. *Environmental Research*, 110, 658–663.

Karpowicz J, de Miguel-Bilbao S, Ramos V, Falcone F, Gryz K, Leszko W, Zradziński P. 2017. The evaluation of stationary and mobile components of radiofrequency electromagnetic exposure in the public accessible environment, *IEEE Conference Publications: 2017 International Symposium on Electromagnetic Compatibility - EMC EUROPE (IEEE Xplore)*, pp. 1–4, doi: 10.1109/EMCEurope.2017.8094751.

Karpowicz J, Gryz K. 2007. Practical aspects of occupational EMF exposure assessment. *Environmentalist*, 27:525–31, http://dx.doi.org/10.1007/s10669-007-9067-y.

Karpowicz J, Gryz K. 2010. *Electromagnetic Hazards in the Workplace, Handbook of Occupational Safety and Health.* Koradecka, D. (ed.) CRC Press, Taylor & Francis Group, 199–218.

Karpowicz J, Šimunić D. 2009. Mechanisms of interaction of electromagnetic fields with human body, 2009 2nd International Symposium on Applied Sciences in Biomedical and Communication Technologies, *IEEE Conference Publications: 2nd International Symposium on Applied Sciences in Biomedical and Communication Technologies*, ISABEL 2009. (IEEE Xplore), pp. 1–4, doi: 10.1109/ISABEL.2009.5373605.

Lopez-Iturri P, de Miguel-Bilbao S, Aguirre E, Azpilicueta L, Falcone F, Ramos V. 2015. Estimation of Radiofrequency Power Leakage from Microwave Ovens for Dosimetric Assessment at Nonionizing Radiation Exposure Levels, *BioMed. Research International* 2015(2015), Article ID 603260, 14 pages. Doi: 10.1155/2015/603260.

Neubauer G, Cecil S, Giczi W, Petric B, Preiner P, Frohlich J, Röösli M. 2010. The Association between exposure determined by radiofrequency personal exposimeters and human exposure; A Simulation Study. *Bioelectromagnetics*, 31(7), 535–545.

Pantchenko OS, Seidman SJ, Guag JW, Witters DW, Sponberg CL. 2011. Electromagnetic compatibility of implantable neurostimulators to RFID emitters. *BioMedical Engineering On Line*, 10:50.

Precautionary Policies and Health Protection: Principles and Applications, Rome, Italy, May 2001. See: http://www.euro.who.int/document/e75313

Reilly PJ. 1998. *Applied Bioelectricity. From Electrical Stimulation to Electropathology.* New York, Springer-Verlag.

Röösli M, Frei P, Bolte J, Neubauer G, Cardis E, Feychting M, Gajsek P, Heinrich S, Wout J, Mann S, Martens L, Mohler E, Parslow R, Harbo Poulsen A, Radon K, Schüz J, Thuroczy G, Viel J-F, Vrijheid M. 2010. Conduct of a personal radiofrequency electromagnetic field measurement study: proposed study protocol. *Environmental Health*, 9:23, 14.

SCENIHR (Scientific Committee on Emerging and Newly Identified Health Risks). 2009. Health Effects of Exposure to EMF, Opinion adopted at the 28th plenary on 19 January 2009, Brussels, http://ec.europa.eu/health/ph_risk/committees/04_scenihr/docs/scenihr_o_022.pdf.

SCENIHR (Scientific Committee on Emerging and Newly Identified Health Risks). 2015. *Oopinion on potential health effects of exposure to electromagnetic fields 15 (EMF), SCENIHR approved this opinion at the 9th plenary meeting on 27 January 2015.*

Šimunić D. 2001. Measurements of near and far fields, in Biological Effects, Health Consequences and Standards for Pulsed Radiofrequency Fields. In: Matthes R., Bernhardt J.H., Repacholi M.H. (eds) Oberschleissheim, ICNIRP, pp. 89–101.

Stam R. 2011. Comparison of international policies on electromagnetic fields (power frequency and radiofrequency fields) *Bilthoven, Netherlands: National Institute for Public Health and the Environment*; 2011 May. Available from: http://ec.europa.eu/health/electromagnetic_fields/docs/emf_comparision_policies_en.pdf.

Szmigielski S. 2013. Cancer risks related to low-level RF/MW exposures, including cell phones. *Electromagnetic Biology and Medicine*. 32(3), 273–280, doi: 10.3109/15368378.2012.701192.

van Deventer E, Šimunić D, Repacholi M. 2006. EMF Standards for Human Health. In: *CRC Handbook of Biological Effects of Electromagnetic Fields*, Barnes, F., Greenbaum, B. (eds.) CRC, 3rd edition.

Vangelova K, Deyanov C, Israel M. 2006. Cardiovascular risk in operators under radiofrequency electromagnetic radiation. *Int. J. Hyg. Environ. Health*, 209, 133–138.

Vesselinova L. 2013. Biosomatic effects of the electromagnetic fields on view of the physiotherapy personnel health. *Electromagnetic Biology and Medicine*, 32(2):192–199.

WHO (World Health Organization) 1993. Environmental Health Criteria 137, Electromagnetic Fields (300 Hz – 300 GHz). 1993, http://www.inchem.org/documents /ehc/ehc/ehc137.htm

Zradziński P. 2013. The Properties of Human Body Phantoms used in Calculations of Electromagnetic Fields Exposure by Wireless Communication Handsets or Hand Operated Industrial Devices. *Electromagnetic Biology and Medicine*, 32(2):192–199.

Zradziński P. 2015a. The examination of virtual phantoms with respect to their involvement in a compliance assessment against the limitations of electromagnetic hazards provided by European Directive 2013/35/EU. *Int J Occup Med Environ Health*. 28(5):781–792.

Zradziński P. 2015b. Difficulties in applying numerical simulations to an evaluation of occupational hazards caused by electromagnetic fields. *Int J Occup Saf Ergon.* 21(2):213–220.

6 Low-Level Thermal Signals
An Understudied Aspect of Radio Frequency Field Exposures with Potential Implications on Public Health

Lucas A. Portelli

CONTENTS

6.1 INTRODUCTION

In the last 100 years, devices and methodologies with the novel capability of artificially depositing substantial amounts of energy in biological systems in nonconventional ways have been introduced. Two vehicles used to inject such energy are electromagnetic fields (i.e., Radio Frequency [RF], light) and ultrasound. Exposures are performed in the civil (environmental sources and personal devices), industrial (occupational sources), medical (e.g., Magnetic Resonance Imaging (MRI), High Intensity Focused Ultrasound (HIFU), Hyperthermia), security (e.g., airport scanners), and military (e.g., Active Denial System, or similar nonlethal weapons) contexts.

While the energy deposited can engage in complex interactions with cellular systems, a common denominator is the generation of heat in the tissue. Some experiments have shown that excessive thermal exposures can be deleterious to cellular systems, depending on their duration, specific temperature, and the tissue type in particular (e.g., neural tissue is more sensitive than muscle tissue). Because of this, scientists, industry executives, and regulators have generated safety standards which contain sets of recommendations to limit the energy deposition with the intention to keep tissue temperatures within what is currently considered as "safe" margins. In the case of exposures to RF fields, safety standards with such recommendations have been in place since the 60s. However, although these standards are a reasonably good start for safety, they have been built and maintained around the same paradigm since their inception: *tissue damage only occurs after temperature thresholds have been breached for certain amounts of time.*

An immediate consequence of such assumption is the disregard of the possibility of any substantial biological relevance of thermal transients. Yet, thermal transients are ubiquitous to RF field exposures in real situations (and therefore chronic in nature). For example, consider an RF field exposure within the allowed limits, which is generally modulated (e.g., on-off-on-off…). This intermittence invariably results in thermal transients in the tissue because of the heat being passively (or actively) redistributed in the tissue and the surrounding environment. Therefore, at the cellular level, this fundamental "heat-in-heat-out" process generates in the exposed tissue what is described in the title of this chapter: a ***thermal signal***. As a result, cells in the exposed tissue are unavoidably exposed to a combination of the original energy injected (e.g., RF electromagnetic field) and its associated heat component (i.e., the RF-induced *thermal signal*) in unison.

Therefore, given this possibility alone, the study of small thermal signals becomes necessary to guarantee human safety in the context of RF exposures, including mobile communications. Nevertheless, to this day, the mere idea of the potential biological relevance of thermal signals in general is not considered by the scientific community or by safety experts and the experimental data exploring the effects of thermal signals are surprisingly scarce. Since this is the case, one might ask: What could be the true relevance of these thermal signals from the cellular and physiological point of view? How could the information contained in thermal signals transduce into biochemical, biological, and ultimately good (or bad) health effects?

This chapter will analyze the current paradigm that the current RF safety standards are built upon. Additionally, a brief review of our current knowledge on thermal sensitivity of biological systems is put into context of thermal signals in an attempt to provide a basis for contemplating their potential biological relevance. Finally, some recommendations on ways to further our currently weak understanding of the true biological relevance of thermal signals are presented.

6.2 THE CURRENT RF SAFETY PARADIGM

Over the years, several groups of international experts including scientists, industry executives, and regulators have generated guidelines and recommendations with the intention to avoid RF exposure hazards (RF meaning c.a. 100 KHz–300 GHz). For this, a fundamental realization made by experts is that a direct consequence of the absorption of energy in biological tissue is the instantaneous generation of heat resulting in a rise in temperature *in situ*. As a result, tissues are unavoidably exposed to a combination of the RF (electric and magnetic) fields and their associated thermal components simultaneously. These two distinct physical exposures have led to grouping the potentially hazardous biological effects of low-level RF exposures into corresponding categories to assess their potential health hazards: ***thermal effects*** and ***nonthermal effects*** (Barnes et al., 2015; Barnes, 2017; Foster, 2000, 2017; Markov, 2006; Sheppard et al., 2008).

Historically, the existence or relevance of ***nonthermal effects*** has been challenged by a part of the scientific community questioning the quality of the evidence on effects of low-level electric and magnetic fields on biochemical reactions or structures (Portelli, 2018). As a result, protection from potential hazards of ***nonthermal effects*** has not been a basis for the delineation of safety guidelines and recommendations. Instead, new scientific developments in this area have only been monitored and catalogued by the experts for the last ~50 years. On the other hand, the recognition that: *excessive thermal doses can be potentially deleterious to several aspects of the biological systems in the human body* has been widely accepted. Thus, protection from ***thermal effects*** has been the common denominator that underlies the conception and improvement of the multiple guidelines and recommendations in today's safety standards for RF exposures.

Good examples of safety standards are those prepared by the International Commission on Nonionizing Radiation Protection (ICNIRP), the institute of Electrical and Electronics Engineers (IEEE) and the International Electrotechnical Commission (IEC) from which most national limits are primarily derived (Ahlbom et al., 1998; ICNIRP, 2009; IEC, 2013; IEEE, 2005). Several differences between standards can be pointed out and the recommendations are undergoing constant revision, actualization, and complementation through expert recommendations (Colombi et al., 2015; Foster et al., 2017; Hashimoto et al., 2017; Lin, 2006; Morimoto et al., 2016; Kodera et al., 2018). Interestingly, the metric of choice by the regulators is not based on the currently recognized biologically-relevant quantity itself: RF-induced temperature and time-of-exposure of tissues (hence, ***thermal dose***). Instead, safety standards provide limited "basic restrictions" for energy deposition in tissues in terms of specific absorption rate (***SAR***) or incident power density (***IPD***) (f > 3–10 GHz) to indirectly observe ***thermal dose*** limits recommendations. **SAR** (measured in (J/s)/Kg or W/Kg) is a conventional way to characterize energy deposition in tissues in terms of the proportion to the localized electric field magnitude and on the tissue physical characteristics at the site of exposure. Such a relation is shown in Equation 1:

$$\mathbf{SAR} = \alpha \mathbf{E}_{\mathbf{rms}}^2; \quad \alpha = \mathbf{s}/\rho \tag{6.1}$$

where **s** (S/m) is the conductivity, ρ (Kg/m³) is the mass density, and $\mathbf{E}_{\mathbf{rms}}$ (V/m) is the electric field magnitude (Foster et al., 1998). As a first approximation, the temperature rate-of-change (**ΔT/dt**) in tissue due to RF exposures can be expressed in terms of SAR as follows:

$$\mathbf{\Delta T/dt} = \sigma \mathbf{E}_{\mathbf{rms}}^2/\mathbf{c} = \mathbf{SAR/c} = \beta \mathbf{SAR}; \quad \beta = 1/\mathbf{c} \tag{6.2}$$

where ***c*** is the tissue specific heat capacity (J/Kg · °C). However, in a real situation, the tissue temperature (and therefore ***thermal dose***) is only partially related to the energy deposited, and therefore, to ***SAR***. This is because during and after the thermal energy is deposited, it is redistributed and dissipated dynamically via a number of active and passive mechanisms inherent to physical (conduction, convection, radiation, evaporation) and biological systems (thermogenesis, thermoregulation) which depend on many factors (Charkoudian, 2003; Moros, 2012). Therefore, estimations of the dynamics of heat distribution at the surface of and inside a biological system subjected to thermal energy deposition is routinely done via improved versions of the bio-heat equation, initially proposed by Pennes in 1948 (Pennes, 1948). However, just as the accuracy of SAR estimations depends on trueness of the determination of the *in situ* electric fields and on the electrical properties of tissues, the accuracy of thermal estimations depends on the trueness of the representation of the thermoregulatory factors and heat redistribution mechanisms present (i.e., blood circulation, basal metabolism, clothing insulation, vasodilation response, etc.). For humans, a contemporary and practical list of such factors is well described by Laakso et al. (2011).

To determine the SAR limits that keep local and global thermal doses within the currently agreed safe limits, steady-state analyses are performed from which correlations between the thermal dose and SAR can be extracted (Hashimoto et al., 2017). In some cases, numerical simulations prepared for dose determination can have more realistic dynamic introduction of such parameters depending on the physical variables in the model (e.g., increasing the local perfusion by a function which depends on temperature (Foster et al., 2016; Kellogg, 2006; Kodera et al., 2018)) (Murbach et al., 2017). However, it is important to understand that ***deleterious thermal dose effects are interpreted, analyzed, and catalogued from a "threshold" perspective only*** below which no deleterious effects are expected to occur (according to the present expert consensus, see "The thermal dose model" section below). Therefore, time-dependent temperature changes (***thermal transients***) are not considered relevant to human safety as long as thermal doses do not exceed such thresholds. Nevertheless, as mentioned before, such transients are an integral part of RF exposures.

6.2.1 The Genesis of Localized Thermal Signals in Biological Tissue

An unavoidable result of the antagonistic thermal processes occurring in a human body exposed to RF (energy in versus energy out) is the generation of thermal

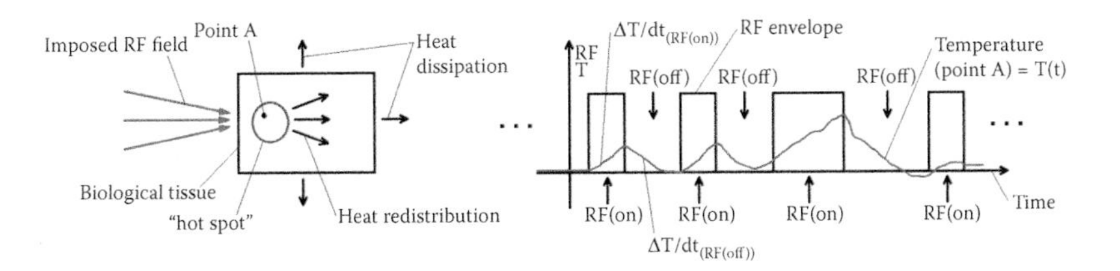

FIGURE 6.1 Imposition of RF signals in tissue is inherently accompanied by a related thermal signal *in situ*. (a) Conceptual representation of the "heat-in-heat-out" process that exists as a result of imposition of modulated RF fields in tissue. (b) Conceptual representation of the localized and time-dependent thermal signal resulting from intermittent RF field exposure. Its characteristics are subject to the dynamics which are involved in energy deposition, redistribution, and dissipation.

transients (or, perhaps more appropriately, ***thermal signals***). Consider the generic case of a simple intermittent RF signal (e.g., on-off-on-off…) imposed on a human tissue (see Figure 6.1). Depending on the intensity and duty-cycle of the imposed RF field, a modulated thermal signal is set to appear on the exposed tissue as a result of the energy deposition and the active and passive heat redistribution by physical and physiological means.

These RF-induced thermal signals are always part of the exposures from the cellular perspective to one degree or another, even if the exposures are within what is considered safe limits, and their magnitudes in biological tissue can be substantial from the microdosimetric point of view.

6.2.2 Current Models and Approximations and the Microdosimetric Perspective

Currently, exposure restrictions rely on models which are based on certain (presumably adequate) degree of spatio-temporal approximations. These approximations are certainly convenient from the practical point-of-view of computation and measurements since they substantially simplify or avoid many technical difficulties. Nevertheless, these approximations can obscure some important microdosimetric aspects of energy deposition (i.e., localized hot-spots and thermal transients are smoothed out). This results in exposure assessments reporting levels of exposure which can be many times below the true exposures as they are "low-pass filtered" in time and space (Lin, 2006). In the case of spatial approximations, these are introduced by model simplifications and by averaging. Regulatory restrictions are based on averages of the energy deposited over volumes (e.g., over any 10 g of tissue (10gSAR), head (hdSAR), whole body (wbSAR) or areas (IPD) depending on frequency) which are numerically correlated with the temperature elevation (Morimoto et al., 2016). However, such averaging (in the order of several mm) can "smooth out" thermal variations contained within these domains.

However, energy deposited in biological tissue is inherently inhomogeneous because of several factors. One of them is the field inhomogeneities introduced by details in the sources (plane waves, dipoles, arrays, Planar Inverted-F Antennas (PIFAs), and other complex antennas, see Figure 6.2) (Douglas et al., 2016; El Halaoui et al., 2017). Also, the inhomogeneities introduced by frequencies, polarizations, and spatial differentials when near the complex structures of the human body (e.g., phone against the head in different locations and positions) can be substantial. Due to this complexity alone, fields can vary greatly from point-to-point in the body generating minute hot-spots where energy deposition can be many times greater (and usually is) than the averaged SAR value reported to the authorities (Bernardi, 2000; Laakso et al., 2017). Additionally, volumes with increased levels of complexity (such as the pinna) sometimes result in such averages being done over volumes which do not contain any tissue. In other cases, the complicated tissues are radically simplified by removing these structures from the model altogether (Morimoto et al., 2016). As a result, a certain device may meet the compliance requirement while still inducing hot-spots (and steep gradients) inside the tissue which are many times greater (e.g., 20X) than the reported value and outside the allowed limits. Therefore, it would be common that a mobile phone may report SAR

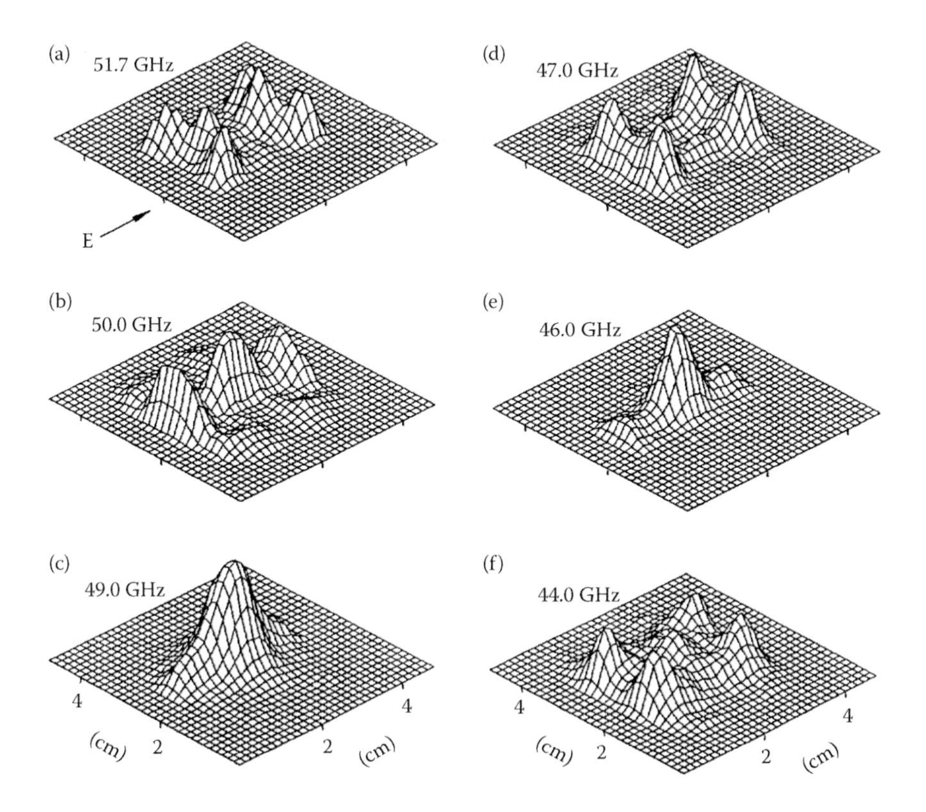

FIGURE 6.2 RF exposures in tissue are inherently inhomogeneous. These examples (a–f) show the frequency-dependent relative heating rate distribution resulting from irradiating a flat surface with a 17 × 26 mm^2 rectangular horn antenna. The area of each frame is 32 × 32 mm^2. (From Khizhnyak EP, Ziskin MC 1994. IEEE Transactions on Biomedical Engineering 41(9):865–73.)

under 2 W/Kg (restriction for the general public) while having hot spots as high as 40 W/Kg in substantial amounts of tissue (Lin, 2006; Schmid, 2015). Nevertheless, one should note that the real exposures may be much larger than this example (20X factor) given the fact that all numerical estimations are based on models which are simplified approximations of the real structures involved. In fact, biological tissues which have architectures with mm and sub-mm complexities are usually represented as homogeneous when modeled numerically. Yet, energy absorption differences only become apparent when the models are refined to accommodate the necessary level of detail (e.g., substantial reflections due to differences between the minuscule layers of the skin (Alekseev et al., 2008; Zhadobov et al., 2015), differential absorption by helical sweat glands (Betzalel et al., 2017; Feldman et al., 2008), etc.; See Figure 6.3).

In the case of temporal approximations, regulatory restrictions are based on averages over time (e.g., over several minutes to 10 seconds on the higher end (300 GHz), with many details depending on frequency and on the specific standard). Roughly, these times are based on simplified numerical models exposed to standard RF exposures until the temperature within the hot-spot of greatest exposure reaches a steady-state (step-response) (Bernardi, 2000). Additionally, in the case of exposures shorter than the averaging time, limits which are several times higher are accepted (e.g., ×1000 IPD for occupational exposure) (Laakso et al., 2017). However, in practice, even within these limits, thermal transients (>0.1°C/s) can be achieved by exposures within the limits proposed by the standards. A thorough deduction can be found in an excellent review by Foster et al. in which they distinguish the mechanisms and rates by which the heat is redistributed in homogeneous tissue when exposed to microwaves, deriving simple models and time constants which are relevant depending on the time of observation. They note that, for the first seconds of exposure, the energy is only slowly redistributed almost exclusively by conduction to the nearest tissues. This process is relatively independent of physiological changes (i.e., blood perfusion, etc.), resulting in a global heat distribution process which can be much slower than the sharp rate at which energy is deposited (even when within the allowed exposure limits) (Foster et al., 1998, 2017). Coincidently, such sharp transients were observed by Morimoto et al., utilizing complex numerical 3D models for frequencies from 1 to 30 GHz (Morimoto et al., 2017). Larger transients were predicted by Laakso et al. on an extended frequency range (up to 300 Ghz). By utilizing human models with some structural complexity, they clearly show absorption hot-spots with sharp temperature rise times whose magnitudes are at least three times higher than the mean temperature. Furthermore, these patterns of temperature rise were highly nonuniform, as expected, with frequency and polarization dependence (Laakso et al., 2017). Therefore, from the microdosimetric perspective, the appearance of hot-spots and transients is clearly dependent on model complexity, getting more pronounced as the model's complexity becomes closer to the true biological architectures.

While these artifacts (hot-spots and transients) can be many times greater than the stipulated safety limits within the "restrictions for the general public," they can be even more pronounced under specialized applications (i.e., industrial (occupational, military, medical) simply because safety limits are much greater (if there are any limits at all). For example, RF exposures on medical imaging applications can be an order of magnitude higher than occupational exposure and

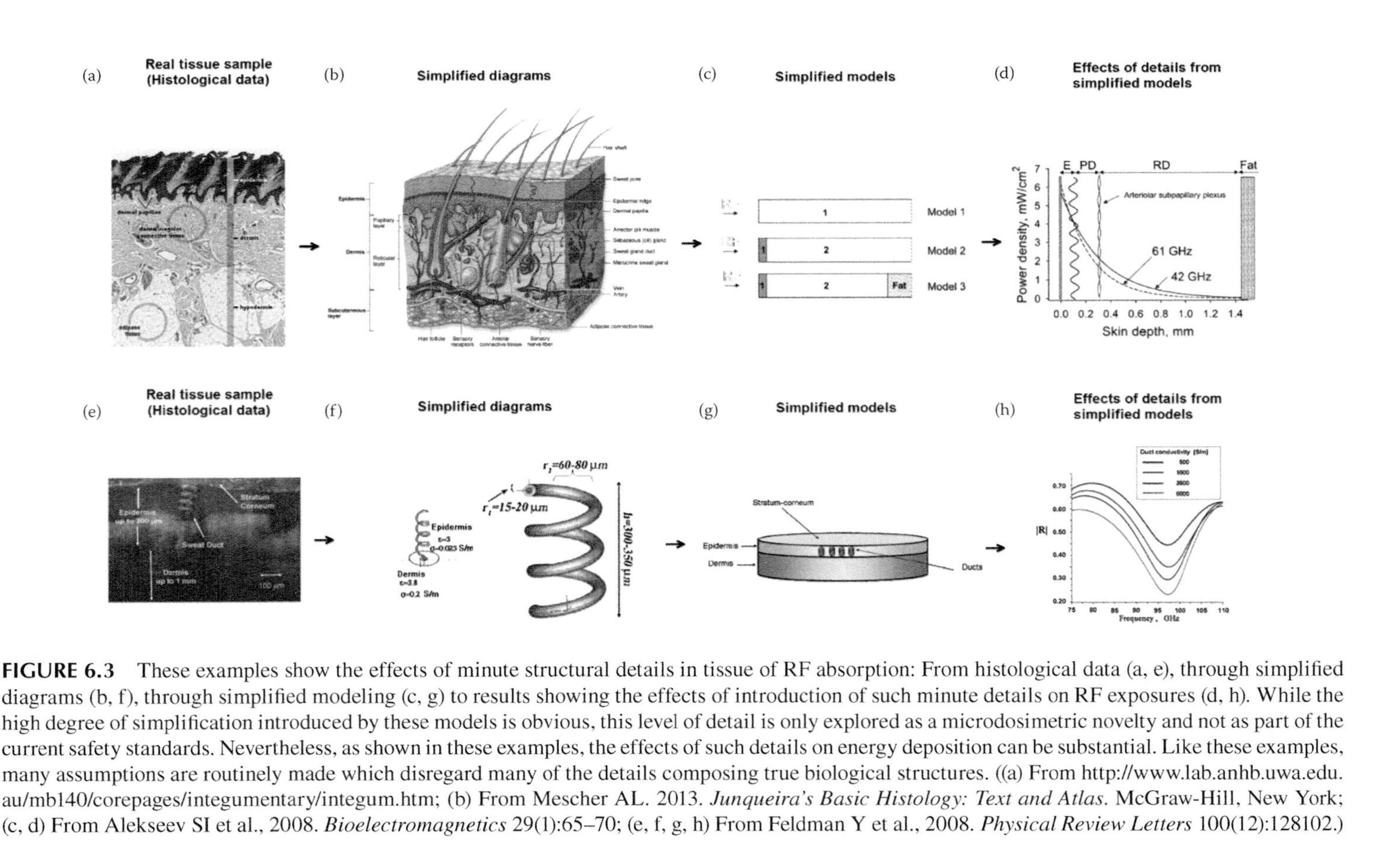

FIGURE 6.3 These examples show the effects of minute structural details in tissue of RF absorption: From histological data (a, e), through simplified diagrams (b, f), through simplified modeling (c, g) to results showing the effects of introduction of such minute details on RF exposures (d, h). While the high degree of simplification introduced by these models is obvious, this level of detail is only explored as a microdosimetric novelty and not as part of the current safety standards. Nevertheless, as shown in these examples, the effects of such details on energy deposition can be substantial. Like these examples, many assumptions are routinely made which disregard many of the details composing true biological structures. ((a) From http://www.lab.anhb.uwa.edu.au/mb140/corepages/integumentary/integum.htm; (b) From Mescher AL. 2013. *Junqueira's Basic Histology: Text and Atlas*. McGraw-Hill, New York; (c, d) From Alekseev SI et al., 2008. *Bioelectromagnetics* 29(1):65–70; (e, f, g, h) From Feldman Y et al., 2008. *Physical Review Letters* 100(12):128102.)

nearly 50 times higher than the guidelines for the general public (Murbach et al., 2015). In addition, signals can be substantially amplified by other factors like the presence of metallic implants which can collect RF energy along its conductive structure, modifying the imposed fields (Lekner, 2013) and depositing localized heat at the implant-tissue interface. Such implants can be active (e.g., cardiac pacemakers and defibrillators, deep brain stimulators, generic neurostimulators) or passive (e.g., stents, screws, plates, shoulder, knee, hip replacements, etc.) and the resulting thermal deposition would depend on the multiple geometric and material details of the imposed field, implant, and subject in question (Acikel et al., 2011; Murbach et al., 2015; Shellock et al., 2000). Numerical and practical assessments of SAR levels in the vicinity of simple generic implants have shown spatial gradients on the order of 5–6 dB/mm (320%–400%/mm). More complex spatial distributions (likely with larger gradients) are possible in the case of real implants with multiple electrodes (Nordbeck et al., 2009; Yao et al., 2017). Furthermore, while assessments are typically made for Continuous Wave RF exposures, gradient coils can also introduce significant eddy-current-induced heating which is oscillatory as a result of the coils' intermittent switching ($\Delta t \approx 125$ μS) (Brühl et al., 2017; Graf et al., 2007; Zilberti et al., 2015, 2017).

Based on the premises presented, it is not hard to imagine that tissues exposed to a modulated RF signal which exists within the allowed regulations are also exposed to a related thermal signal in the order of several hundredths of °C with periods in the order of seconds or less (depending on the specificities of the exposure and physiological factors). In addition, significantly large energy depositions (hence also large $\Delta T/dt$) are certainly possible when purposely operating outside of the safety standards. For example, characterization of hyperthermia experimental setups shows $\Delta T/dt$ in the order of c.a. 0.001–1°C/sec *in vivo* (Griffiths et al., 1986; Lara et al., 2017; Raaijmakers et al., 2017) and up to 3°C/sec with more focused modalities (i.e., nanoparticles) (Cherukuri et al., 2010; Deatsch et al., 2014). In the case of superficial energy deposition, enough intensities can generate pain (activate cutaneous nociceptor neurons) in only a few seconds (94 GHz (CW), $\Delta T/dt = 3.3$°C/s) (Walters et al., 2000). Today, military applications such as the "active denial system" described by Kenny et al. can use this principle to elicit a reflexive reaction (Kenny et al., 2008). Naturally, much larger transients and inhomogeneities are routinely generated in applications whose purpose is ablation (>20°C/s) (Rijkhorst et al., 2011; Worthington et al., 2016) or *in vitro* experimentation with small volumes (50°C/sec) (Mihran et al., 1990) with technologies involving ultrasound. Lasers can introduce enough focused energy to induce temperature transients some orders of magnitude larger in smaller volumes. (Izzo et al., 2008; Shapiro et al., 2012).

6.2.3 The Thermal Dose Model

In the same way as structural, spatial, and temporal approximations can obscure potentially important microdosimetric details, approximations and assumptions from the biological perspective can obscure potentially important physiological reactions. In this regard, there are several assumptions which are made in order to conveniently summarize the biological responses to a presumably adequate degree.

As mentioned before, safety standard recommendations are based on restricting the ***thermal dose.*** A proposed model describing the known limits for thermal damage is the *isoeffect dose cumulative equivalent min 43* (**CEM43** or $\mathbf{t_{43}}$) that comes from the consolidation of results from animal experimental data. This model assumes first-order kinetics (Arrhenius relation, see Equation 6.3), assuming, in principle, that thermal damage increases linearly with time and exponentially with temperature (Dewhirst et al., 2003).

$$\mathbf{CEM43 = tR^{43-T_c}} \tag{6.3}$$

where **t** is the time of exposure at temperature $\mathbf{T_c}$ and **R** is a constant. Therefore, each tissue can be assigned a **CEM43** which represents the maximum ***thermal dose*** (time-temperature combination) above which such tissue could sustain damage. Some established therapies (i.e., the several hyperthermia modalities), for example, make use of such deleterious thermal ranges as a treatment of malignant diseases. This is done by exposing specific tissues to steady-state temperatures above 37°C at specifically prescribed times-of-exposure, solo or as an adjuvant to other therapies (Hildebrandt et al., 2002; van Rhoon et al., 2013; van der Zee et al., 2017).

6.2.4 The Thermal Dose Model Limitations: Low-Levels of Thermal Damage and the Thermal Damage Threshold Perspective

There are multiple traditional concerns with this model, and a good review of such concerns was eloquently presented by Foster and colleagues (Foster et al., 2011) and briefly reiterated more recently (Sienkiewicz et al., 2016). A concern of specific interest to this chapter is the apparently large uncertainty about the effects of chronic exposures to low-level thermal doses. In this regard, one must notice that the CEM43 model, in principle: ***identifies thermal doses producing a specified amount of damage***, instead of a threshold below which no damage occurs. Therefore, the possibility that such a threshold may not exist, and damage may not stop but it may occur in lesser degree as the thermal dose is lower could be substantial.

In this regard, animal and human data for low-levels of thermal dosage is surprisingly scarce. In fact, most of the data supporting this model comes from experiments in which tissues have been almost exclusively heated above 41°C and sometimes above 43°C in rather acute exposures. Additionally, the data utilized is based on animals of several species which have substantially different physiologies and thermoregulatory capabilities leading to not only inherently different thermal set-points (e.g., mouse is 37°C while guinea pig is 39.0–39.5°C), but also significantly different sensitivities to heat across different tissues and organs which are not necessarily representative of those of humans (especially at lower levels). As a result, extrapolating CEM43 to low-levels of thermal exposure (or low-levels of thermal damage) could introduce substantial levels of uncertainty since it is unsupported by data. This makes the prediction power of CEM43 doubtful for low-levels of thermal damage at low thermal doses, even if the assumption that the first-order kinetics followed by all tissues at low thermal doses is correct (which may not be true (Pawar et al., 2016)). Coincidently, CEM43 has been unsuccessful in describing secondary physiological responses of thermal damage (e.g., edema or *ex vivo* thermal coagulation) (Dewey, 1994, 2009). Therefore, while it is a likely possibility that the current thermal dose model is not only inadequate to predict low-levels of thermal damage, it is a certainty that its inception does not contemplate the possibility of chronic physiological effects which depend on the properties of intermittent thermal signals within (or outside) the currently recommended "safe" limits.

6.3 FROM THERMAL DAMAGE TO THERMAL SIGNALING: A NEW PARADIGM

The approximations and assumptions described before in which dosimetric and biological models are based on are certainly useful and convenient for guaranteeing safety under the classical thermal hazard paradigm, which establishes rather acute hazard thresholds. On the other hand, thermal signals are an unavoidable reality in the context of RF interactions with the human body and the current safety perspective could inevitably limit our ability to determine existing harmful (and perhaps useful) effects of low-level (and chronic) thermal exposures. In this regard, the existence of thermal transients is recognized by leaders in the expert community and recommendations for the limitation of their existence have been published (Foster et al., 2017; Laakso et al., 2017). However, such recommendations emerge from the same original paradigm of limiting temperature from reaching certain levels (hence doses) which are known to (or that could) be deleterious in the traditional, rather acute sense. This is understandable and adequate in the sense that the mere concept of "low-level thermal signals" is not considered by the scientific community as something of (potential) biological importance. As a result, neither biological nor health effects have been established from which recommendations for human safety (or therapeutics) can be made. Nevertheless, it is an undeniable fact that such thermal signals are always present, to some degree or another, in RF exposures. Therefore, should the current paradigm be complemented to accommodate the possibility that sufficiently relevant biological and/or health effects may emerge from exposure to such signals?

In order to start answering such a question, one may want to consider the question of how a biological or health effect could come into existence from such apparently subtle signals. Could such signals be (biologically) amplified? Could they substantially modulate biochemical or physiological processes from the biological perspective? In principle, cellular systems are perhaps the most complex (and minute) sensors we know with almost incredible abilities for amplification. Based on these building blocks, biological organisms can sense and respond to minute stimuli to guard their (and the entire system's) homeostatic state, making amplification of subtle environmental (and biochemical) signals fundamental for complex biological system survival. To anchor this perspective, consider that at the cellular level, for example, an action potential (or subthreshold oscillations) can be generated following contact with only a few molecules of neurotransmitter or the oxidative burst introduced by immune cells after an encounter with signs of invasion (Dahlgren et al., 1999; Kandel et al., 2000). These amplification capabilities become greatly enhanced when considering collections of cells which can work in harmony. In such cases, extremely small signals captured by a single or small number of cells can be followed by substantial cascades of biochemical responses (hormones, neurotransmitters, etc.) at the level of the entire organism within seconds. This is evident, for example, in the thermoregulatory processes. Although local and systemic thermoregulatory effects (e.g., vasodilation, etc.) are delayed by physical and physiological restrictions (several seconds to minutes), the sensory and regulatory signals (e.g., neural, hormonal) are in fact triggered immediately via extremely sensitive physiological sensors and can last for much longer times. Cells with amplification capabilities are also densely packed in astonishingly small volumes. For example, consider a 10gSAR cube (the current standard SAR averaging standard) situated in the face of an average human. Within the projection of the area of such a cube (c.a. 4.6 cm^2), the human face would contain tens of thousands of neural ramifications (only in the skin) (Nolano et al., 2013). The same is true for the external part of the ear (pinna) which is usually disregarded in numerical models, measurements and some safety standards (Morimoto et al., 2016; Kodera et al., 2018). In fact, most cellular structures (μm-range) are at least 3–4 orders of magnitude smaller (Iggo, 1974) than this area where differential absorption can generate very localized "hot spots," as shown in the previous section, which may be large (and fast) enough to be of relevance to biological processes.

Therefore, from a sensory perspective, how sensitive are biological systems to subtle thermal challenges? With this in mind, the next section will try to compile existing information to question the possible biological relevance of small thermal signals.

6.4 BIOLOGICAL SYSTEMS THERMAL SENSITIVITY AND REGULATION UNDER THERMAL CHALLENGES

Temperature is one of the fundamental macroscopic properties of matter as it describes the average kinetic energy of its fundamental particles. As such, its concept permeates basically all aspects of every form of living organism playing a fundamental role in many (if not all) of the physicochemical phenomena that lead to life (Precht; 2013; Schrödinger; 1944).

At a fundamental level, chemical (and bio-chemical) reaction rates are governed by forms of the Arrhenius equation, where the temperature dependency is exponential (Arrhenius, 1889; Dewey, 1994; Jorjani et al., 1999; van't Hoff, 1884). This results in living organisms' basic biochemical machinery being particularly sensitive to small temperature changes. Additionally, the kinetics of the cellular complement of proteins (proteome) and cellular structures function within very narrow temperature ranges as a result of their fundamental tendency towards optimization (Sen et al., 2014). In fact, optimization levels can be such that the organism death may be only a few degrees away from its optimal physiological set-point (e.g., humans c.a. $\geq$ 1.5°C from set-point (core = 36.5–37.5°C)) (Dill et al., 2011). In addition, as thermodynamically open systems, living organisms must continuously exchange energy and matter with the surrounding environment which is variable and inhomogeneous (Walleczek et al., 2006). This has pressured organisms to develop various methods for compensation for such unpredictable variations and inhomogeneities to maintain their temperature, however, at great expense (Somero et al., 1971; Ruoff et al., 2003). For example, homeotherms maintain their core temperature in tight ranges either autonomously (endotherms, i.e., most mammals, birds), by significantly intensifying metabolic rates (thermogenesis) or behaviorally (ectotherms, i.e., most hibernators, estivators, kleptotherms) by migrating to locations where the environment provides temperature ranges at which their basal metabolism is sufficient to maintain body temperature (thermoneutrality) (Kokolus et al., 2013). Interestingly, the modern human is a special case of homeotherm, which has partially shifted thermoregulatory control from its body to the artificial environment (temperature regulated dwellings) behaviorally, demanding c.a. 9 to 28 times more energy at a high environmental cost (Hill et al., 2013; Nedergaard et al., 2007). In contrast, some of the complex mesophyles (Poikilotherms, i.e., most fish, amphibians) can function at wider core temperature ranges (spending c.a. 15–30 times less energy than homeotherms), but at the cost of supplementary and redundant cellular and molecular feedback systems (mostly neural) (Abrams et al., 1982; Caplan et al., 2014; Rinberg et al., 2013; Robertson et al., 2012; Sen et al., 2014; Soofi et al., 2014; Warzecha et al., 1999). Some animals have evolved in curious ways around conserving their original thermoregulatory mechanisms. For example, the whale has evolved to still maintain 37°C but minimized a surface area-to-volume ratio (gigantothermy) (Meekan, 2017). Costs of chronic exposure to subthermoneutral temperatures can be substantial. For example, chronic exposures were shown to induce stress with measurable biological consequences like enhanced tumor growth in mice (Eng et al., 2015; Kokolus et al., 2013).

Within the complexity of a biological system, some tissues are more sensitive to thermal differentials than others. In the case of most homeotherms, the shell temperature (skin, subcutaneous tissue, skeletal muscle) is considerably less strictly controlled (e.g., possible variability > 3°C) than the core temperature (abdominal, thoracic, and cranial cavities). Core temperature differentials as low as 1 to 2°C have been widely regarded as harmful under various conditions (i.e., fever, hypothermia). Of the tissues residing in the core, the neural systems appear to be the most thermally regulated (Busto et al., 1987; Childs, 2008). Within the spatio-temporal limitations of current temperature measurement instrumentation and techniques, core thermoregulatory processes (especially within neural systems) have been shown to regulated in the vicinities of 0.1°C with great capability for amplification against movements from the set-point for humans (Adair, 2008; Kräuchi, 2002; Lim et al., 2008). Such regulation capability is dependent on the high sensitivity of thermal regulation systems of core temperatures. Blood flow changes can happen in the order of seconds and the brain thermal response is slower (several tens of seconds). Brain temperature inhomogeneity (colder in the peripherals) is kept within tight ranges (c.a. 0.001–0.2°C) by quick and localized blood flow injections in the event of increased metabolic heat production tied to augmented functional activity. During active periods, the compensation introduced depends on the location in the brain (deep regions cool down while peripheral regions heat up) as a result of arterial blood inflow, the main purpose of which (besides oxygenation) is thermal regulation (McElligott et al., 1967; Sukstanskii et al., 2006; Werner et al., 1988). This behavior has many times been associated with specialized neural structures within the brain which are generally also in charge of the detection of other environmental cues like salt, light, CO_2, and pheromones (Biron et al., 2008; Boulant et al., 1986; Bretscher et al., 2011; Saito et al., 2014; Warzecha et al., 1999). This great capacity for core thermal regulation happens, in part, by help of the shell (skin, etc.) working as a buffer with greater thermal sensitivity, tolerance, and flexibility to rapidly sense, adapt, and counteract changes with time constants in the tens of seconds (Kellogg, 2006). This is consistent with the behavioral thermoregulation data available for hundreds of animal species (including humans) showing distinctive animal sensitivity to environmental temperature (Dell et al., 2011, 2013).

Additionally, biological systems present many times oscillatory behavior. This can be partly due to their need to maintain homeostatic levels, making them reliable on feedback control loops at the molecular, cellular, organ, and system levels. Coincidently, sustained autonomous temperature oscillations around their optimal set-point are known to exist (under steady environmental conditions) for many organisms from cyanobacteria and plants to humans (Morf, 2013; Yoshida et al., 2009). In humans, for example, circadian (i.e., daily c.a. 24 h $\pm$ 0.5°C) and circamensal (i.e., menstrual c.a. 28 d $\pm$ 0.5–1.0°C) as well as circannual (i.e., seasonal c.a. $\pm$ 0.3/0.4°C) cycles have been identified which are directly affected by endogenous (i.e., health, reproductive) as well as exogenous (i.e., weather, environment) status (Hammel et al., 1968; Keatinge et al., 1986; Kelly, 2006, 2007; Kräuchi et al., 2014; Rubin et al., 1987; Shiraki et al., 1986; Webb, 1992). Other mammals also present circadian fluctuations with magnitudes that can be much greater than $\pm$1°C, depending on species (Brown et al., 2002; Giannetto et al., 2012; Refinetti, 1995, 1999, 2016). This is also true at the organ level. For example, rhythmic subcortical fluctuations are inherent to the mammalian (cat) brain (0.001–0.003°C @ 5–12 cycles/min) which are not correlated to breathing rate or blood pressure (McElligott et al., 1967). Other oscillations of the same order are also observed in the brain of monkeys (Hayward et al., 1968). More recently, some authors pointed out that some animals' bodies (including humans) are able to purposely generate and maintain thermal gradients by creating small regions of lower temperature with important biological purpose. For example, differences in the order of 0.5°C have been recorded *in vivo* to tissues surrounding follicles at distinguishable developmental stages (Ye et al., 2007). Also, the existence of intracellular gradients has been proposed by several authors using more nonconventional methods (Benit et al., 2017).

6.4.1 Potential Biological Relevance of Thermal Signals

Under the premises presented in the previous section, it is clear that we know that a multiplicity of biological structures from the molecular to the organ level are sensitive to small thermal differentials (Ezquerra-Romano et al., 2017). However, the capabilities for sensitivity and regulation presented were focused under "conventional" thermal challenges (ΔT) and not under thermal variabilities like those that can be generated with modulation or intermittence of the heating source. However, it is clear that from the cells' perspective that RF exposures are accompanied by thermal signals which are localized in space and are time-dependent. Therefore, while an issue of potential importance to basic science and public health is to estimate how small of a thermal transient ($\Delta T/dt$) (and therefore thermal signal T(t)) can have biological relevance, only a minuscule fraction of thermobiology experiments were directed towards exploring these effects.

Nevertheless, a good start for answering this question is to look at the potential mechanisms which are rooted on the underlying physicochemical properties and interactions of matter under transient thermal conditions. One such interaction is given by the Nernst Equation which describes the relationship between chemical concentrations and electrical potentials across a semipermeable membrane (Vidal-Iglesias et al., 2012). For potassium concentrations, this equation would look like this:

$$[\mathbf{K}_{in}] = [\mathbf{K}_{out}]\mathbf{e}^{\frac{qV}{kT}} \tag{6.4}$$

where $[\mathbf{K}_{in}]$ is the concentration of potassium inside the cell, $[\mathbf{K}_{out}]$ is the concentration of potassium outside of the cell, **q** is the charge of the electron, **V** is the voltage across the membrane, **k** is Boltzmann's constant, and **T** is the absolute temperature. Interestingly, little work is needed to show these parameters' dependence on $\Delta T/dt$. This was done by Prof. Frank Barnes in 1984 (Barnes, 1984). Using the same equation and assuming some approximate values for pacemaker cells from *Aplysia*, he was able to predict current flow through cell membrane in the order of 5 nA as a result of imposing $\Delta T/\Delta t = 0.1°C/sec$. Additionally, as a reference, he stated that experiments previously performed had shown that currents as small as 2 nA injected through a microelectrode would bias such pacemaker cells from cutoff to saturation, and that currents of tenths of nA would change their firing rate. While many more details can be considered in order to predict such dependencies more accurately (Rabbitt et al., 2016), this simple calculation not only showed that, in principle, phyisico-chemical potentials should be affected by thermal transients which are well within technical feasibility, but also that biological relevance of such transients was quite likely.

Coincidently, practical experiments showed changes in the firing rate of pacemaker cells from the ganglion of *Aplysia Califorrnica* induced by $\Delta T/dt$ of about 1°C/sec and that such changes were comparable to the injection of about 1 nA into the cell. Interestingly, the total ΔT in such experiments were little as 0.1°C, hinting to a real dependence of the effect on $\Delta T/dt$ rather than on just ΔT (Barnes et al., 2007; Chalker, 1982). Similar observations were made for the large parietal ganglion of the central nervous system of *Limnea stagnalis* where a substantially slower increase in temperature (1°C/min or slower) increased the firing rate of the pacemaker cell and a rapid increase in temperature (0.1°C/sec or faster), decreased or stopped the firing (Bol'shakov et al., 1986). This hints at further underlying mechanistic complexity which can be perhaps explained by the existence of competing chemical reactions at different rates (Barnes, 1974; Barnes et al., 2018). Later, an excellent cohort of experimental reports came from Ziskin laboratory dealing with the study of biological effects of low-intensity mm waves (30–300 GHz). As a control for their experiments on mm waves (which induce heating), Zisking, Alekseev, and colleagues exposed neurons to changing rates of temperature by conductive heat transfer. With this method they determined the lower threshold for causing recordable changes in the firing rate of the pacemaker neuron of *Lymnaea* (snail) to be in the vicinities of 0.0025°C/sec (Alekseev et al., 1997).

In mammals, early on, experiments by Iggo et al. demonstrated sensitivities for monkey (and human) neurons in the order of 0.05°C/sec (Iggo, 1962). Interestingly, a well performed group of experiments by Blick et al., later revisited by Riu et al., appear to suggest lower thresholds on human sensitivity. While they interpreted these results as being a result of the net temperature change (ΔT), thresholds can be calculated in the order of 0.005–0.013°C/sec (depending on penetration depth) (Blick et al., 1997; Riu et al., 1997). More recently, further evidence of neural activation was presented by Green et al., showing effects on transitions at 0.5 and 4.0 °C/s on human sensation. Here, neural activation was suspected to be linked to certain involvement of various temperature sensitive ion channels (TRP) which were highly rate sensitive (Green et al., 2010). Further evidence supporting the involvement of ion channels sensitive to temperature (Patapoutian et al., 2003) was proposed some groups. For example, a method of stimulation called magneto-thermal genetic stimulation was tested for the first time in freely behaving rats. In this method, heat is delivered to the neural cell membranes with high specificity by imposing alternating magnetic fields with membrane-bound synthesized superparamagnetic nanoparticles. The $\Delta t/dt$ introduced ranged from 0.1 to 1.0°C/s depending on the area density of nanoparticles on the genetically modified cells inducing differential changes in action potentials *in vitro* and multiple distinguishable behavioral changes *in vivo* depending on the area of the brain stimulated (Munshi et al., 2017). More interestingly, a group of experiments on *Drosophila* larvae showed the possible interaction of Ca^{2+} with TRP channels on sensing rates in the order of 0.02–0.5°C/s. Of special interest is that more marked responses were shown as rates were increased (high-pass filter behavior) providing a signal which correlates to the size of the needed reaction (Luo et al., 2017). Interestingly, nonexcitable cells are also known to respond to spatio-temporal thermal gradients (Shapiro et al., 2012). For example, human fibrosarcoma cell cultures (HT1080) were shown to have proliferation effects (>20%) when cultured at an oscillating temperature (max. $\Delta t/dt = 0.6$°C/s) (Portelli et al., 2017).

It is perhaps important to note that while all these effects are observed, the understanding of their reasons is still limited due to the complexity of the many microscopic events occurring simultaneously in the cell. Traditionally, the electrophysiological model used to explain nerve activity modulation is given by the Hodgkin and Huxley model which considers voltage-dependent conductances (Hodgkin et al., 1952; Kandel et al., 2000). In essence, this model is only based on a simplified lumped-element model built on empirical observations rather than on basic thermodynamics (which some might call "curve fitting" in a relaxed academic environment). In contrast, many other physicochemical phenomena are observed in real cells during action potentials. For example, mechanical and thermal transients (0.00002–0.04°C/s, depending on technical details) have been observed to operate as part of a passing action potential in *in vitro* experiments on olfactory nerves (Böckmann et al., 1996; Tasaki et al., 1989, 1992) accompanied by minute mechanical perturbations in the medium. This being the case, there have been multiple attempts to reconcile these details with the Hodgkin and Huxley model. However, progress has been limited due to the inherent limitations imposed by the model not being based on fundamental thermodynamics (i.e., not considering changes in temperature, lateral tension, pH, etc.). Some efforts have been made to derive such expressions from thermodynamic perspectives to integrate thermal sensitivities with little success (Forrest, 2014). Fortunately, much more complex models which include the details and concepts to reconcile the multiplicity of simultaneous thermal and nonthermal phenomena known to be associated with neural activity have been proposed. The most prominent of these is perhaps the Heimburg–Jackson model which proposes the action potential propagation to be of the nature of a piezo electric wave (a localized density excitation that propagates in the axon bilipid membrane without any distortion (soliton wave)). While several aspects of theory are currently under scientific scrutiny (Appali et al., 2012; Hasani et al., 2015), its fundamentals are able to explain many observed phenomenon like the transient and reversible lipid channel formation, mechanical change in thickness of nerves, change in temperature, and even the reason for the anesthetics effects in the medical practice (Andersen et al., 2009; Blicher et al., 2009; Heimburg et al., 2007, 2015; Heimburg, 2008, 2010; Laub et al., 2012; Mosgaard et al., 2012, 2013). Although much work is still necessary, one can surmise that under such a model, the temperature dependence (ΔT and $\Delta T/dt$) of the factors involved in action potential generation and propagation becomes obvious.

In view of the facts presented, one can see that sensitivity to temperature changes is an inherent aspect of classical physicochemical theory. Since the cell is a collection of dynamic biochemical reactions and structures, it would not be surprising that signals formed by collections of temperature changes (ΔT and $\Delta T/dt$) can have some degree of influence on the dynamics or function of such biochemical reactions and structures, and therefore, on the biological system as a whole. Therefore, in essence, every biochemical reaction can be seen as a thermal transducer which can act as a handle into the cellular processes.

6.4.2 From Thermal Signal into Biological and Health Effects

An interesting example of biological amplification via transduction of thermal signals in the skin resulting in biological and health effects relevant to this discussion is the therapeutic application of mm waves by therapists in Eastern Europe and the former Soviet Union (Betskii et al., 2004; Pakhomov et al., 2000). In short, 15–30 min exposures on body points of high neural density (sometimes associated with acupuncture points) have shown stimulation of the nervous system and immune activation followed by endogenous opioid release in animals and humans, resulting in analgesic and multiple immune effects at an organism level (Egot-Lemaire et al., 2011; Ziskin, 2013). The many empirical observations of the therapeutic potential of such exposures led Dr. Marvin Ziskin and his colleagues in the west to perform many experiments (for 25 years) to unveil the mechanism of action. Their results suggested that the effects observed are mostly thermally-mediated through the absorption in water at the most external skin layers (<0.5 mm thick) (Haas et al., 2017; Ziskin, 2013), perhaps with only some exceptions (Habauzit et al., 2014). They noted that stimulation most likely occurred at free nerve endings extending into the epidermis as well as residing immunocompetent cells (i.e., Langerhans, keratinocytes).

These experiments propose the potential for amplification of thermal signals at the levels of the skin into full body responses. In practice, exposures can be much longer and include areas with higher neural density (face, hands), potentially inducing similar or greater responses. While this is perhaps the only set of data along these lines, its existence is intriguing and compelling for further investigation, not only for its potential therapeutic applications, but also for its relevance to the widespread use of mobile communications and must be pursued further.

From the last section, it is evident that thermal signals are always, to some degree or other, an inseparable aspect of RF exposures. Therefore, in view of the effects described above, and without making any assumption of the true biological relevance of RF fields themselves (a topic that is known as "nonthermal effects") one can hypothesize that these secondary thermal signals associated with RF exposure may work at the cellular level as a signaling vehicle for information transfer. Therefore, one may hypothesize that under certain conditions, exposures to such signals may artificially force physiological responses of relevance (e.g., stress) which may add up over time.

6.4.3 Resonance and Other Forms of Interaction with Dynamic Biochemical Systems

In the case where thermal signals are transferring information to the cell (meaning that the amount of energy is infinitesimally small), one may consider other ways in which such information is amplified into the biological effects observed. In this regard, many examples of such amplification potential can be found at the molecular, cellular, organ, and organism levels. One of such ways may be through resonant processes. As one may surmise, thermal oscillatory behavior present in most complex organisms (discussed earlier in this chapter) is driven or in close relationship to underlying biochemical oscillations. Such oscillations appear to be fundamental to life. In fact, a growing body of evidence indicates that biochemical signaling encodes information in oscillatory signals rather than in constant ones (Dolmetsch et al., 1998; Tostevin et al., 2012). Examples of biochemical oscillations can be observed from scales that vary from complete organism and usually slow oscillations (lasting hours to days) (e.g., circadian) to more rapid ones (e.g., insulin, heart, brain chemical oscillations) all the way down to the cellular and even intracellular level in the second and subsecond range (action potentials, intracellular ion concentrations, subthreshold neural oscillations, etc.) (Bergsten, 2002; Brasen et al., 2010; Buzsáki et al. 2004; Ehrengruber et al., 1996; Falcke et al., 2003; Koshiya et al., 1999; Matsumoto et al., 2016; Maroto et al., 2008; Novák et al., 2008; Rapp, 1979; Slaby et al., 2009; Smelder et al., 2014; Stark et al., 2007).

Substantial effects on such oscillatory systems can be caused with an infinitesimal amount of energy given that it is delivered timely (resonance). For example, Wachtel showed how neural firing patterns of pacemaker cells can be synchronized (entrained) with relatively weak and periodic electrical stimuli. In addition, Wachtel showed how increasing amounts of intracellular and intercellular current were needed when the frequency of the periodic electrical signal differed from the natural frequency of the cells (Wachtel, 1985). This phenomenon is expected according to the properties of synchronization (or injection locking and pulling) of autonomous oscillators whose properties have been widely studied because of their relevance to various physical and chemical systems (Adler, 1946; Paciorek, 1965; Razavi, 2004). In essence, any oscillatory system has a frequency (or group of frequencies) at which it oscillates best, or in other words, the frequency at which the energy input needed to make it osculate is minimum (we call this the natural frequency, see Figure 6.4). Consequently, pressing the system to oscillate at another frequency, although possible, would take more input energy than at its natural frequency to account for the extra strain imposed in the system. Nonlinearities in the oscillating system can introduce dependencies on the amplitude of the driving signal (Donoso et al., 2012).

Interestingly, artificially generated environments with oscillating thermal signals have been shown to entrain and synchronize the autonomous circadian oscillators in plants (Eckardt, 2005), nematodes (Van der Linden et al., 2010), and insects (Glaser et al., 2005). Similarly, several reports have shown that interaction with unorganized cellular cultures is possible by introducing thermal oscillations of the same order as those generated *in vivo* (e.g., as low as ±0.3/0.4°C for humans) (Hammel et al., 1968; Keatinge et al., 1986; Kelly, 2006, 2007; Kräuchi et al., 2014; Rubin, 1987; Shiraki et al., 1986; Webb, 1992). Some hypothesize that this responsiveness may come from the absence of synchronizing biochemical signals found *in vivo*, making these (unorganized) cells in culture more susceptible to those of thermal origin. For example, cultures of peripheral cells (human fibroblasts) autonomous oscillators have been shown to be able to be synchronized *in vitro* by small temperature fluctuations (c.a. ± 0.5°C) mimicking daily body temperature fluctuations as effectively as with other chemical signals (Saini et al., 2012). Similar results were observed for rats' suprachiasmatic nucleus cells (c.a. ± 0.75°C), rat fibroblasts (c.a. ± 1.25°C), mice fibroblasts (c.a. ± 1.5°C), and even cyanobacteria (c.a. ± 7.5°C) (Herzog et al., 2003; Sladek et al., 2013; Yoshida et al., 2009). Furthermore, thermal signals (c.a. ± 1.25°C, 1/7–1/25 Hz) have been shown to inhibit growth rates of human fibrosarcoma cells in culture in a frequency dependent manner, hinting at a possible interaction with ongoing

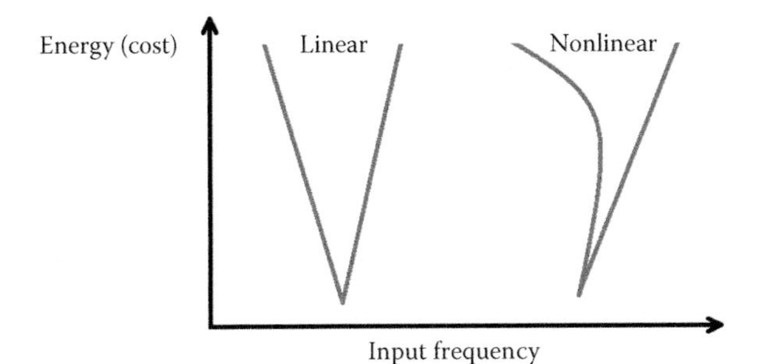

FIGURE 6.4 Energy cost for driving an oscillator with an external signal. The energy needed for driving the oscillator (cost) is minimized at the oscillator natural frequencies. Nonlinearities may also make the natural oscillation amplitude (and sequence) dependent.

oscillatory biochemical signals (Portelli et al., 2017). Furthermore, the intrinsic complexity and nonlinearity of biological systems (especially neural networks) can show special nonlinear resonance traits by responding to special combinations and sequences of stimuli (Hayashi, 2014; Izhikevich et al., 2003). Another way of transduction of thermal transients into biological systems may be through interaction with competing chemical reactions which have different time constants. Such a case can lead to substantial biochemical differences induced by long versus short thermal transients (Barnes, 1974).

Therefore, in similar ways to those shown by these examples, the injection of periodic thermal signals could, under the specific conditions necessary, resonate, entrain, synchronize, interrupt or disturb biochemical oscillators resulting in substantial biological effects which could be of enough magnitude to elicit health effects. This makes the potential scientific relevance of these stimuli substantial.

6.4.4 Other Factors of Potential Biological Relevance

One has to consider that in practice, there are several factors which determine the ultimate thermal signals delivered at the cell level (e.g., clothing, humidity, etc.). In the case of cellular phones, Straume and colleagues have measured superficial temperatures increases by several degrees as a result of direct contact (and pressure) from the phone on the skin. They note that this effect resulted from reduced cooling from air circulation as well as heat conduction due to power dissipation within the phone (Straume et al., 2005). Therefore, in such cases, the total thermal signal delivered to the outer tissues of the human head and face will result in a complex spatiotemporal combination of this factor, the RF-induced heat and the redistribution and dissipation of such heat via active and passive physical and physiological mechanisms. Therefore, a SAR or IPD restriction may indeed be insufficient to guarantee safe thermal levels of such superficial tissues under the current paradigm.

Another factor of potential interest is how fast the energy is deposited. This factor could have some potential biological relevance via the ***Thermoacoustic Effect*** in which transient tissue volume differentials are introduced by the rate-of-change of the energy deposition (**ΔSAR/dt**). In other words, this will result in a pressure wave (sound) deposited into the biological system generated as a result of a sudden change in temperature (Xia et al., 2014). As a reference, a simple thermodynamics calculation shows that a maximum SAR deposition of 0.25 W/Kg achieved in 1 μS ($\mathbf{t_{slope(on)\text{-}RF}}$ in Figure 6.5) yields an instantaneous pressure transient with magnitudes around 20 Pascals (in soft tissue) and frequencies in the range of a few hundred kilohertz. Interestingly, this would be enough to allow thermoacoustic tomography on an MRI scanner as it is about 20 dB above thermal noise. In practice, much higher pressures are possible depending on the commercial equipment in use (Winkler et al., 2017) or other energy deposition modalities (light, ultrasound). As a comparison, note that neuromodulation has been achieved *in vitro* and *in vivo* in animals and humans with high spatial specificity (mm range) although with significantly larger intensities (Lee et al., 2016; Mehić et al., 2014; Mueller et al., 2014). Nevertheless, just as with thermal signals themselves, one might wonder how low these signals should be before their

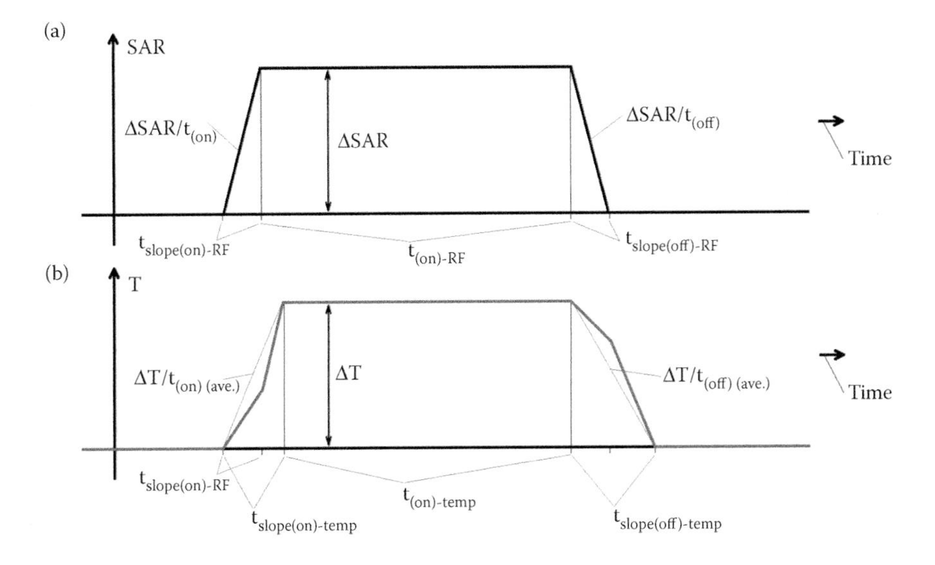

FIGURE 6.5 Thermoacoustic effect principle. (a) SAR resulting from imposing a pulsed RF electromagnetic field in tissue. (b) Corresponding thermal signal (T(t)) in tissue). Notice how the rate-of-change of SAR can also influence the thermal rate-of-change, modifying the resulting thermal signal. The representation of the thermal transients is an approximation for reference and is not to scale. Real transients are typically more complex with nonlinear transitions.

biological effects are negligible from a physiological point of view, considering low-level chronic exposures.

6.5 GETTING STARTED: ESTABLISHING THE TRUE *IN VITRO* AND *IN VIVO* BIOLOGICAL RELEVANCE OF THERMAL SIGNALS

The study of thermal signals may open a myriad of possibilities. Noninvasive, nonchemical interaction with biochemical signals could be a fantastic tool for cellular manipulation and signaling. One such possibility is the synchronization or entrainment of cellular cycles or other biochemical processes (e.g., metabolic, ionic concentrations, sub-threshold oscillations, etc.) which may lead to the improvement or generation of new tools in the scientific, industrial or therapeutic arenas (Katriel, 2008; Kuramoto, 1975). However, experimentation with thermal signals *in vitro* is not easy. One of the common obstacles is the thermal transients and oscillations which are inherent to laboratory rooms and equipment (incubators, etc.). Such oscillations and transients can be of the same order (or much larger) than the signals whose effects are summarized in the past section (i.e., $\Delta T > 1°C$) (Portelli, 2017). In fact, these variations are such that one may contemplate this being one of the reasons behind the irreproducibility of much of the published biological research (Begley et al., 2012; Freedman et al., 2014).

In such variable baseline conditions, it is practically impossible to study the effect of small thermal signals without specialized equipment. However, designing, building, calibrating, and operating the necessary equipment require extraordinary effort and expertise. One may contemplate that this combination of factors may very well have discouraged research in this area. Nevertheless, the methods responsible for the results presented in this chapter are useful to continue and expand this novel branch of Thermobiology.

In essence, a system that can generate thermal signals is based in two factors: *getting the heat in and getting the heat out of certain target volume*. In this regard, an advantage of *in vitro* experimentation is the malleability of the thermal properties of the sample which can be orders of magnitude different from those found *in vivo*, allowing to mobilize heat more efficiently. For example, choosing a small thermal capacity of a culture container makes it susceptible to rapid temperature changes without the need for much energy. However, to achieve rapid changes, there needs to be a good heat transfer coefficient between this container and the driving heat (cold) source. Additionally, real time monitoring from the culture perspective during the entire experiment (not only exposure) is fundamental, since cells respond to their immediate environment, even during times of normal incubation (which may far exeed the experimental exposures (Portelli, 2018). Therefore, specialized incubation applications are needed that minimize the residual thermal variations below the levels being studied.

An example of such a system was proposed by Portelli and colleagues in which multiple cultures are placed on a Peltier-based system which can induce or extract heat from the culture. An important feature of such a system is the ability to monitor cells' temperatures at the culture level and to control the thermal signal delivered depending on the direction of the applied electric current (with a thermal constant of c.a. 2 seconds) (Portelli et al., 2010, 2011, 2017). Along the same lines, mm wave exposures are an attractive method for studying transient and periodic temperature effects. By also using microscale thermocouples, Zhadobov and colleagues have recently produced such an exposure system which is suitable for studying short pulses on adherent cell cultures (in monolayer), demonstrating good agreement with numerical models (Zhadobov et al., 2017). Other embodiments of mm wave exposure systems can be found in the work by Ziskin, Alekseev, and colleagues (Ziskin, 2013). Previous systems proposed are capable of introducing pulsed heat via an intermittent pulse of microwaves into water pipe generating a heated block of flowing water which feeds the culture container water jacket, transferring the heat transient into the cells (Chalker, 1982; Barnes, et al., 2007). Recently, some work has gone into miniaturization of resistive and semiconductor thermal devices (50–1 mm) which could potentially sustain cultures in smaller areas or in a lab-on-chip context (Fernandes et al., 2016; Reverter et al., 2014).

On a related note, the effect of thermal signals might be one of the reasons behind the irreproducibility of low-level RF experimental reports which is commonplace in the field of bioelectromagnetics (Foster et al., 2011; Portelli, 2017). This argument may be that as a part of the uncertainty of RF exposure, systems and conditions would also lead to large uncertainties in the thermal signal imposed on cells due to differentials in heat deposition and removal of the specific exposure systems and methods utilized. In this regard, some authors have performed numerical simulations on RF-exposed culture containers showing sufficient differentials in energy deposition warranting convection within the liquid medium. Such flow, for example, might create local concentrations of nutrients affecting cultures in a differential way (Paffi et al., 2015a,b).

Interestingly, several authors have worked in characterizing, cataloguing, comparing, and explaining the exposures and effects of pulsed light and ultrasound exposures, generating exposure systems and methods which may be of importance to study the effects of thermal signaling. In the case of light pulses, microstimulation with such systems has the ability to introduce very localized (mm range) thermal transients of the order of several tens to thousands of °C/s (Chu et al., 2015; Ibsen et al., 2015; Luan et al., 2014; Ter Haar et al., 2013; Urdaneta et al., 2017). Recently, optical neuromodulation is a field gaining momentum in the scientific community both as a scientific novelty and also as a wishful alternative to electrical stimulation and its associated limitations. In fact, nondestructive action potential generation and phase-locking are some commonly achieved effects in culture. In this regard, there is a sufficient amount of research with reasonable agreement with the hypothesis that the effects correspond to charge redistributions that are thermally-mediated ($\Delta T/dt$) by water energy absorption (Duke et al., 2012, 2013; Izzo et al., 2008; Norton et al., 2013; Rabbitt et al., 2016; Shapiro et al., 2012; Thompson et al., 2014; Wells et al., 2007). Similar effects can be elicited by ultrasound pulses where less localized thermal transients on the order of 50 °C/s can be achieved in culture. However, in this case, the source of the effects observed are perhaps also dependent on the mechanical aspect of this stimulus (Mihran et al., 1990).

Finally, just as with any other form of biological research, the downside of *in vitro* experimentation is its possible low relevance to *in vivo* situations. While some *in vivo* effects have been already exposed by the extensive work initially performed at Ziskin laboratory on thermal stimulus at the levels of the skin (Ziskin, 2013), much remains to be done in this area to fully explain the mechanisms and explore optimal exposure modalities. In the case of stimulation of deeper tissues, an obvious possibility is the intermittent use of hyperthermia exposures. Characterization of hyperthermia experimental setups shows $\Delta T/dt$ in the order of c.a. 0.001–1°C/sec *in vivo* (Griffiths et al., 1986; Lara et al., 2017; Raaijmakers et al., 2017) and up to 3°C/sec with more focused modalities (i.e., nanoparticles) (Cherukuri et al., 2010; Deatsch et al., 2014). Another possibility is the use of focused ultrasound in the same intermittent way (Lee et al., 2016; Mehić et al., 2014; Mueller et al., 2014; Ter Haar, 2013). Nevertheless, to this day, there are no studies looking at the potential benefits (or deleterious effects) of intermittent hyperthermia exposures in any modality.

6.6 CONCLUSIONS

It is an undeniable fact that complex biological systems, from the molecular to the full organism level, are built around very rigorous thermal specifications making them very sensitive and responsive to small temperature changes in their internal or external vicinity. Hence, thermal signals which are invariably linked to the imposition of RF fields have the potential to be accompanied by compensatory biochemical responses from tissue at a local or global level in the organism. Such thermal signals might initially have modest effects on biochemical reactions and structures, however, these effects may then be amplified by the biological system into relevant biological and health effects.

From the public health perspective, a necessary question to answer is: what are the biological effects of chronic exposures to low-level thermal signals and what are the relative health risks? (i.e., compared to a smoking certain number of cigarettes a day, for example). However, to date, our currently poor understanding about the true biological relevance of thermal signals is insufficient to draw useful scientific conclusions which can affect decisions, recommendations, and policy to protect the public from potential hazards. In fact, the amount of data available is much less than would be considered the bare minimum. How "small" a thermal signal is can only be judged from a biological system perspective by generating the appropriate set of experiments and interpreting them from a paradigm that includes this possibility. While, in essence, the characteristics of this thermal signal will be a result of the antagonistic thermal processes (heat-in versus heat-out) specific to the details of the exposure, the need for consideration of the effects from the cellular spatio-temporal scale might require significant amounts of effort and complications. However, such apparent complications, in return, may hold substantial scientific, industrial, and therapeutic potential at best or understanding of realistic safety thresholds at worst.

Therefore, in view of the pervasiveness and potential relevance of low-level thermal signals, the paradigm centered around the notion of a "thermal damage threshold" on which the current safety standards and recommendations for mobile communications are currently based might be incomplete. For this reason alone, basic research in this area is imperative. Therefore, scientists and executives who are seriously concerned about the implications of mobile communications on public health must consider directing their scientific resources towards unveiling the true biological relevance of RF-induced small thermal signals to such a degree as these are directed towards the study of RF-induced "thermal" and "nonthermal" effects. In this regard, thermal signals may not only appear as a secondary effect in other instances of intermittent energy deposition (ultrasound or light), but it could also be purposely generated to achieve therapeutic levels, should these exist.

Moving forward, perhaps we must only recognize one simple but righteous universal truth: things will be as simple as they are instead of as simple as we need them to be. Or in other words: the fact that the conventional approximations and models we utilize from the dosimetric and biological points of view are convenient and apparently adequate for our purposes or technical limitations does not mean that they are sufficiently representative of the complex reality of biological systems and their response to subtle and chronic physical stimuli.

ACKNOWLEDGMENTS

This work was only funded by my own personal resources and based on experience and discussions which were acquired thanks to the interactions with the work of multiple scientists and friends over the years. Many of them are part of the references. To all of them, thank you.

REFERENCES

Abrams TW, Pearson KG 1982. Effects of temperature on identified central neurons that control jumping in the grasshopper. *Journal of Neuroscience* 2(11):1538–53.

Acikel V, Atalar E 2011. Modeling of radio-frequency induced currents on lead wires during MR imaging using a modified transmission line method. *Medical Physics* 38(12):6623–32.

Adair ER 2008. Reminiscences of a journeyman scientist: Studies of thermoregulation in non-human primates and humans. *Bioelectromagnetics* 29(8):586–97.

Adler R 1946. A study of locking phenomena in oscillators. *Proceedings of the IRE* 34(6):351–7.

Ahlbom A, Bergqvist U, Bernhardt JH, Cesarini JP, Grandolfo M, Hietanen M, Mckinlay AF et al. 1998. Guidelines for limiting exposure to time-varying electric, magnetic, and electromagnetic fields (up to 300 GHz). *Health Physics* 74(4):494–521.

Alekseev SI, Radzievsky AA, Logani MK, Ziskin MC 2008. Millimeter wave dosimetry of human skin. *Bioelectromagnetics* 29(1):65–70.

Alekseev SI, Ziskin MC, Kochetkova NV, Bolshakov MA 1997. Millimeter waves thermally alter the firing rate of the Lymnaea pacemaker neuron. *Bioelectromagnetics* 18(2):89–98.

Andersen SS, Jackson AD, Heimburg T 2009. Towards a thermodynamic theory of nerve pulse propagation. *Progress in Neurobiology* 88(2):104–13.

Appali R, van Rienen U, Heimburg T 2012. A comparison of the Hodgkin-Huxley model and the soliton theory for the action potential in nerves. *Advances in Planar Lipid Bilayers and Liposomes* 16:275–99.

Arrhenius S 1889. Über die Reaktionsgeschwindigkeit bei der Inversion von Rohrzucker durch Säuren. *Zeitschrift für physikalische Chemie* 4:226–48.

Barnes FS 1974. Biological damage resulting from thermal pulses. In: Wolbarsht ML (ed) *Laser Applications in Medicine and Biology* (pp. 205–221). Springer, New York.

Barnes FS 1984. Cell membrane temperature rate sensitivity predicted from the Nernst equation. *Bioelectromagnetics* 5(1):113–5.

Barnes FS 2017. External electric and magnetic fields as a signaling mechanism for biological systems. In: Markov M (ed) *Dosimetry in Bioelectromagnetics*. CRC Press, Boca Raton, FL, 157–170.

Barnes FS, Greenebaum B (eds) 2007. *Biological and Medical Aspects of Electromagnetic Fields*. CRC Press, Boca Raton, FL.

Barnes FS, Greenebaum B 2015. The effects of weak magnetic fields on radical pairs. *Bioelectromagnetics* 36(1):45–54.

Barnes FS, Kandala S. 2018. Effects of time delays on biological feedback systems and electromagnetic field exposures. *Bioelectromagnetics* (in press).

Begley CG, Ellis LM 2012. Drug development: Raise standards for preclinical cancer research. *Nature* 483(7391):531–3.

Benit P, Ha HH, Keipert S, El-Khoury R, Chang YT, Jastroch M, Jacobs H, Rustin P, Rak M 2017. Mitochondria Are Physiologically Maintained At Close To 50 C. bioRxiv, p.133223.

Bergsten P 2002. Role of oscillations in membrane potential, cytoplasmic Ca2+, and metabolism for plasma insulin oscillations. *Diabetes* 51(suppl 1):S171–6.

Bernardi P, Cavagnaro M, Pisa S, Piuzzi E 2000. Specific absorption rate and temperature increases in the head of a cellular-phone user. *IEEE Transactions on Microwave Theory and Techniques* 48(7):1118–26.

Betskii OV, Lebedeva NN 2004. Low-intensity millimeter waves in Biology and Medicine. In: Rosch P, Markov M (eds) *Clinical Application of Bioelectromagnetic Medicine*, New-York, USA; Marcel Dekker Inc 741–760.

Betzalel N, Feldman Y, Ishai PB 2017. The Modeling of the Absorbance of Sub-THz Radiation by Human Skin. *IEEE Transactions on Terahertz Science and Technology* 7(5):521–8.

Biron D, Wasserman S, Thomas JH, Samuel AD, Sengupta P 2008. An olfactory neuron responds stochastically to temperature and modulates Caenorhabditis elegans thermotactic behavior. *Proceedings of the National Academy of Sciences* 105(31):11002–7.

Blicher A, Wodzinska K, Fidorra M, Winterhalter M, Heimburg T 2009. The temperature dependence of lipid membrane permeability, its quantized nature, and the influence of anesthetics. *Biophysical Journal* 96(11):4581–91.

Blick DW, Adair ER, Hurt WD, Sherry CJ, Walters TJ, Merritt JH 1997. Thresholds of microwave-evoked warmth sensations in human skin. *Bioelectromagnetics* 18(6):403–9.

Böckmann M, Hess B, Müller SC 1996. Temperature gradients traveling with chemical waves. *Physical Review E* 53(5):5498.

Bol'shakov MA, Alekseyev SI 1986. Change in the electrical activity of the pacemaker neurons of L. stagnalis with the rate of their heating. *Biophysics* 31:569–71.

Boulant JA, Dean JB 1986. Temperature receptors in the central nervous system. *Annual Review of Physiology* 48(1):639–54.

Brasen JC, Barington T, Olsen LF 2010. On the mechanism of oscillations in neutrophils. *Biophysical Chemistry* 148(1):82–92.

Bretscher AJ, Kodama-Namba E, Busch KE, Murphy RJ, Soltesz Z, Laurent P, de Bono M 2011. Temperature, oxygen, and salt-sensing neurons in C. elegans are carbon dioxide sensors that control avoidance behavior. *Neuron* 69(6):1099–113.

Brown SA, Zumbrunn G, Fleury-Olela F, Preitner N, Schibler U 2002. Rhythms of mammalian body temperature can sustain peripheral circadian clocks. *Current Biology* 12(18):1574–83.

Brühl R, Ihlenfeld A, Ittermann B 2017. Gradient heating of bulk metallic implants can be a safety concern in MRI. *Magnetic Resonance in Medicine* 77(5):1739–40.

Busto R, Dietrich WD, Globus MY, Valdés I, Scheinberg P, Ginsberg MD 1987. Small differences in intraischemic brain temperature critically determine the extent of ischemic neuronal injury. *Journal of Cerebral Blood Flow & Metabolism* 7(6):729–38.

Buzsáki G, Draguhn A 2004. Neuronal oscillations in cortical networks. *Science* 304(5679):1926–9.

Caplan JS, Williams AH, Marder E 2014. Many parameter sets in a multicompartment model oscillator are robust to temperature perturbations. *Journal of Neuroscience* 34(14):4963–75.

Chalker RB 1982. The effect of microwave absorption and associated temperature dynamics on nerve cell activity in Aplysia, M.S. thesis. University of Colorado Boulder.

Charkoudian N 2003. Skin Blood Flow in Adult Human Thermoregulation: How It Works, When It Does Not, and Why. *Mayo Clin Proc* 78:603–12.

Cherukuri P, Curley SA 2010. Use of nanoparticles for targeted, noninvasive thermal destruction of malignant cells. In: Grobmyer S, Moudgil B. (eds) *Cancer Nanotechnology. Methods in Molecular Biology (Methods and Protocols)*, vol 624. Humana Press.

Childs C 2008. Human brain temperature: Regulation, measurement and relationship with cerebral trauma: Part 1. *British Journal of Neurosurgery* 22(4):486–96.

Chu PC, Liu HL, Lai HY, Lin CY, Tsai HC, Pei YC 2015. Neuromodulation accompanying focused ultrasound-induced blood-brain barrier opening. *Scientific Reports* 5:15477.

Colombi D, Thors B, Törnevik C 2015. Implications of EMF exposure limits on output power levels for 5G devices above 6 GHz. *IEEE Antennas and Wireless Propagation Letters* 14:1247–9.

Dahlgren C, Karlsson A 1999. Respiratory burst in human neutrophils. *Journal of Immunological Methods* 232(1):3–14.

Deatsch AE, Evans BA 2014. Heating efficiency in magnetic nanoparticle hyperthermia. *Journal of Magnetism and Magnetic Materials* 354:163–72.

Dell AI, Pawar S, Savage VM 2011. Systematic variation in the temperature dependence of physiological and ecological traits. *Proceedings of the National Academy of Sciences* 108(26):10591–6.

Dell AI, Pawara S, Savagea VM 2013. The thermal dependence of biological traits. *Landscape* 36:37.

Dewey WC 1994. Arrhenius relationships from the molecule and cell to the clinic. *International Journal of Hyperthermia* 10(4):457–83.

Dewey WC, Diederich CJ 2009. Hyperthermia classic commentary: Arrhenius relationships from the molecule and cell to the clinic'by William Dewey. *International Journal of Hyperthermia* 25(1):21–4.

Dewhirst MW, Viglianti BL, Lora-Michiels M, Hanson M, Hoopes PJ 2003. Basic principles of thermal dosimetry and thermal thresholds for tissue damage from hyperthermia. *International Journal of Hyperthermia* 19(3):267–94.

Dill KA, Ghosh K, Schmit JD 2011. Physical limits of cells and proteomes. *Proceedings of the National Academy of Sciences* 108(44):17876–82.

Dolmetsch RE, Xu K, Lewis RS 1998. Calcium oscillations increase the efficiency and specificity of gene expression. *Nature* 392(6679):933–6.

Donoso G, Ladera CL 2012. Nonlinear dynamics of a magnetically driven Duffing-type spring–magnet oscillator in the static magnetic field of a coil. *European Journal of Physics* 33(6):1473.

Douglas MG, Portelli L, Carrasco E, Christ A, Jain N, Kuster N 2016. Comprehensive validation and uncertainty evaluation of new SAR measurement technologies. In *Proceedings of the 10th European Conference on Antennas and Propagation (EuCAP 2016)*, Davos, Switzerland, April 11–15, 2016.

Duke AR, Jenkins MW, Lu H, McManus JM, Chiel HJ, Jansen ED 2013. Transient and selective suppression of neural activity with infrared light. *Scientific Reports* 3: Article no. 2600.

Duke AR, Peterson E, Mackanos MA, Atkinson J, Tyler D, Jansen ED 2012. Hybrid electro-optical stimulation of the rat sciatic nerve induces force generation in the plantarflexor muscles. *Journal of Neural Engineering* 9(6):066006.

Eckardt NA 2005. Temperature entrainment of the Arabidopsis circadian clock. *The Plant Cell* 17(3):645–7.

Egot-Lemaire SJ, Ziskin MC 2011. Dielectric properties of human skin at an acupuncture point in the 50–75 GHz frequency range: A pilot study. *Bioelectromagnetics* 32(5):360–6.

Ehrengruber MU, Deranleau DA, Coates TD 1996. Shape oscillations of human neutrophil leukocytes: Characterization and relationship to cell motility. *Journal of Experimental Biology* 199(4):741–7.

El Halaoui M, Kaabal A, Asselman H, Ahyoud S, Asselman A 2017. Multiband Planar Inverted-F Antenna with Independent Operating Bands Control for Mobile Handset Applications. *International Journal of Antennas and Propagation*. 2017: 13 pages. Article ID 8794039. https://doi.org/10.1155/2017/879403.

Eng JW, Reed CB, Kokolus KM, Pitoniak R, Utley A, Bucsek MJ, Ma WW, Repasky EA, Hylander BL 2015. Housing temperature-induced stress drives therapeutic resistance in murine tumour models through β2-adrenergic receptor activation. *Nature Communications* 6:6426.

Ezquerra-Romano I, Ezquerra A 2017. Highway to thermosensation: A traced review, from the proteins to the brain. *Reviews in the Neurosciences* 28(1):45–57.

Falcke M, Malchow D (eds) 2003. *Understanding Calcium Dynamics: Experiments and Theory*. Springer, New York.

Feldman Y, Puzenko A, Ishai PB, Caduff A, Agranat AJ 2008. Human skin as arrays of helical antennas in the millimeter and submillimeter wave range. *Physical Review Letters* 100(12):128102.

Fernandes J, Dinis H, Gonçalves LM, Mendes PM 2016. *Microcooling Solution Development and Performance Assessment for Thermal Neuromodulation Applications.* IFESS La Grande Motte, France.

Forrest MD 2014. Can the thermodynamic Hodgkin-Huxley model of voltage-dependent conductance extrapolate for temperature? *Computation* 2(2):47–60.

Foster KR 2000. Thermal and nonthermal mechanisms of interaction of radio-frequency energy with biological systems. *IEEE Transactions on Plasma Science* 28(1):15–23.

Foster KR, Lozano-Nieto A, Riu PJ, Ely TS 1998. Heating of tissues by microwaves: A model analysis. *Bioelectromagnetics* 19(7):420–8.

Foster KR, Morrissey JJ 2011. Thermal aspects of exposure to radiofrequency energy: Report of a workshop. *International Journal of Hyperthermia* 27(4):307–19.

Foster KR, Ziskin MC, Balzano Q 2016. Thermal response of human skin to microwave energy: A critical review. *Health Physics.* 111(6):528–41.

Foster KR, Ziskin MC, Balzano Q 2017. Thermal modeling for the next generation of radiofrequency exposure limits: Commentary. *Health Physics* 113(1):41–53.

Freedman LP, Inglese J 2014. The increasing urgency for standards in basic biologic research. *Cancer Research* 74(15):4024–29.

Giannetto C, Fazio F, Vazzana I, Panzera M, Piccione G 2012. Comparison of cortisol and rectal temperature circadian rhythms in horses: The role of light/dark cycle and constant darkness. *Biological Rhythm Research* 43(6):681–7.

Glaser FT, Stanewsky R 2005. Temperature synchronization of the Drosophila circadian clock. *Current Biology* 15(15):1352–63.

Graf H, Steidle G, Schick F 2007. Heating of metallic implants and instruments induced by gradient switching in a 1.5-Tesla whole-body unit. *Journal of Magnetic Resonance Imaging* 26(5):1328–33.

Green BG, Akirav C 2010. Threshold and rate sensitivity of low-threshold thermal nociception. *European Journal of Neuroscience* 31(9):1637–45.

Griffiths H, Ahmed A, Smith CW, Moore JL, Kerby IJ, Davies RM 1986. Specific absorption rate and tissue temperature in local hyperthermia. *International Journal of Radiation Oncology* Biology* Physics* 12(11):1997–2002.

Haas AJ, Le Page Y, Zhadobov M, Sauleau R, Dréan YL, Saligaut C 2017. Effect of acute millimeter wave exposure on dopamine metabolism of NGF-treated PC12 cells. *Journal of Radiation Research* 24:1–7.

Habauzit D, Le Quément C, Zhadobov M, Martin C, Aubry M, Sauleau R, Le Dréan Y 2014. Transcriptome analysis reveals the contribution of thermal and the specific effects in cellular response to millimeter wave exposure. *PloS One* 9(10):e109435.

Hammel HT, Pierce JB 1968. Regulation of internal body temperature. *Annual Review of Physiology* 30(1):641–710.

Hasani MH, Gharibzadeh S, Farjami Y, Tavakkoli J 2015. Investigating the Effect of Thermal Stress on Nerve Action Potential Using the Soliton Model. *Ultrasound in Medicine & Biology* 41(6):1668–80.

Hashimoto Y, Hirata A, Morimoto R, Aonuma S, Laakso I, Jokela K, Foster KR 2017. On the averaging area for incident power density for human exposure limits at frequencies over 6 GHz. *Physics in Medicine and Biology* 62(8):3124.

Hayashi C 2014. *Nonlinear Oscillations in Physical Systems.* Princeton University Press, New Jersey.

Hayward JN, Baker MA 1968. Role of cerebral arterial blood in the regulation of brain temperature in the monkey. *American Journal of Physiology—Legacy Content* 215(2):389–403.

Heimburg T 2008. *Thermal Biophysics of Membranes.* John Wiley & Sons, Hoboken, NJ.

Heimburg T 2010. Lipid ion channels. *Biophysical Chemistry* 150(1):2–2.

Heimburg T, Jackson AD 2007. On the action potential as a propagating density pulse and the role of anesthetics. *Biophysical Reviews and Letters* 2(01):57–78.

Heimburg T, Jackson AD 2015. On soliton propagation in biomembranes and nerves. *Proceedings of the National Academy of Sciences of the United States of America* 102(28):9790–5.

Herzog ED, Huckfeldt RM 2003. Circadian entrainment to temperature, but not light, in the isolated suprachiasmatic nucleus. *Journal of Neurophysiology* 90(2):763–70.

Hildebrandt B, Wust P, Ahlers O, Dieing A, Sreenivasa G, Kerner T, Felix R, Riess H 2002. The cellular and molecular basis of hyperthermia. *Critical Reviews in Oncology/Hematology* 43(1):33–56.

Hill RW, Muhich TE, Humphries MM 2013. City-scale expansion of human thermoregulatory costs. *PloS One* 8(10):e76238.

Hodgkin AL, Huxley AF 1952. A quantitative description of membrane current and its application to conduction and excitation in nerve. *The Journal of Physiology* 117(4):500–44.

Ibsen S, Tong A, Schutt C, Esener S, Chalasani SH 2015. Sonogenetics is a non-invasive approach to activating neurons in Caenorhabditis elegans. *Nature Communications* 6: 8264.

Iggo A 1962. An electrophysiological analysis of afferent fibres in primate skin. *Acta neurovegetativa* 24(1–4):225–40.

Iggo A 1974. Cutaneous receptors. In: Hubbard JI (ed) *The Peripheral Nervous System*. Springer, Boston, MA, 347–404.

Institute of Electrical and Electronics Engineers (IEEE) 2005. *Standard for Safety Levels with Respect to Human Exposure to Radio Frequency Electromagnetic Fields, 3 kHz–300 GHz*. IEEE, Piscataway, NJ, C95.1.

International Commission on Non-Ionizing Radiation Protection (ICNIRP) 2009. ICNIRP statement on the "guidelines for limiting exposure to time-varying electric, magnetic, and electromagnetic fields (up to 300 ghz)". *Health Physics* 97(3):257–8.

International Electrotechnical Commission (IEC) 2013. Medical electrical equipment - Part 2–33: Particular requirements for the basic safety and essential performance of magnetic resonance equipment for medical diagnosis. IEC Standard 60601–2–33, Edition 3.1.

Izhikevich EM, Desai NS, Walcott EC, Hoppensteadt FC 2003. Bursts as a unit of neural information: Selective communication via resonance. *Trends in Neurosciences* 26(3):161–7.

Izzo AD, Walsh JT, Ralph H, Webb J, Bendett M, Wells J, Richter CP 2008. Laser stimulation of auditory neurons: Effect of shorter pulse duration and penetration depth. *Biophysical Journal* 94(8):3159–66.

Jorjani P, Ozturk SS 1999. Effects of cell density and temperature on oxygen consumption rate for different mammalian cell lines. *Biotechnology and Bioengineering* 64(3):349–56.

Kandel E.R., Schwartz J.H., Jessell T.M. (eds) 2000. *Principles of Neural Science*. McGraw-Hill, New York.

Katriel G 2008. Synchronization of oscillators coupled through an environment. *Physica D: Nonlinear Phenomena* 237(22):2933–44.

Keatinge WR, Mason AC, Millard CE, Newstead CG 1986. Effects of fluctuating skin temperature on thermoregulatory responses in man. *The Journal of Physiology* 378(1):241–52.

Kellogg DL 2006. In vivo mechanisms of cutaneous vasodilation and vasoconstriction in humans during thermoregulatory challenges. *Journal of Applied Physiology* 100(5):1709–18.

Kelly GS 2006. Body temperature variability (Part 1): A review of the history of body temperature and its variability due to site selection, biological rhythms, fitness, and aging. *Alternative Medicine Review* 11(4):278.

Kelly GS 2007. Body temperature variability (Part 2): Masking influences of body temperature variability and a review of body temperature variability in disease. *Alternative Medicine Review* 12(1):49.

Kenny JM, Ziskin M, Adair B, Murray B, Farrer D, Marks L, Bovbjerg V 2008. *A Narrative Summary and Independent Assessment of the Active Denial System*. Applied Research Laboratory, Penn State.

Khizhnyak EP, Ziskin MC 1994. Heating patterns in biological tissue phantoms caused by millimeter wave electromagnetic irradiation. *IEEE Transactions on Biomedical Engineering* 41(9):865–73.

Kodera S, Gomez-Tames J, Hirata A 2018. Temperature elevation in the human brain and skin with thermoregulation during exposure to RF energy. *BioMedical Engineering* Online 17:1.

Kokolus KM, Capitano ML, Lee CT, Eng JW, Waight JD, Hylander BL, Sexton S et al. 2013. Baseline tumor growth and immune control in laboratory mice are significantly influenced by subthermoneutral housing temperature. *Proceedings of the National Academy of Sciences* 110(50):20176–81.

Koshiya N, Smith JC 1999. Neuronal pacemaker for breathing visualized in vitro. *Nature* 400(6742):360–633.

Kräuchi K 2002. How is the circadian rhythm of core body temperature regulated?. *Clinical Autonomic Research* 12(3):147–9.

Kräuchi K, Konieczka K, Roescheisen-Weich C, Gompper B, Hauenstein D, Schoetzau A, Fraenkl S, Flammer J 2014. Diurnal and menstrual cycles in body temperature are regulated differently: A 28-day ambulatory study in healthy women with thermal discomfort of cold extremities and controls. *Chronobiology International* 31(1):102–13.

Kuramoto Y 1975. Self-entrainment of a population of coupled non-linear oscillators. In: Araki H. (ed) *International Symposium on Mathematical Problems in Theoretical Physics*. Lecture Notes in Physics, vol 39. Springer, Berlin Heidelberg, 420–422.

Laakso I, Hirata A 2011. Dominant factors affecting temperature rise in simulations of human thermoregulation during RF exposure. *Physics in Medicine and Biology* 56(23):7449.

Laakso I, Morimoto R, Heinonen J, Jokela K, Hirata A 2017. Human exposure to pulsed fields in the frequency range from 6 to 100 GHz. *Physics in Medicine & Biology* 62(17):6980.

Lara NC, Haider AA, Wilson LJ, Curley SA, Corr SJ 2017. Unique heating curves generated by radiofrequency electric-field interactions with semi-aqueous solutions. *Applied Physics Letters* 110(1):013701.

Laub KR, Witschas K, Blicher A, Madsen SB, Lückhoff A, Heimburg T 2012. Comparing ion conductance recordings of synthetic lipid bilayers with cell membranes containing TRP channels. *Biochimica et Biophysica Acta (BBA)-Biomembranes* 1818(5):1123–34.

Lee W, Kim HC, Jung Y, Chung YA, Song IU, Lee JH, Yoo SS 2016. Transcranial focused ultrasound stimulation of human primary visual cortex. *Scientific Reports* 6:34026.

Lekner J 2013. Conducting cylinders in an external electric field: Polarizability and field enhancement. *Journal of Electrostatics* 71(6):1104–10.

Lim CL, Byrne C, Lee JK 2008. Human thermoregulation and measurement of body temperature in exercise and clinical settings. *Annals Academy of Medicine Singapore* 37(4):347.

Lin JC 2006. A new IEEE standard for safety levels with respect to human exposure to radio-frequency radiation. *IEEE Antennas and Propagation Magazine* 48(1):157–9.

Luan S, Williams I, Nikolic K, Constandinou TG 2014. Neuromodulation: Present and emerging methods. *Frontiers in Neuroengineering* 7:27.

Luo J, Shen WL, Montell C 2017. TRPA1 mediates sensation of the rate of temperature change in Drosophila larvae. *Nature Neuroscience* 20(1):34–41.

Markov M 2006. Thermal vs. nonthermal mechanisms of interactions between electromagnetic fields and biological systems. In: Ayrapetyan SN, Markov MS (eds) *Bioelectromagnetics Current Concepts*. NATO Security through Science Series, vol 5. Springer, Dordrecht.

Maroto M, Monk N (eds) 2008. *Cellular Oscillatory Mechanisms*. Springer, New York.
Matsumoto N, Okamoto K, Takagi Y, Ikegaya Y 2016. 3-Hz subthreshold oscillations of CA2 neurons In vivo. *Hippocampus*. 26(12):1570–1578.
McElligott JG, Melzack R 1967. Localized thermal changes evoked in the brain by visual and auditory stimulation. *Experimental Neurology* 17(3):293–312.
Meekan M 2017. Why do whale sharks get so big?. *Australasian Science* 38(3):34.
Mehić E, Xu JM, Caler CJ, Coulson NK, Moritz CT, Mourad PD 2014. Increased anatomical specificity of neuromodulation via modulated focused ultrasound. *PLoS One* 9(2):e86939.
Mescher AL. 2013. *Junqueira's Basic Histology: Text and Atlas*. McGraw-Hill, New York.
Mihran RT, Barnes FS, Wachtel H 1990. Temporally-specific modification of myelinated axon excitability in vitro following a single ultrasound pulse. *Ultrasound in Medicine & Biology* 16(3):297–309.
Morf J, Schibler U 2013. Body temperature cycles: Gatekeepers of circadian clocks. *Cell Cycle* 12(4):539.
Morimoto R, Hirata A, Laakso I, Ziskin MC, Foster KR 2017. Time constants for temperature elevation in human models exposed to dipole antennas and beams in the frequency range from 1 to 30 GHz. *Physics in Medicine and Biology* 62(5):1676.
Morimoto R, Laakso I, De Santis V, Hirata A 2016. Relationship between peak spatial-averaged specific absorption rate and peak temperature elevation in human head in frequency range of 1–30 GHz. *Physics in Medicine and Biology* 61(14):5406.
Moros E (ed) 2012. *Physics of Thermal Therapy: Fundamentals and Clinical Applications*. CRC Press, Boca Raton, FL.
Mosgaard LD, Jackson AD, Heimburg T 2012. Low-Frequency Sound Propagation in Lipid Membranes. In: Aleš I. (ed) *Advances in Planar Lipid Bilayers and Liposomes*. Academic Press, New York, 6, 51–74.
Mosgaard LD, Jackson AD, Heimburg T 2013. Fluctuations of systems in finite heat reservoirs with applications to phase transitions in lipid membranes. *The Journal of Chemical Physics* 139(12):09B646_1.
Mueller J, Legon W, Opitz A, Sato TF, Tyler WJ 2014. Transcranial focused ultrasound modulates intrinsic and evoked EEG dynamics. *Brain Stimulation* 7(6):900–8.
Munshi R, Qadri SM, Zhang Q, Rubio IC, del Pino P, Pralle A 2017. Magnetothermal genetic deep brain stimulation of motor behaviors in awake, freely moving mice. *Elife* 6:e27069.
Murbach M, Neufeld E, Samaras T, Córcoles J, Robb FJ, Kainz W, Kuster N 2017. Pregnant women models analyzed for RF exposure and temperature increase in 3 T RF shimmed birdcages. *Magnetic Resonance in Medicine* 77(5):2048–56.
Murbach M, Zastrow E, Neufeld E, Cabot E, Kainz W, Kuster N 2015. Heating and Safety Concerns of the Radio-Frequency Field in MRI. *Current Radiology Reports* 3(12):45.
Nedergaard J, Bengtsson T, Cannon B 2007. Unexpected evidence for active brown adipose tissue in adult humans. *American Journal of Physiology-Endocrinology and Metabolism* 293(2):E444–52.
Nolano M, Provitera V, Caporaso G, Stancanelli A, Leandri M, Biasiotta A, Cruccu G, Santoro L, Truini A 2013. Cutaneous innervation of the human face as assessed by skin biopsy. *Journal of Anatomy* 222(2):161–9.
Nordbeck P, Weiss I, Ehses P, Ritter O, Warmuth M, Fidler F, Herold V et al. 2009. Measuring RF-induced currents inside implants: Impact of device configuration on MRI safety of cardiac pacemaker leads. *Magnetic Resonance in Medicine* 61(3):570–8.
Norton BJ, Bowler MA, Wells JD, Keller MD 2013. Analytical approaches for determining heat distributions and thermal criteria for infrared neural stimulation. *Journal of Biomedical Optics* 18(9):098001.
Novák B, Tyson JJ 2008. Design principles of biochemical oscillators. *Nature Reviews Molecular Cell Biology* 9(12):981–91.
Paciorek LJ 1965. Injection locking of oscillators. *Proceedings of the IEEE* 53(11):1723–7.

Paffi A, Apollonio F, Liberti M, Sheppard A, Bit-Babik G, Balzano Q 2015a. Culture medium geometry: The dominant factor affecting in vitro RF exposure dosimetry. *International Journal of Antennas and Propagation*. 2015: 10 pages. Article ID 438962. http://dx.doi.org/10.1155/2015/438962.

Paffi A, Liberti M, Apollonio F, Sheppard A, Balzano Q 2015b. In vitro exposure: Linear and non-linear thermodynamic events in Petri dishes. *Bioelectromagnetics* 36(7):527–37.

Pakhomov AG, Murthy PR 2000. Low-intensity millimeter waves as a novel therapeutic modality. *IEEE Transactions on Plasma Science* 28(1):34–40.

Patapoutian A, Peier AM, Story GM, Viswanath V 2003. ThermoTRP channels and beyond: Mechanisms of temperature sensation. *Nature Reviews Neuroscience* 4(7):529–39.

Pawar S, Dell AI, Savage VM, Knies JL 2016. Real versus artificial variation in the thermal sensitivity of biological traits. *The American Naturalist* 187(2):E41–52.

Pennes HH 1948. Analysis of tissue and arterial blood temperatures in the resting human forearm. *Journal of Applied Physiology* 1(2):93–122.

Portelli LA. 2018. Overcoming the irreproducibility barrier: Considerations to improve the quality of experimental practice in the effects of Low-Level electric and magnetic fields on in vitro biological systems. In: Barnes FS, Greenebaum B (eds). *Handbook of Biological Effects of Electromagnetic Fields*, 4 ed. CRC Press, Boca Raton, FL.

Portelli L, Kausik A, Barnes F, Martino C 2011. Study of the effects of pulsed temperature stimulus on fibrosarcoma HT1080 cells. *The Bioelectromagnetics Society (BEMS) Annual Meeting Halifax*, Canada.

Portelli L, Rengnath L, Martino C, Barnes F 2010. Study of the effects of pulsed temperature stimulus on fibrosarcoma HT1080 cells. In *Proceedings of the 32nd Annual Meeting of the Bioelectromagnetics Society*.

Portelli LA 2017. Uncertainty sources associated with low-frequency electric and magnetic field experiments on cell cultures. In: Markov M (ed) *Dosimetry in Bioelectromagnetics*. CRC Press, Boca Raton, FL, 25–68.

Portelli LA, Kausik A, Barnes FS 2017. Effects of small and rapid temperature oscillations on adherent cell cultures: Exposure system, experimental method and a pilot study on human cancer cells. In *EMBEC & NBC* 2017 (pp. 707–710). Springer, Singapore.

Precht H 2013. *Temperature and life*. Springer Science & Business Media, New York, NY.

Raaijmakers EAL, Mestrom RMC, Sumser K, Salim G, van Rhoon GC, Essers J, Paulides MM 2017. An MR-compatible antenna and application in a murine superficial hyperthermia applicator. *International Journal of Hyperthermia* 1–7. DOI: 10.1080/02656736.2017.1369.

Rabbitt RD, Brichta AM, Tabatabaee H, Boutros PJ, Ahn J, Della Santina CC, Poppi LA, Lim R 2016. Heat pulse excitability of vestibular hair cells and afferent neurons. *Journal of Neurophysiology* 116(2):825–43.

Rapp P 1979. An atlas of cellular oscillators. *Journal of Experimental Biology* 81(1):281–306.

Razavi B 2004. A study of injection locking and pulling in oscillators. *IEEE Journal of Solid-State Circuits* 39(9):1415–24.

Refinetti R 1995. Rhythms of temperature selection and body temperature are out of phase in the golden hamster. *Behavioral Neuroscience* 109(3):523.

Refinetti R 1999. Amplitude of the daily rhythm of body temperature in eleven mammalian species. *Journal of Thermal Biology* 24(5):477–81.

Refinetti R 2016. *Circadian Physiology*. CRC Press, Boca Raton, FL.

Reverter F, Prodromakis T, Liu Y, Georgiou P, Nikolic K, Constandinou T 2014. Design considerations for a CMOS Lab-on-Chip microheater array to facilitate the in vitro thermal stimulation of neurons. In *2014 IEEE International Symposium on Circuits and Systems (ISCAS)* (pp. 630–633), Melbourne, Australia. IEEE.

Rijkhorst EJ, Rivens I, Haar GT, Hawkes D, Barratt D 2011. Effects of respiratory liver motion on heating for gated and model-based motion-compensated high-intensity focused ultrasound ablation. In *Proceedings of the 14th International Conference on Medical Image Computing and Computer-Assisted Intervention-Volume Part I* (pp. 605–612), New York, Springer-Verlag.

Rinberg A, Taylor AL, Marder E 2013. The effects of temperature on the stability of a neuronal oscillator. *PLoS Computational Biology* 9(1):e1002857.

Riu PJ, Foster KR, Blick DW, Adair ER 1997. A thermal model for human thresholds of microwave-evoked warmth sensations. *Bioelectromagnetics* 18(8):578–83.

Robertson RM, Money TG 2012. Temperature and neuronal circuit function: Compensation, tuning and tolerance. *Current Opinion in Neurobiology* 22(4):724–34.

Rubin SA 1987. Core temperature regulation of heart rate during exercise in humans. *Journal of Applied Physiology* 62(5):1997–2002.

Ruoff P, Christensen MK, Wolf J, Heinrich R 2003. Temperature dependency and temperature compensation in a model of yeast glycolytic oscillations. *Biophysical Chemistry* 106(2):179–92.

Saini C, Morf J, Stratmann M, Gos P, Schibler U 2012. Simulated body temperature rhythms reveal the phase-shifting behavior and plasticity of mammalian circadian oscillators. *Genes & Development* 26(6):567–80.

Saito S, Banzawa N, Fukuta N, Saito CT, Takahashi K, Imagawa T, Ohta T, Tominaga M 2014. Heat and noxious chemical sensor, chicken TRPA1, as a target of bird repellents and identification of its structural determinants by multispecies functional comparison. *Molecular Biology and Evolution* 31(3):708–22.

Schmid G, Kuster N 2015. The discrepancy between maximum in vitro exposure levels and realistic conservative exposure levels of mobile phones operating at 900/1800MHz. *Bioelectromagnetics* 36(2):133–48.

Schrödinger E 1944. *What Is Life? the Physical Aspect of the Living Cell and Mind.* Cambridge University Press, Cambridge.

Sen S, Murray RM 2014. Negative Feedback Facilitates Temperature Robustness in Biomolecular Circuit Dynamics. *bioRxiv.* 007385.

Shapiro MG, Homma K, Villarreal S, Richter CP, Bezanilla F 2012. Infrared light excites cells by changing their electrical capacitance. *Nature Communications* 3:736.

Shellock FG 2000. Radiofrequency energy-induced heating during MR procedures: A review. *Journal of Magnetic Resonance Imaging* 12(1):30–6.

Sheppard AR, Swicord ML, Balzano Q 2008. Quantitative evaluations of mechanisms of radiofrequency interactions with biological molecules and processes. *Health Physics* 95(4):365–96.

Shiraki KE, Konda NO, Sagawa SU 1986. Esophageal and tympanic temperature responses to core blood temperature changes during hyperthermia. *Journal of Applied Physiology* 61(1):98–102.

Sienkiewicz Z, van Rongen E, Croft R, Ziegelberger G, Veyret B 2016. A closer look at the thresholds of thermal damage: Workshop report by an ICNIRP task group. *Health Physics* 111(3):300.

Slaby O, Lebiedz D 2009. Oscillatory NAD (P) H waves and calcium oscillations in neutrophils? A modeling study of feasibility. *Biophysical Journal* 96(2):417–28.

Sládek M, Sumová A 2013. Entrainment of spontaneously hypertensive rat fibroblasts by temperature cycles. *PloS One* 8(10):e77010.

Smedler E, Uhlén P 2014. Frequency decoding of calcium oscillations. *Biochimica Et Biophysica Acta (BBA)-General Subjects.* 1840(3):964–9.

Somero GN, Hochachka PW 1971. Biochemical adaptation to the environment. *American Zoologist* 11(1):159–67.

Soofi W, Goeritz ML, Kispersky TJ, Prinz AA, Marder E, Stein W 2014. Phase maintenance in a rhythmic motor pattern during temperature changes in vivo. *Journal of Neurophysiology* 111(12):2603–13.

Stark J, Chan C, George AJ 2007. Oscillations in the immune system. *Immunological Reviews* 216(1):213–31.

Straume A, Oftedal G, Johnsson A 2005. Skin temperature increase caused by a mobile phone: A methodological infrared camera study. *Bioelectromagnetics* 26(6):510–9.

Sukstanskii AL, Yablonskiy DA 2006. Theoretical model of temperature regulation in the brain during changes in functional activity. *Proceedings of the National Academy of Sciences* 103(32):12144–9.

Tasaki I, Byrne PM 1992. Heat production associated with a propagated impulse in bullfrog myelinated nerve fibers. *The Japanese Journal of Physiology* 42(5):805–13.

Tasaki I, Kusano K, Byrne P 1989. Rapid mechanical and thermal changes in the garfish olfactory nerve associated with a propagated impulse. *Biophysical Journal* 55(6):1033–40.

Ter Haar G 2013. Safety first: Progress in calibrating high-intensity focused ultrasound treatments. *Imaging in Medicine.* 5(6):567.

Thompson AC, Stoddart PR, Jansen ED 2014. Optical stimulation of neurons. *Current Molecular Imaging* 3(2):162–77.

Tostevin F, Ronde W, Wolde PR 2012. Ten. Reliability of Frequency and Amplitude Decoding in Gene Regulation. *Phys Rev Lett.* 108(10):108104.

Urdaneta ME, Koivuniemi AS, Otto KJ 2017. Central nervous system microstimulation: Towards selective micro-neuromodulation. *Current Opinion in Biomedical Engineering* 4:65–77.

Van der Linden AM, Beverly M, Kadener S, Rodriguez J, Wasserman S, Rosbash M, Sengupta P 2010. Genome-wide analysis of light-and temperature-entrained circadian transcripts in Caenorhabditis elegans. *PLoS Biology* 8(10):e1000503.

van der Zee, J. van Rhoon, GC 2017. Hyperthermia with radiotherapy and with systemic therapies. In: Veronesi U, Goldhirsch A, Veronesi P, Gentilini O, Leonardi M (eds) *Breast Cancer* (pp. 855–862). Springer, Cham.

Van Rhoon GC, Samaras T, Yarmolenko PS, Dewhirst MW, Neufeld E, Kuster N 2013. CEM43° C thermal dose thresholds: A potential guide for magnetic resonance radiofrequency exposure levels? *European Radiology* 23(8):2215–27.

van't Hoff JH 1884. *Etudes de Dynamique Chemique.* Muller & Co., Amsterdam.

Vidal-Iglesias FJ, Solla-Gullón J, Rodes A, Herrero E, Aldaz A 2012. Understanding the Nernst Equation and other electrochemical concepts: An easy experimental approach for students. *Journal of Chemical Education* 89(7):936–9.

Wachtel H 1985. Synchronization of neural firing patterns by relatively weak ELF fields. In: Grandolfo M, Michaelson SM, Rindi A (eds) *Biological Effects and Dosimetry of Static and ELF Electromagnetic Fields* (pp. 313–328). Ettore Majorana International Science Series. Springer, Boston, MA.

Walleczek J (ed). 2006. *Self-Organized Biological Synamics and Nonlinear Control: Toward Understanding Complexity, Chaos and Emergent Function in Living Systems.* Cambridge University Press, New York.

Walters TJ, Blick DW, Johnson LR, Adair ER, Foster KR 2000. Heating and pain sensation produced in human skin by millimeter waves: Comparison to a simple thermal model. *Health Physics* 78(3):259–67.

Warzecha A, Horstmann W, Egelhaaf M 1999. Temperature-dependence of neuronal performance in the motion pathway of the blowfly Calliphora erythrocephala. *Journal of Experimental Biology* 202(22):3161–70.

Webb P 1992. Temperatures of skin, subcutaneous tissue, muscle and core in resting men in cold, comfortable and hot conditions. *European Journal of Applied Physiology and Occupational Physiology* 64(5):471–6.

Wells J, Kao C, Konrad P, Milner T, Kim J, Mahadevan-Jansen A, Jansen ED 2007. Biophysical mechanisms of transient optical stimulation of peripheral nerve. *Biophysical Journal* 93(7):2567–80.

Werner J, Buse MO 1988. Temperature profiles with respect to inhomogeneity and geometry of the human body. *Journal of Applied Physiology* 65(3):1110–8.

Winkler SA, Picot PA, Thornton MM, Rutt BK 2017. Direct SAR mapping by thermoacoustic imaging: A feasibility study. *Magnetic Resonance in Medicine* 78(4):1599–606.

Worthington A, Peng P, Rod K, Bril V, Tavakkoli J 2016. Image-Guided High Intensity Focused Ultrasound System for Large Animal Nerve Ablation Studies. *IEEE Journal of Translational Engineering in Health and Medicine* 4:1–6.

Xia J, Yao J, Wang LV 2014. Photoacoustic tomography: Principles and advances. *Electromagnetic waves (Cambridge, Mass.).* 147:1.

Yao A, Zastrow E, Kuster N 2017. Robust experimental evaluation method for the safety assessment of implants with respect to RF-induced heating during MRI. *32nd URSI GASS, Montreal*, Canada.

Ye J, Coleman J, Hunter MG, Craigon J, Campbell KH, Luck MR 2007. Physiological temperature variants and culture media modify meiotic progression and developmental potential of pig oocytes in vitro. *Reproduction* 133(5):877–86.

Yoshida T, Murayama Y, Ito H, Kageyama H, Kondo T 2009. Nonparametric entrainment of the in vitro circadian phosphorylation rhythm of cyanobacterial KaiC by temperature cycle. *Proceedings of the National Academy of Sciences* 106(5):1648–53.

Zhadobov M, Alekseev SI, Le Dréan Y, Sauleau R, Fesenko EE 2015. Millimeter waves as a source of selective heating of skin. *Bioelectromagnetics* 36(6):464–75.

Zhadobov M, Alekseev SI, Sauleau R, Le Page Y, Le Dréan Y, Fesenko EE 2017. Microscale temperature and SAR measurements in cell monolayer models exposed to millimeter waves. *Bioelectromagnetics* 38(1):11–21.

Zilberti L, Arduino A, Bottauscio O, Chiampi M 2017. The underestimated role of gradient coils in MRI safety. *Magnetic Resonance in Medicine* 77(1):13–5.

Zilberti L, Bottauscio O, Chiampi M, Hand J, Lopez HS, Brühl R, Crozier S 2015. Numerical prediction of temperature elevation induced around metallic hip prostheses by traditional, split, and uniplanar gradient coils. *Magnetic Resonance in Medicine.* 74(1):272–9.

Ziskin MC 2013. Millimeter waves: Acoustic and electromagnetic. *Bioelectromagnetics* 34(1):3–14.

7 How Cancer Can Be Caused by Microwave Frequency Electromagnetic Field (EMF) Exposures

EMF Activation of Voltage-Gated Calcium Channels (VGCCs) Can Cause Cancer Including Tumor Promotion, Tissue Invasion, and Metastasis via 15 Mechanisms

Martin L. Pall

CONTENTS

7.1 INTRODUCTION

Twenty nine different reviews [1–29], 24 of which were peer reviewed, provide a massive amount of evidence and opinion that microwave frequency EMFs are carcinogenic. Such EMFs not only produce initiation of the process of carcinogenesis, but also act as tumor promoters [2,3,14,16], a process also supported by two recent studies [30,31]. This vast amount of evidence and opinion on carcinogenicity of microwave frequency EMFs should, in the author's opinion, be definitive. However, if there are any questions about this, such questions should have been resolved by the 25 million dollar National Institute of Toxicology study on cancer causation by 2G cell phone radiation in rats [32]. This study showed that such radiation causes both gliomas and normally quite rare heart schwannomas as well as cellular DNA damage which may act as initiators of the process of carcinogenesis.

Despite all of this evidence and opinion, the National Cancer Institute [33] stated that "No mechanism by which ELF-EMFs or radiofrequency radiation could cause cancer has been identified" and industry-friendly organizations have even claimed there could not be such mechanisms. Similarly, the 2014 Canadian Report on Electromagnetic Fields [34] included cancer in their statement that, "At present, there is no scientific basis for the occurrence of acute, chronic and/ or cumulative adverse health risks from RF field exposure at levels below the limits outlined in Safety Code 6." This issue of mechanism is the focus of this review. But before getting to that issue, we need to consider how such EMFs act in the cells of our bodies in order to determine what downstream effects of such action can be carcinogenic.

7.2 MICROWAVE/LOWER FREQUENCY EMFS ACT VIA ACTIVATION OF VOLTAGE-GATED CALCIUM CHANNELS (VGCCs) LEADING TO DOWNSTREAM EFFECTS

There is a large literature showing that EMF exposures produce large changes in calcium fluxes and large increases in calcium signaling [35,36]. This led to the suggestion by W.R. Adey that the main target of the EMFs is in the plasma membrane of cells, producing such calcium changes as follows: "Collective evidence points to cell membrane receptors as the probable site of first tissue interactions with both extremely low frequency and microwave fields for many neurotransmitters, hormones, growth-regulating enzyme expression, and cancer-promoting chemicals. In none of these studies does tissue heating appear to be involved causally in the responses" (from a talk at the Royal Society of Physicians, London May 16–17, 2002, quoted in Reference 37).

The main EMF target was identified by the author initially from two studies cited in Reference 35 and then later 24 [38] and then 26 [39] studies. Each of these 26 studies showed that EMF effects could be blocked by calcium channel blockers, drugs that are specific for blocking the voltage-gated calcium channels (VGCCs). Five distinct classes of blockers were used in these studies, each class with a distinct structure and binding to a distinct site when acting as a calcium channel blocker. Each of the five is thought to be highly specific for blocking the VGCCs. When a blocker blocked or greatly lowered one effect it also blocked or greatly lowered other effects that were measured in the same study [38]. It follows from these various studies that EMFs act via activation of the voltage-gated calcium channels and that channel activation produces most if not all of the effects seen. Among the EMFs shown to act in this way are not only microwave frequency EMFs, such as those produced by various wireless communications devices which are the focus of this review, but also extremely low frequency EMFs such as 50 or 60 Hz EMFs from our power wiring [38]. It follows that effects in common produced by both types of EMFs, including cancer, may be explained as being caused by downstream mechanisms triggered by VGCC activation.

Such downstream mechanisms are produced by VGCC activation starting with increased intracellular calcium [Ca2+]i (Figure 7.1) [38–43]. The downstream mechanism that is most relevant to the cellular DNA damage produced by EMF exposure is the peroxynitrite pathway (lower right) producing reactive free radicals which attack the DNA. This pathway has been shown in four studies cited in reference 38 to be elevated following EMF exposure, such that 3-nitrotyrosine levels, a marker for peroxynitrite, are elevated. Other carcinogenic effects of EMF exposure are thought to involve both this pathway and also excessive [Ca2+]i signaling (down-facing arrow, near center of Figure 7.1), as discussed below.

Before leaving this issue, it is important to discuss why the VGCCs are so sensitive to activation by these low-intensity EMFs. The VGCCs have a voltage sensor which is made up of 4 alpha helixes in the plasma membrane, with each helix having 5 positive

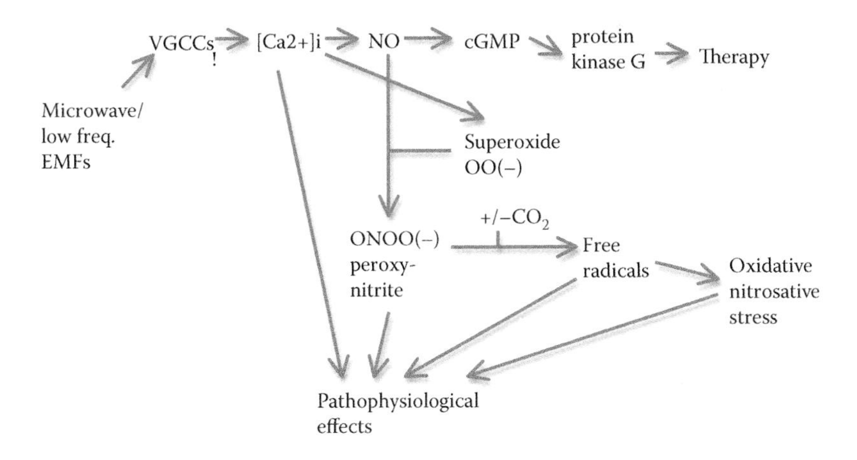

FIGURE 7.1 EMFs act via downstream effects of VGCC activation to produce pathophysiological and therapeutic effects. (Modified from Pall ML 2015. *Rev Environ Health* 30:99–116. With permission.)

charges on it, for a total of 20 positive charges [39]. Each of these charges is within the lipid bilayer part of the plasma membrane. The electrical forces on the voltage sensor are very high for three distinct reasons [39,42,43]. (1) The 20 charges on the voltage sensor make the forces on voltage sensor 20 times higher than the forces on a single charge. (2) Because these charges are within the lipid bilayer section of the membrane where the dielectric constant is about 1/120th of the dielectric constant of the aqueous parts of the cell, the law of physics called Coulomb's law predicts that the forces will be approximately 120 times higher than the forces on charges in the aqueous parts of the cell. (3) Because the plasma membrane has a high electrical resistance whereas the aqueous parts of the cell are highly conductive, the electrical gradient across the plasma membrane is estimated to be concentrated about 3000-fold. The combination of these effects means that comparing the forces on the voltage sensor with the forces on singly charged groups in the aqueous parts of the cell, the forces on the voltage sensor is approximately $20 \times 120 \times 3000 = 7.2$ million times higher [39]. The physics predicts, therefore, extraordinarily strong forces activating the VGCCs via the voltage sensor. It follows that the biology tells us that the VGCCs are the main target of the EMFs and the physics tells us why they are the main target. Thus the physics and biology are pointing in the same direction.

EMFs have been shown to act in plants very similarly to how they act in animals, via activation of calcium channels in the plasma membrane of cells [43]. Although the plant channels are somewhat different from the animal VGCCs, they are thought to be channels regulated by a similar voltage sensor, such that the voltage sensor may well be the universal target of the low intensity EMFs [43].

7.3 MICROWAVE AND LOWER FREQUENCY EMFs CAUSE SINGLE STRAND AND DOUBLE STRAND BREAKS IN CELLULAR DNA

Single strand breaks in cellular DNA are primarily detected through what are sometimes called alkaline comet assays of the DNA, a method that can give a measure of such breaks when they occur in large numbers even in single cells. Double strand breaks in cellular DNA are detected by their ability to produce chromosome breaks and rearrangements, including the production of micronuclei.

Reviews of studies of single strand breaks in cellular DNA [38,39,44–49] and double strand breaks in cellular DNA [39,44–50] have been published earlier and no further review of the primary literature will be given here.

Breaks in cellular DNA produce large increases in polyADP-ribose polymerase (PARP) activity, which has roles in repairing these breaks. While to my knowledge there have been only three studies of PARP following microwave frequency EMF exposure [51–53], each of them found such increased PARP activity.

In Reference 38, a number of studies are discussed where a particular research group using a consistent methodology and the same EMF found that different cell types differed from one another in whether EMF exposure produced detectable increases in single strand DNA breaks. On p. 106 of Reference 39, it was found that studies of other types of EMF-dependent DNA damage also showed variations from one cell type to another. Studies discussed in Reference 38 also showed that free radical scavengers and other agents that act through gene regulation to lower levels of peroxynitrite and also free radicals enzymatically, greatly lower the production of single stranded breaks in cellular DNA following EMF exposure. These provide substantial evidence that the DNA strand breaks are produced by free radical attack on the DNA backbone. It will be argued below that these regulatory responses protecting the DNA from the EMF effects is Nrf2 [54], where raising Nrf2 lowers peroxynitrite and free radicals produced from peroxynitrite and also increases the repair of lesions produced by some free radical attacks on DNA. These studies support the view that the DNA strand breaks are produce through free radical attack on the DNA. Specifics will follow.

In addition, in some but not other studies, pulsed EMFs were shown to be much more active than are nonpulsed (also known as continuous wave) EMFs. This is consistent with many studies reviewed earlier, showing the pulsed EMFs are, in most cases, more biologically active than are continuous wave EMFs [39,55–61]. This effect of pulsations is very important because wireless communication devices communicate via pulsations with "smarter" devices and communicate more information, therefore producing still greater pulsations and therefore, being, at least potentially, much more dangerous.

7.3.1 How DNA Strand Breaks Are Produced by Peroxynitrite and Free Radicals and How This Leads to Cancer

DNA strand breaks and also DNA base changes are produced by peroxynitrite [62–64], acting through free radical breakdown products with the chemistry discussed in References 62–68. As shown in the peroxynitrite/free radical/oxidative stress pathway (see Figure 7.1), both peroxynitrite and its CO_2 adduct, nitrosoperoxycarbonate, break down and release free radicals. Peroxynitrite breaks down to release the hydroxyl radical and NO_2 radical. Nitrosoperoxycarbonate breaks down to produce the carbonate radical and NO_2 radical. Strand breaks in DNA occur due to hydrogen extraction from deoxyribose sugars in the DNA backbone. Most such extraction is performed by the hydroxyl radicals, but the carbonate radicals have some activity as well [68]. In contrast, carbonate radicals are more active in producing the base changes in the DNA [68], which are considered in the next section.

Double strand breaks are linked to cancer, in part because mutations that produce deficiencies in double strand breaks repair and produce cancer-prone phenotypes [69]. Double strand breaks have carcinogenesis roles in producing specific chromosomal rearrangements, including the Philadelphia chromosome, including many less specific rearrangements, deletions of tumor suppressor genes, gene amplification (including of oncogenes), copy number of mutations via aberrant recombination, and deletion or aberrant DNA replication processes leading to duplications and various other aberrations. Single strand breaks are less well understood but may cause copy number mutations via aberrant recombination.

7.4 DNA BASE CHANGES FOLLOWING EMF EXPOSURE

There is one base change that has been shown to occur following EMF exposure, as well as several other such changes that are expected to occur but have not been studied or not been adequately studied. The change that has been shown to occur is the oxidation of the guanine base in the DNA to form either 8-hydroxydeoxyguanosine (often abbreviated 8-OHdG) or 8-oxo-dihydrodeoxyguanosine (often abbreviated 8-oxodG). These two are rapidly interconvertible such that they flip back and forth from one form to another. I will refer to them both, therefore, as 8-OHdG although you will see these other designations in the literature and sometimes they are both referred to by the base rather than the deoxynucleoside. When the 8-OHdG is formed in the DNA, much of it, but not all, is rapidly excised from the DNA via a DNA repair mechanism, so that free 8-OHdG can be measured either in the blood or cerebrospinal fluid or in tissue fluids. Elevated 8-OHdG in these fluids is considered to be both an indication of oxidative stress and also as an indication of oxidative attack on the cellular DNA. Some studies following EMF exposure have shown elevated 8-OHdG in the cellular DNA [70–74] and other studies have shown elevated levels of free 8-OHdG in the body fluids [73,75–84]. One of these studies [70] also detected formamidopyrimidine elevation in the DNA following EMF exposure and Reference 85 also detected these oxidized bases in cellular DNA following EMF exposure. Reference 86 detected elevated levels of two of these formamidopyrimidine bases and also 8-OHdG following extremely low frequency EMF exposure. Because such extremely low frequency EMFs also act via VGCC activation [38] as do the microwave frequency EMFs, it is to be expected that similar EMF responses may be found. In summary, we have 16 studies each showing increased 8-OHdG following microwave frequency EMF exposure. 8-OHdG in cellular DNA should be considered to be an established effect of EMF exposure. The rate limiting step in the formation of 8-OHdG is hydrogen extraction from the guanine base in the DNA and this extraction is thought to be produced by the carbonyl radical [68], derived from the CO_2 adduct of peroxynitrite, nitrosoperoxycarbonate. We have, then, a plausible mechanism for the formation of this compound following EMF exposure.

There are other DNA base changes that are produced by peroxynitrite, but we will only discuss one of these. 8-nitrodG is produced by peroxynitrite breakdown products and is thought to have a major role in inflammatory carcinogenesis. It has never been tested for following EMF exposure to my knowledge. However, because 8-nitrotyrosine levels, considered a marker of peroxynitrite elevation, has been shown to be elevated following EMF exposures [38], and the chemistry of formation of 3-nitrotyrosine is almost identical to the chemistry of formation of 8-nitrodG, it is my opinion that it is highly likely that 8-nitrodG will be found to be elevated following suitable EMF exposures. Both 8-OHdG and 8-nitrodG are known to be mutagenic, producing both transition mutations and also the usually functionally more damaging transversion mutations, it may be expected that each of them contributes mutationally to EMF cancer causation.

7.5 ROLE OF EMF-INDUCED ORNITHINE DECARBOXYLASE IN CAUSING CANCER

Ornithine decarboxylase (ODCase) is an enzyme where increased activity has an important role in cancer [87–90]. Studies have shown that difluoromethylornithine and other ODCase inhibitors have substantial anticancer activity [88–90]. Studies have also shown that pulsed microwave frequency EMFs raise ODCase [91–95]. Two reviews included studies on EMFs raising ODCase [15,96].

Four of these studies of the EMF-ODCase connection have suggested that EMF-caused increased ODCase has an important role in EMF cancer causation [15,91,94,96], including specifically that ODCase may have a role in cell phone caused cancer [96]. It is quite possible, therefore, that increased ODCase activity following EMF exposure has an important role in EMF cancer causation.

ODCase activity is rapidly increased by oxidative stress, a process antagonized by antioxidants [97–100], suggesting that EMF exposures can increase ODCase activity via oxidative stress (see Figure 7.1).

7.6 ROLE OF EMF-INDUCED MELATONIN DEFICIENCY IN CAUSING CANCER

Melatonin has been shown to be useful for both cancer prevention and cancer treatment [101–104]. Melatonin levels, which are usually high at night, have a role in producing sleep coordinated with the circadian rhythm. It has been shown to be often depleted at night by microwave and lower frequency EMF exposures [95,96,105–111]. These findings argue, therefore, that melatonin depletion, as suggested previously [95,96], is likely to have a role in EMF-caused carcinogenesis.

How then might melatonin act to help prevent or treat cancer? It is the author's opinion that melatonin probably acts both by raising both Nrf2 activity [112,113] and by raising adenosine monophosphate-activated protein kinase (AMPK) activity [114,115]. Nrf2 has important cancer preventive activity [116,117] and AMPK has important cancer treatment activity [118,119].

How then might EMFs act via VGCC activation to lower nocturnal melatonin levels? Probably by raising intracellular calcium [Ca2+]i which both increases the release of melatonin precursor serotonin [120] from the pineal gland and also by disrupting the circadian rhythm control [121,122].

7.7 EMF PRODUCED ELEVATED NF-KAPPA B ACTIVITY IS INVOLVED IN MULTIPLE MECHANISMS OF CANCER CAUSATION

Studies have shown that microwave frequency EMF exposures can produce substantial increases in nuclear factor-kappaB (NF-kappaB) activity [123–127]. This should not be surprising because it has been known for over 25 years that oxidative stress produces increases in NF-kappa B activity [128]. NF-kappa B produces proliferation of pre-malignant and malignant cells, prevents apoptosis of cancer cells, promotes angiogenesis of solid tumors, and stimulates invasion including metastasis [129–133]. Consequently, the rise in NF-kappa B activity following EMF exposure may be a major pathway of action of cancer causation produced by EMF exposures.

NF-kappa B activity may explain part of the findings in the two previous sections on ODCase and cancer and also on melatonin and cancer. Part of the activity of oxidative stress in raising ODCase is mediated by the role of oxidative stress in raising NF-kappa B, which raises, in turn, ODCase [99,134]. Melatonin, as you may recall, produces much of its anticancer effects by raising the levels of both Nrf2 and

AMPK. Both Nrf2 and AMPK lower the activity of NF-kappa B, providing a partial further explanation for the anticancer activities of melatonin.

7.8 EMF CAUSED TUMOR PROMOTION VIA DISRUPTION OF GAP JUNCTIONS

The overall hypothesis being explored here is that gap junction disruption has an important role in tumor promotion and that free radicals and other oxidants activate AP-1 which increases transcription of matrix metalloproteinase (MMP) genes, leading to degradation of both gap junctions and tight junctions.

Many reviews have documented the role of gap junctions in preventing tumor promotion [135–140] and therefore the role of gap junction disruption in causing tumor promotion. MMPs have important roles in degrading the proteins making up gap junctions [135–140] and also tight junctions [141,142]. AP-1 is a transcription factor activated by free radicals and other oxidants which acts to increase transcription of MMP-9 and other MMPs [136–140,143,144]. Such MMP increases may well explain the breakdown of the blood-brain barrier that occurs following EMF exposures [141,142,145]. It follows from the above in this paragraph, that the each of the mechanisms in our overall hypothesis here is well documented, such that we can explain how EMFs, acting via the peroxynitrite/free radical/oxidative stress pathway, outlined in Figure 7.1 can lead, to tumor promotion via gap junction disruption.

Gap junction and tight junction disruption also have an important role in tissue invasion including metastasis [135–140,146], thus producing other important types of dysfunction that help cause tumor progression.

7.9 DOUBLE STRAND BREAKS, TUMOR PROMOTION, AND GENE AMPLIFICATION

Gene amplification of oncogenes has been known for about 40 years to have a role in carcinogenesis. It is thought that gene amplification has a role in tumor promotion [147–152]. Tumor promoters including phorbol ester tumor promoters stimulate gene amplification [148–152]. These findings suggest that other effects that stimulate gene amplification that are produced by EMF exposures, including double strand DNA breaks (reviewed in References 153–155) and possibly single strand DNA breaks [156], can also act to stimulate tumor promotion following EMF exposure.

7.10 OTHER CALCIUM MEDIATED ACTIONS IN CANCER

Because VGCC activation acts in the cell predominantly via excessive [Ca2+]i, reviews on cancer and calcium can be used to search for additional types of evidence arguing that such activation can have roles in cancer causation. Elevated [Ca2+]i has been shown to have such roles in a broad range of activities in tumorigenesis and progression including tumor initiation, aberrant proliferation, cell migration, progression, metastasis, and angiogenesis [157–164].

Genetic evidence also implicates excessive [Ca2+]i in carcinogenesis, including cancer causation due to mutations activating T-type VGCCs [165]. Other such gene mutations that raise [Ca2+]i and cause cancer include mutations in the TRP superfamily of receptors, Orai channels, and calcium ATPase pumps in both the sarcoplasmic reticulum (SERCA) and the plasma membrane (ATP2A2 and ATP2C1) and store-operated calcium channels [166–169]. Each of these types of cancer causing mutations produce increases in [Ca2+]i, showing that elevated [Ca2+]i has a key role in carcinogenesis.

Specific, cancer causing mechanisms produced as downstream effects of excessive [Ca2+]i are described in Table 7.1.

7.11 SUMMARY: 15 DISTINCT EMF-INITIATED CAUSES OF CANCER

This paper is based on three important findings. First, that microwave and lower frequency EMFs act via activation of VGCCs. Second, 29 different reviews have concluded that such EMFs cause cancer, raising the question of how VGCC activation can cause cancer. Third, because VGCC activation acts mainly via increased [Ca2+]i, it is reasonable to assume that cancer causation occurs via increased calcium signaling and via other downstream effects of [Ca2+]i. This paper finds that there are multiple mechanisms that fit each of these two descriptions that cause cancer based on the cancer literature. Many of them come from the downstream effects involving the peroxynitrite/free radical/oxidative stress pathway and one of the important consequences of that pathway, elevated NF-kappa B. Those downstream effects are similar or identical to the effects that are central to inflammatory carcinogenesis in the literature. But, in addition, there are cancer causing effects that are caused by excessive calcium signaling and these are also discussed here.

These mechanisms are listed below. Mechanisms 1–6 are all reported to be raised following EMF exposures and are, therefore, particularly plausibly involved in EMF-caused carcinogenesis. Each of these 15 is produced as a consequence of either the peroxynitrite/free radical/oxidative stress pathway of action of as a consequence of excessive calcium signaling. Each is, therefore, highly plausible because each of these pathways of action are well documented downstream effects of EMF exposures.

1. Formation of single strand breaks in cellular DNA and
2. Double strand breaks in cellular DNA. The double strand breaks have multiple roles in carcinogenesis. The single strand breaks may generate chromosomal rearrangements and copy number mutations via aberrant recombination events. Double strand breaks are known to help cause gene amplification events and single strand breaks may also have roles in gene amplification.
3. Oxidized bases, of which 8-OHdG has been by far the most studied, which produce point mutations including transversion mutations. 8-OHdG is produced via peroxynitrite breakdown product free radicals including hydroxyl and carbonate radicals. These same free radicals have roles in

TABLE 7.1
Additional [Ca2+]i-Mediated Cancer-Related Activities

Citation(s)	Cancer-Related Activity
[170,171]	Calcium-dependent phosphatidylserine flippase activity; this calcium-dependent enzyme activity controls, in turn, many different cancer cell surface markers, while placing substantial levels of phosphatidylserine on the outer surface of the plasma membrane specifically in cancer cells. This, in turn, makes the cancer cells resistant to immune surveillance.
[172–179]	The calcium/calmodulin-dependent protein kinase, CaMKII controls the progress through the cell cycle in many different types of cancer.
[180–182]	CaMKII activity is also stimulated by oxidation of methionine residues in the enzyme to methionine sulfoxide, a process that is greatly increased in oxidative stress. It follows that the cell cycling activated by CaMKII (see immediately above) can also be increased by oxidative stress.
[183–192]	c-src, viewed as being one of the most important cellular oncogenes causing human cancer, is activated by calcium binding to calmodulin [183–185]. c-src a tyrosine protein kinase, phosphorylates a tyrosine residue on L-type VGCCs, leading to large increases in the sensitivity of the VGCCs to activation [186–188]. This suggests that these mechanisms may constitute a positive feedback loop, leading to excessive [Ca2+]i levels that may be substantially higher than those obtained by the direct impact of EMFs on the VGCCs. A second somewhat similar positive feedback loop occurs as a consequence of reactive oxygen species that are elevated under oxidative stress, also activates the L-type VGCCs [189–192]. It may be suggested, therefore, that these mechanisms may not only contribute to cancer causation, but also to electromagnetic hypersensitivity (EHS).
[159]	In a much broader pattern than the c-src connection, immediately above, Marchi and Pinton [159] reviewed various studies showing that calcium up-regulates multiple cellular oncogenes and down-regulates multiple tumor suppressor genes, thus stimulating large numbers of mechanisms involved in causing cancer.
[193,194]	Calpains are calcium-activated, cysteine proteases which are viewed, therefore, as calcium receptors. An excellent review of calpains and cancer [193] describes the complex and often divergent roles of calpains in cancer—roles that are sufficiently complex and divergent, that in most cases, this reviewer cannot summarize them. The one exception to that is the role [193] where "the positive role played by calpains in tumor cell migration and invasion has been well established" often leading to metastasis. Investigations show that calpain activity is correlated with invasion and that calpain inhibition leads to lowered cell migration and invasion. Calpains function in this role by increasing the activity of several proteins involved in cell movement as well as degrading the extracellular matrix. In the latter function, calpains act along with the matrix metalloproteinases (MMPs) which are discussed above in this paper. The role of calpains in tissue invasion and metastasis is confirmed in a recent review [194] on calpains in breast cancer.

generating both single strand breaks and double strand breaks in cellular DNA.

4. Increased ODCase produced following EMF exposures is an additional mechanism likely to be involved in EMF-caused carcinogenesis. Increased ODCase is caused by oxidative stress.

5. Lowered melatonin levels follow EMF exposures. Melatonin has anti-cancer activities which are thought to be produced primarily via melatonin-mediated increases in Nrf2 activity and increases in AMPK activity. Nrf2 helps prevent cancer and AMPK helps treat cancer.
6. Increased NF-kappaB activity is produced by oxidative stress which occurs following EMF exposure. NF-kappaB has multiple roles in cancer causation. NF-kappa B produces proliferation of premalignant and malignant cells, prevents apoptosis of cancer cells, promotes angiogenesis of solid tumors, and stimulates invasion including metastasis. NF-kappaB also helps explain 4 and 5 above. NF-kappaB acts to raise ODCase. Part of the cancer prevention or cancer treating actions of Nrf2 and AMPK is that they both act to lower NF-kappaB.
7. EMF-induced tumor promotion via gap-junction disruption, where oxidative activation of AP-1 induces increased proteolysis of both gap-junction and tight junction proteins, leading to gap-junction disruption and tumor promotion.
8. EMF-induced disruption of gap-junctions and tight junctions (see 7 immediately above) also has a key role in increasing tumor invasion and metastasis.
9. Tumor promotion via double strand breaks in cellular DNA and consequent gene amplification of cellular oncogenes. The other mostly calcium-linked mechanisms all come from Table 7.1.
10. The calcium-dependent enzyme, phosphatidylserine flippase, produces substantial levels of phosphatidylserine on the outer surface of cancer cells, producing many cancer-specific cell surface markers and resistance of the cancer cells to immune surveillance.
11. The calcium/calmodulin dependent protein kinase, CaMKII, controls progress through the cell cycle in many types of cancer cells.
12. CaMKII activity is stimulated by oxidation of methionine residues in the protein, caused by oxidative stress; it follows that this critically important activity in cancer cells is both produced directly by elevated [Ca2+]i, and also oxidative stress.
13. The cellular oncoprotein c-src is activated by calcium binding to calmodulin and it acts in turn to raise the sensitivity of the L-type VGCCs to voltage activation. It follows that this may produce a positive feedback loop, leading to amplified [Ca2+]i levels. Oxidants also sensitize the VGCCs to activation, suggesting an additional positive feedback loop.
14. March and Pinton [159] reviewed a broad pattern of calcium effects, where calcium raised the activity of cellular oncoproteins and, in addition, lowered the activity of tumor suppressor proteins.
15. Calpains, calcium-activated cysteine proteases, increase tumor cell migration and tissue invasion leading to metastasis.

We have, then, 15 well-documented mechanisms by which EMFs acting via VGCC activation can cause cancer. It is complete and utter to nonsense, therefore, to claim there are no such mechanisms.

7.12 THE AUTHOR DECLARES NO CONFLICTS OF INTEREST

All time and financial costs in the writing of this paper are being donated by the author and no reimbursement will be sought or accepted for these costs. Therefore, the author declares no conflict of interest.

REFERENCES

1. Dwyer MJ, Leeper DB. 1978. A Current Literature Report on the Carcinogenic Properties of Ionizing and Nonionizing Radiation. DHEW Publication (NIOSH) 78-134, March 1978.
2. Adey WR. 1988. Cell membranes: The electromagnetic environment and cancer promotion. *Neurochem Res* 13:671–677.
3. Adey WR. 1990. Joint actions of environmental nonionizing electromagnetic fields and chemical pollution in cancer promotion. *Environ Health Perspect* 86:297–305.
4. Goldsmith JR. 1995. Epidemiological evidence of radiofrequency radiation (microwave) effects on health in military, broadcasting and occupational settings. *Int J Occup Environ Health* 1:47–57.
5. Goldsmith JR. 1997. Epidemiologic evidence relevant to radar (microwave) effects. *Env Health Perspect* 105(Suppl 6):1579–1587.
6. Kundi M, Kild K, Hardell L, Mattsson M. 2004. Mobile telephones and cancer—A review of the epidemiological evidence. *J Toxicol Env Health, Part B* 7:351–384.
7. Kundi M. 2004. Mobile phone use and cancer. *Occup Env Med* 61:560–570.
8. Behari J, Paulraj R. 2007. Biomarkers of induced electromagnetic field and cancer. *Indian J Exp Biol* 45:77–85.
9. Hardell L, Carlberg M, Soderqvist F, Hansson Mild K. 2008. Meta-analysis of long-term mobile phone use and the association with brain tumors. *Int J Oncol* 32:1097–1103.
10. Khurana VG, Teo C, Kundi M, Hardell L, Carlberg M. 2009. Cell phones and brain tumors: A review including the long-term epidemiologic data. *Surg Neurol* 72:205–214.
11. Desai NR, Kesari KK, Agarwal A. 2009. Pathophysiology of cell phone radiation: Oxidative stress and carcinogenesis with focus on the male reproductive system. *Reproduct Biol Endocrinol* 7:114.
12. Yakymenko I, Sidorik E. 2010. Risks of carcinogenesis from electromagnetic radiation and mobile telephony devices. *Exp Oncol* 32:729–736.
13. Giuliani L, Soffriti M (eds). 2010. Non-thermal effects and mechanisms of interaction between electromagnetic fields and living matter, Ramazzini Institute Eur. *J. Oncol. Library* Volume 5, National Institute for the Study and Control of Cancer and Environmental Diseases "Bernardino Ramazzini" Bologna, Italy 2010, 400 page monograph.
14. Khurana VG, Hardell L, Everaert J, Bortkiewicz A, Carlberg M, Ahonen M. 2010. Epidemiological evidence for a health risk from mobile phone base stations. *Int J Occup Environ Health* 16, 263–267.
15. Yakymenko I, Sidorik E, Kyrylenko S, Chekhun V. 2011. Long-term exposure to microwave radiation provokes cancer growth: Evidences from radars and mobile communication systems. *Exp Oncol* 33(2), 62–70.
16. Carpenter DO. 2010. Electromagnetic fields and cancer: The cost of doing nothing. *Rev Environ Health* 25:75–80.
17. Biointiative Working Group, David Carpenter and Cindy Sage (eds). 2012. Bioinitiative 2012: A rationale for biologically-based exposure standards for electromagnetic radiation. http://www.bioinitiative.org/participants/why-we-care/

18. Ledoigt G, Belpomme D. 2013. Cancer induction molecular pathways and HF-EMF irradiation. *Adv Biol Chem* 3:177–186.
19. Hardell L, Carlberg M, Hansson Mild K. 2013. Use of mobile phones and cordless phones is associated with increased risk for glioma and acoustic neuroma. *Pathophysiology* 2013;20(2):85–110.
20. Davis DL, Kesari S, Soskolne CL, Miller AB, Stein Y. 2013. Swedish review strengthens grounds for concluding that radiation from cellular and cordless phones is a probable human carcinogen. *Pathophysiology* 20:123–129.
21. Morgan LL, Miller AB, Sasco A, Davis DL. 2015. Mobile phone radiation causes brain tumors and should be classified as a probable human carcinogen (2A). *Int J Oncol* 46(5):1865–1871.
22. Mahdavi M, Yekta R, Tackallou SH. 2015. Positive correlation between ELF and RF electromagnetic fields on cancer risk. *J Paramed Sci* 6(3), ISSN 2008-4978.
23. Carlberg M, Hardell L. 2017. Evaluation of mobile phone and cordless phone use and glioma risk using the Bradford hill viewpoints from 1965 on association or causation. *BioMed Res Int* 2017:9218486. Article ID 9218486, https://doi.org/10.1155/2017/9218486
24. Bortkiewicz A, Gadzicka E, Szymczak W. 2017. Mobile phone use and risk for intracranial tumors and salivary gland tumors—A meta-analysis. *Int J Occup Med Environ Health* 30:27–43.
25. Bielsa-Fernández P, Rodríguez-Martín B. 2017. Association between radiation from mobile phones and tumour risk in adults. *Gac Sanit* Apr 12. pii: S0213-9111(17)30083-3. doi: 10.1016/j.gaceta.2016.10.014. [Epub ahead of print]
26. Alegría-Loyola MA, Galnares-Olalde JA, Mercado M. 2017. Tumors of the central nervous system. *Rev Med Inst Mex Seguro Soc* 55:330–340.
27. Prasad M, Kathuria P, Nair P, Kumar A, Prasad K. 2017. Mobile phone use and risk of brain tumours: A systematic review of association between study quality, source of funding, and research outcomes. *Neurol Sci* Feb 17. doi: 10.1007/s10072-017-2850-8. [Epub ahead of print].
28. Miller A. 2017. References on cell phone radiation and cancer. https://ehtrust.org/references-cell-phone-radio-frequency-radiation-cancer/ (accessed Sprt. 9, 2017)
29. Hardell L. 2017. World Health Organization, radiofrequency radiation and health—A hard nut to crack (Review). *Int J Oncol* 51:405–413.
30. Lerchl A, Klose M, Grote K, Wilhelm AF, Spathmann O, Fiedler T, Streckert J, Hansen V, Clemens M. 2015. Tumor promotion by exposure to radiofrequency electromagnetic fields below exposure limits for humans. *Biochem Biophys Res Commun*. 459:585–590.
31. Soffritti M, Tibaldi E, Padovani M, Hoel DG, Giuliani L, Bua L, Lauriola M et al. 2016. Life-span exposure to sinusoidal-50 Hz magnetic field and acute low-dose γ radiation induce carcinogenic effects in Sprague-Dawley rats. *Int J Radiat Biol* 92:202–214.
32. Wyde M, Cesta M, Blystone C, Blystone C, Elmore S, Foster P, Hooth M, Kissling G, et al. 2016. Report of Partial findings from the National Toxicology Program Carcinogenesis Studies of Cell Phone Radiofrequency Radiation in Hsd: Sprague Dawley® SD rats (Whole Body Exposure). bioRXiv doi: https://doi.org/10.1101/055699
33. National Cancer Insistute. 2015. Electromagnetic Fields and Cancer. https://www.cancer.gov/about-cancer/causes-prevention/risk/radiation/electromagnetic-fields-fact-sheet (accessed September 28, 2017).
34. Canadian Royal Society Expert Panel Report on Radiofrequency Fields. 2014. Available at https://rsc-src.ca/sites/default/files/pdf/SC6_Report_Formatted_1.pdf (accessed September 30, 2017).
35. Walleczek J. 1992. Electromagnetic field effects on cells of the immune system: The role of calcium signaling. *FASEB J* 6:3177–3185.
36. Adey WR. 1993. Biological effects of electromagnetic fields. *J Cell Biochem* 51:410–416.

37. Herbert MR, Sage C. 2013. Autism and EMF? Plausibility of a pathophysiological link—Part I. *Pathophysiology* 20:191–209.
38. Pall, ML. 2013. Electromagnetic fields act via activation of voltage-gated calcium channels to produce beneficial or adverse effects. *J Cell Mol Med* 17:958–965. doi: 10.1111/jcmm.12088.
39. Pall, ML. 2015. Scientific evidence contradicts findings and assumptions of Canadian Safety Panel 6: Microwaves act through voltage-gated calcium channel activation to induce biological impacts at non-thermal levels, supporting a paradigm shift for microwave/lower frequency electromagnetic field action. *Rev Environ Health* 30:99–116. doi: 10.1515/reveh-2015-0001.
40. Pall ML. 2014. Electromagnetic field activation of voltage-gated calcium channels: Role in therapeutic effects. *Electromagn Biol Med* Apr 8. doi: 10.3109/15368378.2014.906447.
41. Pall ML. 2016. Microwave frequency electromagnetic fields (EMFs) produce widespread neuropsychiatric effects including depression. *J Chem Neuroanat* Sep;75(Pt B):43–51. doi: 10.1016/j.jchemneu.2015.08.001. Epub 2015 Aug 21.
42. Pall ML. 2015. How to approach the challenge of minimizing non-thermal health effects of microwave radiation from electrical devices. *International Journal of Innovative Research in Engineering & Management (IJIREM)* September;2(5):71–76. ISSN: 2350-0557.
43. Pall ML. 2016. Electromagnetic fields act similarly in plants as in animals: Probable activation of calcium channels via their voltage sensor. *Curr Chem Biol* 10: 74–82.
44. Hardell L, Sage C. 2008. Biological effects from electromagnetic field exposure and public exposure standards. *Biomed. Pharmacother.* 62:104–109.
45. Ruediger HW. 2009. Genotoxic effects of radiofrequency electromagnetic fields. *Pathophysiology.* 16:89–102.
46. Phillips JL, Singh NP, Lai H. 2009. Electromagnetic fields and DNA damage. *Pathophysiology* 16:79–88.
47. Makker K, Varghese A, Desai NR, Mouradi R, Agarwal A. 2009. Cell phones: Modern man's nemesis? *Reprod Biomed Online* 18:148–157.
48. Batista Napotnik T, Reberšek M, Vernier PT, Mali B, Miklavčič D. 2010. Effects of high voltage nanosecond electric pulses on eukaryotic cells (*in vitro*): A systematic review. *Bioelectrochemistry* 110:1–12.
49. Asghari A, Khaki AA, Rajabzadeh A, Khaki A. 2016. A review on electromagnetic fields (EMFs) and the reproductive system. *Electron Physician.* Jul 25;8(7):2655–2662.
50. Glaser ZR PhD. 1971. *Naval Medical Research Institute Research Report, June 1971.* Bibliography of Reported Biological Phenomena ("Effects") and Clinical Manifestations Attributed to Microwave and Radio-Frequency Radiation. Report No. 2 Revised. https://scholar.google.com/scholar?q=Glaser+naval+medical+microwave+radio-frequency+1972&btnG=&hl=en&as_sdt=0%2C38 (accessed September 9, 2017)
51. Zuo H, Lin T, Wang D, Peng R, Wang S, Gao Y, Xu X et al. 2014. Neural cell apoptosis induced by microwave exposure through mitochondria-dependent caspase-3 pathway. *Int J Med Sci* 11:426–435.
52. He Q, Sun Y, Zong L, Tong J, Cao Y. 2016. Induction of poly(ADP-ribose) polymerase in mouse bone marrow stromal cells exposed to 900 MHz radiofrequency fields: Preliminary observations. *Biomed Res Int* 2016:4918691.
53. He Q, Zong L, Sun Y, Vijaylaxmi, Prihoda TJ, Tong J, Cao Y. 2017. Adaptive response in mouse bone marrow stromal cells exposed to 900 MHz radiofrequency fields: Impact of poly (ADP-ribose) polymerase (PARP). *Mutat Res/Genet Toxicol Environ Metagen* 820:19–25.
54. Pall ML, Levine S. 2015. Nrf2, a master regulator of detoxification and also antioxidant, anti- inflammatory and other cytoprotective mechanisms, is raised by health promoting factors. *Acta Physiologica Sinica* 67:1–18.

55. Osipov YuA, 1965. *Labor Hygiene and the Effect of Radiofrequency Electromagnetic Fields on Workers*. Leningrad Meditsina Publishing House, Leningrand, USSR, 220 pp.
56. Pollack H, Healer J. 1967. *Review of Information on Hazards to Personnel from High-Frequency Electromagnetic Radiation*. Institute for Defense Analyses; Research and Engineering Support Division. IDA/HQ 67-6211, Series B, May 1967.
57. Creighton MO, Larsen LE, Stewart-DeHaan PJ, Jacobi JH, Sanwal M, Baskerville JC, Bassen HE, Brown DO, Trevithick JR. 1987. In vitro studies of microwave-induced cataract. II. Comparison of damage observed for continuous wave and pulsed microwaves. *Exp Eye Res* 45:357–373.
58. Belyaev I. 2005. Non-thermal biological effects of microwaves. *Microwave Rev* 11:13–29.
59. Markov MS. 2007. Pulsed electromagnetic field therapy: History, state of the art and future. *The Environmentalist* 27:465–475.
60. Panagopoulos DJ, Johansson O, Carlo GL. 2015. Real versus simulated mobile phone exposures in experimental studies. *BioMed. Res. Int.* article ID 607053, 8 pages. doi: 10.1155/2015/607053.
61. Belyaev I. 2015. Biophysical mechanisms for nonthermal microwave effects. In: *Electromagnetic Fields in Biology and Medicine*, M.S. Markov, ed, CRC Press, New York, pp. 49–67.
62. Szabo C, Ohshima H. 1997. DNA damage induced by peroxynitrite: Subsequent biological effects. *Nitric oxide* 1:373–385.
63. Szabo G, Bahrle S. 2005. Role of nitrosative stress and poly(ADP-ribose) polymerase activation in myocardial reperfusion injury. *Curr Vasc Pharmacol* 3:215–220.
64. Moon HK, Yang ES, Park JW. 2006. Protection of peroxynitrite-induced DNA damage by dietary antioxidants. *Arch Pharm Res* 29:213–217.
65. Sakihama Y, Maeda M, Hashimoto M, Tahara S, Hashidoko Y, et al. 2012. Beetroot betalain inhibits peroxynitrite-mediated tyrosine nitration and DNA strand damage. *Free Radic Res* 46:93–99.
66. Islam BU, Habib S, Ahmad P, Allarakha S, Moinuddin, Ali A. 2015. Pathophysiological role of peroxynitrite induced DNA damage in human diseases: A special focus on poly(ADP-ribose) polymerase (PARP). *Indian J Clin Biochem* 30:368–385.
67. Ducrocq C, Blanchard B, Pignatelli B, Ohshima H. 1999. Peroxynitrite: An endogenous oxidizing and nitrating agent. *Cell Mol Life Sci* 55:1068–1077.
68. Roginskaya M, Moore TJ, Ampadu-Boateng D, Razskazovskiy Y. 2015. Efficacy and site specificity of hydrogen abstraction from DNA 2-deoxyribose by carbonate radicals. *Free Radic Res* 49:1431–1437.
69. Khanna KK, Jackson SP. 2001. DNA doublwe-strand breaks: Signaling, repair and the cancer connection. *Nature Genet* 27:247–254.
70. Liu CV, Duan W, Xu S, Chen C, He M, Zhang L, Yu Z, Zhou Z. 2013. Exposure to 1800 MHz radiofrequency electromagnetic radiation induces oxidative DNA base damage in mouse spermatocyte-derived cell line. *Toxicol Lett* 218:2–9.
71. Wang X, Liu C, Ma Q, Feng W, Yang L, Lu Y, Zhou Z, Yu Z, Li W, Zhang L. 2015. 8-oxoG DNA glycosylase-1 inhibition sensitizes neuro-2a cells to oxidative DNA base damage induced by 900 MHz radiofrequency electromagnetic radiation. *Cell Physiol Biochem* 37:1075–1088.
72. De Iuliis GN, Newey RJ, King BV, Aitken RJ. 2009. Mobile phone radiation induces reactive oxygen species production and DNA damage in human spermatozoa *in vitro*. *PLoS One* Jul 31;4(7):e6446. doi: 10.1371/journal.pone.0006446.
73. Atasoy HI, Gunal MY, Atasoy P, Elgun S, Bugdayci G. 2013. Immunohistopathologic demonstration of deleterious effects on growing rat testes of radiofrequency waves emitted from conventional Wi-Fi devices. *J Pediatr Urol* 9:223–229.

74. Sun Y, Zong L, Gao Z, Zhu S, Tong J, Cao Y. 2017. Mitochondrial DNA damage and oxidative damage in HL-60 cells exposed to 900MHz radiofrequency fields. *Mutat Res* 797-799:7–14.
75. Sahin D, Ozgur E, Guler G, Tomruk A, Unlu I, Sepici-Dinçel A, Seyhan N. 2016. The 2100 MHz radiofrequency radiation of a 3G-mobile phone and the DNA oxidative damage in brain. *J Chem Neuroanat* 75(Pt B):94–98.
76. Güler G, Ozgur E, Keles H, Tomruk A, Vural SA, Seyhan N. 2016. Neurodegenerative changes and apoptosis induced by intrauterine and extrauterine exposure of radiofrequency radiation. *J Chem Neuroanat* 75(Pt B):128–133.
77. Gürler HŞ, Bilgici B, Akar AK, Tomak L, Bedir A. 2014. Increased DNA oxidation (8-OHdG) and protein oxidation (AOPP) by low level electromagnetic field (2.45 GHz) in rat brain and protective effect of garlic. *Int J Radiat Biol* 90:892–896.
78. Khalil AM, Abu Khadra KM, Aljaberi AM, Gagaa MH, Issa HS. 2014. Assessment of oxidant/antioxidant status in saliva of cell phone users. *Electromagn Biol Med* 33:92–97.
79. Burlaka A, Tsybulin O, Sidorik E, Lukin S, Polishuk V, Tsehmistrenko S, Yakymenko I. 2013. Overproduction of free radical species in embryonal cells exposed to low intensity radiofrequency radiation. *Exp Oncol* 35:219–225.
80. Hanci H, Odaci E, Kaya H, Aliyazicioglu Y, Turan I, Demir S, Colakoglu S. 2013. The effect of prenatal exposure to 900-megahertz electromagnetic field on the 21-old-day rat testicle. *Reprod Toxicol* 42:203–209.
81. Güler G, Tomruk A, Ozgur E, Sahin D, Sepici A, Altan N, Seyhan N. 2012. The effect of radiofrequency radiation on DNA and lipid damage in female and male infant rabbits. *Int J Radiat Biol* 88:367–373.
82. Khalil AM, Gagaa MH, Alshamali AM. 2012. 8-Oxo-7, 8-dihydro-2'-deoxyguanosine as a biomarker of DNA damage by mobile phone radiation. *Hum Exp Toxicol* 31:734–740.
83. Xu S, Zhou Z, Zhang L, Yu Z, Zhang W, Wang Y, Wang X et al. 2010. Exposure to 1800 MHz radiofrequency radiation induces oxidative damage to mitochondrial DNA in primary cultured neurons. *Brain Res* 1311:189–196.
84. Güler G, Tomruk A, Ozgur E, Seyhan N. 2010. The effect of radiofrequency radiation on DNA and lipid damage in non-pregnant and pregnant rabbits and their newborns. *Gen Physiol Biophys* 29:59–66.
85. Duan W, Liu C, Zhang L, He M, Xu S, Chen C, Pi H et al. 2015. Comparison of the genotoxic effects induced by 50 Hz extremely low-frequency electromagnetic fields and 1800 MHz radiofrequency electromagnetic fields in GC-2 cells. *Radiat Res* 183:305–314.
86. Yokus B, Akdag MZ, Dasdag S, Cakir DU, Kizil M. 2008. Extremely low frequency magnetic fields cause oxidative DNA damage in rats. *In J Radiat Biol* 84:789–795.
87. Paz EA, Garcia-Huidobro J, Ignatenko NA. 2011. Polyamines in cancer. *Adv Clin Chem* 54:45–70.
88. Nowotarski SL, Woster PM, Casero RA Jr. 2013. Polyamines and cancer: Implications for chemotherapy and chemoprevention. *Expert Rev Mol Med* Feb 22;15:e3. doi: 10.1017/erm.2013.3.
89. Alexiou GA, Lianos GD, Ragos V, Galani V, Kyritsis AP. 2017. Difluoromethylornithine in cancer: New advances. *Future Oncol* 13:809–819. doi: 10.2217/fon-2016-0266.
90. Olsen RR, Zetter BR. 2011. Evidence of a role for antizyme and antizyme inhibitor as regulators of human cancer. *Mol Cancer Res* 9:1285–93. doi: 10.1158/1541-7786.MCR-11-0178. Epub 2011 Aug 17.
91. Byus CV, Kartun K, Pieper S, Adey WR. 1988. Increased ornithine decarboxylase activity in cultured cells exposed to low energy modulated microwave fields and phorbol ester tumor promoters. *Cancer Res* 48:4222–4226.
92. Litovitz TA, Krause D, Penafiel M, Elson EC, Mullins JM. 1993. The role of coherence time in the effect of microwaves on ornithine decarboxylase activity. *Bioelectromagnetics* 14:395–403.

93. Penafiel LM, Litovitz T, Krause D, Desta A, Mullins JM. 1997. Role of modulation on the effect of microwaves on ornithine decarboxylase activity in L929 cells. *Bioelectromagnetics* 18:132–141.
94. Paulraj R, Behari J, Rao AR. 1999. Effect of amplitude modulated RF radiation on calcium ion efflux and ODCase activity in chronically exposed rat brain. *Indian J Biochem Biophys* 36:337–340.
95. Paulraj R, Behari J. 2012. Biochemical changes in rat brain exposed to low intensity 9.9 GHz microwave radiation. *Cell Biochem Biophys* 63:97–102.
96. K Sri N. 2015. Mobile phone radiation: Physiological & pathophysiologcal considerations. *Indian J Physiol Pharmacol* 59:125–135.
97. Ansar S, Iqbal M. 2016. Antioxidant and nephroprotective potential of butylated hydroxyanisole against ferric nitrilotriacetate-induced oxidative stress and early tumor events. *Hum Exp Toxicol* 35:448–453.
98. Sultana S, Nafees S, Khan AQ. 2013. Perillyl alcohol as a protective modulator against rat hepatocarcinogenesis via amelioration of oxidative damage and cell proliferation. *Hum Exp Toxicol* 32:1179–1192.
99. Smirnova OA, Isaguliants MG, Hyvonen MT, Keinanen TA, Tunitskaya VL, Vepsalainen J, Alhonen L, Kochetkov SN, Ivanov AV. 2012. Chemically induced oxidative stress increases polyamine levels by activating the transcription of ornithine decarboxylase and spermidine/spermine-N1-acetyltransferase in human hepatoma HUH7 cells. *Biochimie.* 94:1876–1883.
100. Otieno MA, Kensler TW. 2000. A role for protein kinase C-delta in the regulation of ornithine decarboxylase expression by oxidative stress. *Cancer Res* 60:4391–4396.
101. Proietti S, Cucina A, Minini M, Bizzarri M. 2017. Melatonin, mitochondria, and the cancer cell. *Cell Mol Life Sci* Aug 7. doi: 10.1007/s00018-017-2612-z.
102. Blask DE, Sauer LA, Dauchy RT. 2002. Melatonin as a chronobiotic/anticancer agent: Cellular, biochemical, and molecular mechanisms of action and their implications for circadian-based cancer therapy. *Curr Top Med Chem* 2:113–132.
103. Jung B, Ahmad N. 2006. Melatonin in cancer management: Progress and promise. *Cancer Res* 66:9789–9793.
104. Lissoni P, Barni S, Mandalà M, Ardizzoia A, Paolorossi F, Vaghi M, Longarini R, Malugani F, Tancini G. 1999. Decreased toxicity and increased efficacy of cancer chemotherapy using the pineal hormone melatonin in metastatic solid tumour patients with poor clinical status. *Eur J Cancer* 35:1688–1692.
105. Halgamuge MN. 2013. Pineal melatonin level disruption in humans due to electromagnetic fields and ICNIRP limits. *Radiat Prot Dosimetr* 154:405–416.
106. Kim HS, Paik MJ, Lee YH, Lee YS, Choi HD, Pack JK, Kim N, Ahn YH. 2015. Eight hours of nocturnal 915 MHz radiofrequency identification (RFID) exposure reduces urinary levels of melatonin and its metabolite via pineal arylalkylamine N-acetyltransferase activity in male rats. *Int J Radiat Biol* 91: 898–907.
107. Cao H, Qin F, Liu X, Wang J, Cao Y, Tong J, Zhao H. 2015. Circadian rhythmicity of antioxidant markers in rats exposed to 1.8 GHz radiofrequency fields. *Int J Environ Res Public Health* 12:2071–2087.
108. Lewczuk B, Redlarski G, Zak A, Ziolkowska N, Przybylska-Gornowicz B, Krawczuk M. 2014. Influence of electric, magnetic, and electromagnetic fields on the circadian system: Current stage of knowledge. *Review. Biomed Res Int* 2014:169459.
109. Trosic I, Pavicic I, Marjanovic AM, Busljeta I. 2012. Non-Thermal Biomarkers of Exposure to Radiofrequency/Microwave Radiation. [review] *Arh Hig Rada Toksikol* 63:67–73.
110. Davanipour Z, Sobel E. 2009. Long-term exposure to magnetic fields and the risks of Alzheimer's disease and breast cancer: Further biological research. *Pathophysiology* 16:149–156.

111. Karasek M, Woldanska-Okonska M. 2004. Electromagnetic fields and human endocrine system. *ScientificWorld Journal* Oct 20;4(Suppl 2):23–28.
112. Vriend J, Reiter RJ. 2016. Melatonin, bone regulation and the ubiquitin-proteasome connection: A review. *Life Sci* 145:152–160.
113. Chen LY, Renn TY, Liao WC, Mai FD, Ho YJ, Hsiao G, Lee AW, Chang HM. 2017. Melatonin successfully rescues hippocampal bioenergetics and improves cognitive function following drug intoxication by promoting Nrf2-ARE signaling activity. *J Pineal Res* Sep;63(2). doi: 10.1111/jpi.12417.
114. Wang X, Xue GX, Liu WC, Shu H, Wang M, Sun Y, Liu X et al. 2017. Melatonin alleviates lipopolysaccharide-compromised integrity of blood-brain barrier through activating AMP-activated protein kinase in old mice. *Aging Cell* 16:414–421.
115. Guven C, Taskin E, Akcakaya H. 2016. Melatonin reverses flow shear stress-induced injury in bone marrow mesenchymal stem cells via activation of AMP-activated protein kinase signaling. *J Pineal Res* 60:228–241.
116. Pall ML, Levine S. 2015. Nrf2, a master regulator of detoxification and also antioxidant, anti- in ammatory and other cytoprotective mechanisms, is raised by health promoting factors. *Acta Physiol Sinica* 67:1–18.
117. Baird L, Dinkova-Kostova AT. 2011. The cytoprotective role of the Keapl-Nrf2 pathway. *Arch Toxicol* 85:241–272.
118. Dowling RJ, Goodwin PJ, Stambolic V. 2011. Understanding the benefit of metformin use in cancer treatment. *BMC Med.* Apr 6;9:33. doi: 10.1186/1741-7015-9-33. Review.
119. Garcia D, Shaw RJ. 2017. AMPK: Mechanisms of cellular energy sensing and restoration of metabolic balance. *Mol Cell* 66:789–800.
120. Fuentes IM, Christianson JA. 2016. Ion channels, ion channel receptors, and visceral hypersensitivity in irritable bowel syndrome. *Neurogastroenterol Motil* 28:1613–1618.
121. Kon N, Fukada Y. 2015. Cognitive Function and Calcium. Ca2+-dependent regulatory mechanism of circadian clock oscillation and its relevance to neuronal function. *Clin Calcium* 25:201–208.
122. Ikeda M. 2004. Calcium dynamics and circadian rhythms in suprachiasmatic nucleus neurons. *Neuroscientist* 10:315–324.
123. Wu H, Wang D, Meng Y, Ning H, Liu X, Xie Y, Cui L, Wang S, Xu X, Peng R. 2017. Activation of TLR signalling regulates microwave radiation-mediated impairment of spermatogenesis in rat testis. *Andrologia* Aug 6. doi: 10.1111/and.12828.
124. Glushkova OV, Khrenov MO, Novoselova TV, Lunin SM, Fesenko EE, Novoselova EG. 2015. The role of CK2 protein kinase in stress response of RAW 264.7 macrophages. *Dokl Biol Sci* 464:260–262.
125. He GL, Liu Y, Li M, Chen CH, Gao P, Yu ZP, Yang XS. 2014. The amelioration of phagocytic ability in microglial cells by curcumin through the inhibition of EMF-induced pro-inflammatory responses. *J Neuroinflammation* Mar 19;11:49. doi: 10.1186/1742-2094-11-49.
126. Khrenov MO, Cherenkov DA, Glushkova OV, Novoselova TV, Lunin SM, Parfeniuk SB, Lysenko EA, Novoselova EG, Fesenko EE. 2007. The role of transcription factors in the response of mouse lymphocytes to low-level electromagnetic and laser radiations [foreign-language]. *Biofizika* 52:888–892.
127. Natarajan M, Vijayalaxmi, Szzliagyl M, Roldan FN, Meltz ML. 2002. NF-kappaB DNA-binding activity after high peak power pulsed microwave (8.2 GHz) exposure of normal human monocytes. *Bioelectromagnetics* 23:271–277.
128. Sies H, Berndt C, Jones DP. 2017. Oxidative Stress. *Annu Rev Biochem* Jun 20;86:715–748.
129. Karin M, Greten FR. 2005. NF-kappaB: Linking inflammation and immunity to cancer development and progression. *Nat Rev Immunol* 5:749–759.
130. Luo JL, Kamata H, Karin M. 2005. IKK/NF-kappaB signaling: Balancing life and death--a new approach to cancer therapy. *J Clin Invest* 115:2625–2632.

131. Bhaumik D, Scott GK, Schokrpur S, Patil CK, Campisi J, Benz CC. 2008. Expression of microRNA-146 suppresses NF-kappaB activity with reduction of metastatic potential in breast cancer cells. *Oncogene* 27:5643–5647.
132. Bassères DS, Baldwin AS. 2006. Nuclear factor-kappaB and inhibitor of kappaB kinase pathways in oncogenic initiation and progression. *Oncogene* 25:6817–6830.
133. Naugler WE, Karin M. 2008. NF-kappaB and cancer-identifying targets and mechanisms. *Curr Opin Genet Dev* 18:19–26.
134. Ali F, Khan BA, Sultana S. 2016. Wedelolactone mitigates UVB induced oxidative stress, inflammation and early tumor promotion events in murine skin: Plausible role of NFκB pathway. *Eur J Pharmacol* 786:253–264.
135. Bissell MJ, Radisky D. 2001. Putting tumours in context. *Nat Rev Canc* 1:46–54.
136. Trosko JE, Ruch RJ. 2002. Gap junctions as targets for cancer chemoprevention and chemotherapy. *Cur Drug Targets* 3:465–482.
137. Cronier L, Crespin S, Strale PO, Defamie N, Mesnil M. 2009. Gap junctions and cancer: New functions for an old story. *Antioxid Redox Signal* 11:323–338.
138. Kessenbrock K, Plaks V, Werb Z. 2010. Matrix metalloproteinases: Regulators of the tumor microenvironment. *Cell* 141:52–67.
139. Noël A, Jost M, Maquoi E. 2008. Matrix metalloproteinases at cancer tumor-host interface. *Semin Cell Dev Biol* 19:52–60.
140. Jabłońska-Trypuć A, Matejczyk M, Rosochacki S. 2016. Matrix metalloproteinases (MMPs), the main extracellular matrix (ECM) enzymes in collagen degradation, as a target for anticancer drugs. *J Enzyme Inhib Med Chem* 31(Suppl 1):177–183.
141. Kurzepa J, Kurzepa J, Golab P, Czerska S, Bielewicz J. 2014. The significance of matrix metalloproteinase (MMP)-2 and MMP-9 in the ischemic stroke. *Int J Neurosci* 124:707–716.
142. Rosenberg GA, Yang Y. 2007. Vasogenic edema due to tight junction disruption by matrix metalloproteinases in cerebral ischemia. *Neurosurg Focus.* May 15;22(5):E4.
143. Hsieh HL, Chi PL, Lin CC, Yang CC, Yang CM. 2014. Up-regulation of ROS-dependent matrix metalloproteinase-9 from high-glucose-challenged astrocytes contributes to the neuronal apoptosis. *Mol Neurobiol* 50:520–533.
144. Shirato K, Takanari J, Ogasawara J, Sakurai T, Imaizumi K, Ohno H, Kizaki T. 2016. Enzyme-treated asparagus extract attenuates hydrogen peroxide-induced matrix metalloproteinase-9 expression in murine skin fibroblast L929 cells. *Nat Prod Commun 2016* 11:677–680.
145. Rempe RG, Hartz AM, Bauer B. 2016. Matrix metalloproteinases in the brain and blood-brain barrier: Versatile breakers and makers. *J Cereb Blood Flow Metab* 36:1481–1507.
146. Brown GT, Murray G. 2015. Current mechanistic insights into the roles of matrix metalloproteinases in tumour invasion and metastasis. *J Pathol* 237:273–281.
147. Pall ML. 1981. Gene-amplification model of carcinogenesis. *Proc Natl Acad Sci U S A* 78:2465–2468.
148. Hayashi K, Makino R, Kakizoe T, Fujiki H, Sugimura T. 1983. Increase in frequency of appearance of cadmium-resistant cells induced by various tumor promoters; evidence for the induction of gene amplification. *Princess Takamatsu Symp* 14:255–259.
149. Hayashi K, Fujiki H, Sugimura T. 1983. Effects of tumor promoters on the frequency of metallothionein I gene amplification in cells exposed to cadmium. *Cancer Res* 43:5433–5436.
150. Herschman HR. 1985. A 12-O-tetradecanoylphorbol-13-acetate (TPA)-nonproliferative variant of 3T3 cells is resistant to TPA-enhanced gene amplification. *Mol. Cell. Biol* 5:1130–1135.
151. Yamagishi H, Kunisada T, Toda M, Ohnishi N, Fujiki H, Sekiguchi T. 1985. Tumor promoters may induce the appearance of extrachromosomal circular DNAs in rodent cell lines. *Biomed Res* 5:405–412.

152. Matz B, Schlehofer JR, Zur Hausen H, Huber B, Fanning E. 1985. HSV- and chemical carcinogen-induced amplification of SV40 DNA sequences in transformed cells is cell-line-dependent. *Int J Cancer* 35:521–525.
153. Alexander JL, Orr-Weaver TL. 2016. Replication fork instability and the consequences of fork collisions from rereplication. *Genes Dev* 30:2241–2252.
154. Mondello C, Smirnova A, Giulotto E. 2010. Gene amplification, radiation sensitivity and DNA double-strand breaks. *Mutat Res* 704:29–37.
155. Myllykangas S, Knuutila S. 2006. Manifestation, mechanisms and mysteries of gene amplifications. *Cancer Lett.* 232:79–89.
156. Morrical SW. 2015. DNA-pairing and annealing processes in homologous recombination and homology-directed repair. *Cold Spring Harb Perspect Biol* Feb 2;7(2):a016444. doi: 10.1101/cshperspect.a016444.
157. White C. 2017. The Regulation of Tumor Cell Invasion and Metastasis by Endoplasmic Reticulum-to-Mitochondrial Ca2+ Transfer. *Front Oncol* Aug 10;7:171. doi: 10.3389/fonc.2017.00171. eCollection 2017.
158. Cui C, Merritt R, Fu L, Pan Z. 2017. Targeting calcium signaling in cancer therapy. *Acta Pharm Sin B* 7:3–17.
159. Marchi S, Pinton P. 2016. Alterations of calcium homeostasis in cancer cells. *Curr Opin Pharmacol* 29:1–6.
160. Chen YF, Hsu KF, Shen MR. 2016. The store-operated Ca(2+) entry-mediated signaling is important for cancer spread. *Biochim Biophys Acta* 1863(6 Pt B):1427–1435.
161. Jardin I, Rosado JA. 2016. STIM and calcium channel complexes in cancer. *Biochim Biophys Acta* 1863(6 Pt B):1418–1426.
162. Moccia F, Zuccolo E, Poletto V, Turin I, Guerra G, Pedrazzoli P, Rosti V, Porta C, Montagna D. 2016. Targeting Stim and Orai proteins as an alternative approach in anticancer therapy. *Curr Med Chem* 23:3450–3480.
163. Déliot N, Constantin B. 2015. Plasma membrane calcium channels in cancer: Alterations and consequences for cell proliferation and migration. *Biochim Biophys Acta* 1848(10 Pt B):2512–2522.
164. Parkash J, Asotra K. 2010. Calcium wave signaling in cancer cells. *Life Sci* 87:587–595.
165. Dziegielewska B, Gray LS, Dziegielewski J. 2014. T-type calcium channels blockers as new tools in cancer therapies. *Pflugers Arch* 466:801–810.
166. Mignen O, Constantin B, Potier-Cartereau M, Penna A, Gautier M, Guéguinou M, Renaudineau Y et al. 2017. Constitutive calcium entry and cancer: Updated views and insights. *Eur Biophys J* 46:395–413.
167. Kania E, Roest G, Vervliet T, Parys JB, Bultynck G. 2017. IP3 Receptor-Mediated Calcium Signaling and Its Role in Autophagy in Cancer. *Front Oncol* Jul 5;7:140. doi: 10.3389/fonc.2017.00140. eCollection 2017.
168. Padányi R, Pászty K, Hegedűs L, Varga K, Papp B, Penniston JT, Enyedi Á. 2016. Multifaceted plasma membrane Ca(2+) pumps: From structure to intracellular Ca(2+) handling and cancer. *Biochim Biophys Acta* 1863(6 Pt B):1351–1363.
169. Bechetti A. 2011. Ion channels and transporters in cancer. 1. Ion channels and cell proliferation in cancer. *Am J Physiol Cell Physiol* 301:C255–C265.
170. Sharma B, Kanwar SS. 2017. Phosphatidylserine: A cancer cell targeting biomarker. *Semin Cancer Biol* Sep 1. pii: S1044-579X(17)30058-5.
171. Birge RB, Boeltz S, Kumar S, Carlson J, Wanderley J, Calianese D, Barcinski M et al. 2016. Phosphatidylserine is a global immunosuppressive signal in efferocytosis, infectious disease, and cancer. *Cell Death Differ* 23:962–978.
172. Gu Y, Zheng W, Zhang J, Gan X, Ma X, Meng Z, Chen T et al. 2016. Aberrant activation of CaMKIIγ accelerates chronic myeloid leukemia blast crisis. *Leukemia* 30:1282–1289.

173. Wang YY, Zhao R, Zhe H. 2015. The emerging role of CaMKII in cancer. *Oncotarget* 6:11725–11734.
174. Marcelo KL, Means AR, York B. 2016. The Ca(2+)/Calmodulin/CaMKK2 Axis: Nature's metabolic CaMshaft. *Trends Endocrinol Metab* 27:706–718.
175. Monaco S, Rusciano MR, Maione AS, Soprano M, Gomathinayagam R, Todd LR, Campiglia P et al. 2015. Ca2+/calmodulin-dependent protein kinase II (CaMKII); CaMKII inhibitor; cancer; cell cycle; therapeutic target. *Cell Signal* 27:204–214.
176. Rusciano MR, Salzano M, Monaco S, Sapio MR, Illario M, De Falco V, Santoro M et al. 2010. The Ca2+-calmodulin-dependent kinase II is activated in papillary thyroid carcinoma (PTC) and mediates cell proliferation stimulated by RET/PTC. *Endocr Relat Cancer* 17:113–123.
177. Hoffman A, Carpenter H, Kahl R, Watt LF, Dickson PW, Rostas JA, Verrills NM, Skelding KA. 2014. Dephosphorylation of CaMKII at T253 controls the metaphase-anaphase transition. *Cell Signal* 26:748–756.
178. Humeau J, Bravo-San Pedro JM, Vitale I, Nuñez L, Villalobos C, Kroemer G, Senovilla L. 2017. Calcium signaling and cell cycle: Progression or death. *Cell Calcium* Jul 25. pii: S0143-4160(17)30061-1.
179. Abd-Rabou AA. 2017. Calcium, a cell cycle commander, drives colon cancer cell diffpoptosis. *Indian J Clin Biochem*. 32:9–18.
180. Anderson ME. 2015. Oxidant stress promotes disease by activating CaMKII. *J Mol Cell Cardiol* 89(Pt B):160–167.
181. Purohit A, Rokita AG, Guan X, Chen B, Koval OM, Voigt N, Neef S et al. 2013. Oxidized Ca(2+)/calmodulin-dependent protein kinase II triggers atrial fibrillation. *Circulation* 128:1748–1757.
182. Gu SX, Blokhin IO, Wilson KM, Dhanesha N, Doddapattar P, Grumbach IM, Chauhan AK, Lentz SR. 2016. Protein methionine oxidation augments reperfusion injury in acute ischemic stroke. *JCI Insight*. 1(7):pii: e86460. Epub 2016 May 19.
183. Anguita E, Villalobo A. 2017. Src-family tyrosine kinases and the Ca2+ signal. *Biochim Biophys Acta* 1864:915–932.
184. Zhao Y, Sudol M, Hanafusa H, Krueger J. 1992. Increased tyrosine kinase activity of c-Src during calcium-induced keratinocyte differentiation. *Proc Natl Acad Sci U S A* 89:8298–8302.
185. Okuda M, Takahashi M, Suero J, Murry CE, Traub O, Kawakatsu H, Berk BC. 1999. Shear stress stimulation of p130(cas) tyrosine phosphorylation requires calcium-dependent c-Src activation. *J Biol Chem* 274:26803–26809.
186. Hu XQ, Singh N, Mukhopadhyay D, Akbarali HI. 1998. Modulation of voltage-dependent Ca2+ channels in rabbit colonic smooth muscle cells by c-Src and focal adhesion kinase. *J Biol Chem* 273:5337–5342.
187. Gui P, Wu X, Ling S, Stotz SC, Winkfein RJ, Wilson E, Davis GE, Braun AP, Zamponi GW, Davis MJ. 2006. Integrin receptor activation triggers converging regulation of Cav1.2 calcium channels by c-Src and protein kinase a pathways. *J Biol Chem* 281:14015–14025.
188. Gulia J, Navedo MF, Gui P, Chao JT, Mercado JL, Santana LF, Davis MJ. 2013. Regulation of L-type calcium channel sparklet activity by c-Src and PKC-α. *Am J Physiol Cell Physiol* 305:C568–C577.
189. Amberg GC, Earley S, Glapa SA. 2010. Local regulation of arterial L-type calcium channels by reactive oxygen species. *Circ Res* 107:1002–1010.
190. Chaplin NL, Nieves-Cintrón M, Fresquez AM, Navedo MF, Amberg GC. 2015. Arterial smooth muscle mitochondria amplify hydrogen peroxide microdomains functionally coupled to L-type calcium channels. *Circ Res* 117:1013–1023.
191. Shaifta Y, Snetkov VA, Prieto-Lloret J, Knock GA, Smirnov SV, Aaronson PI, Ward JP. 2015. Sphingosylphosphorylcholine potentiates vasoreactivity and voltage-gated Ca2+ entry via NOX1 and reactive oxygen species. *Cardiovasc Res* 106:121–130.

192. Howitt L, Kuo IY, Ellis A, Chaston DJ, Shin HS, Hansen PB, Hill CE. 2013. Chronic deficit in nitric oxide elicits oxidative stress and augments T-type calcium-channel contribution to vascular tone of rodent arteries and arterioles. *Cardiovasc Res* 98:449–457.
193. Moretti D, Del Bello B, Allavena G, Maellaro E. 2014. Calpains and cancer: Friends or enemies? *Arch Biochem Biophys* 564:26–36.
194. Storr SJ, Thompson N, Pu X, Zhang Y, Martin SG. 2015. Calpain in breast cancer: Role in disease progression and treatment response. *Pathobiology* 82:133–141.

8 A Summary of Recent Literature (2007–2017) on Neurobiological Effects of Radio Frequency Radiation

Henry Lai

CONTENTS

8.1 INTRODUCTION

Neurological effects are caused by changes in the nervous system. Factors that act directly or indirectly on the nervous system causing morphological, chemical or electrical changes in the nervous system can lead to neurological effects. The final manifestation of these effects can be seen as psychological/behavioral changes, for example, memory, learning, and perception. The nervous system is an electrical organ. Thus, it should not be surprising that exposure to electromagnetic fields could lead to neurological changes. Morphological, chemical, electrical, and behavioral changes have been reported in animals and cells after exposure to nonionizing electromagnetic fields (EMF) across a range of frequencies. The consequences of physiological changes in the nervous system are very difficult to assess. We do not quite understand how the nervous system functions and reacts to external perturbations. The highly flexible nervous system could easily compensate for external disturbances. On the other hand, the consequence of neural perturbation is also situation-dependent. For example, an EMF-induced change in brain electrical activity could lead to different consequences depending on whether a person is watching TV or driving a car.

The following is a summary of the research literature on the neurological effects of exposure to radio frequency radiation (RFR), a part of the EMF spectrum that is used in wireless communications, published between 2007 and 2017. The database came from a survey of the Medline and understandably does not include all the relevant papers published during the period.

8.2 THE STUDIES

There are many new studies on human subjects. Many of them are on changes in brain electrical activities after exposure to cell phone radiation. Bak et al. (2010) (Global System for Mobile Communication [GSM] 935 MHz, 217 Hz pulses, 20 min, 0.0052 mW/cm^2) reported effects on event-related brain potentials. Maganioti et al. (2010) (900 MHz and 1800 MHz, 45 min) further reported that RFR affected the gender-specific components of event-related potentials (see also Hountala et al., 2008). Croft et al. (2008) (GSM 895 MHz, modulated at 217 Hz, 0.11 W/kg over 10 gm tissue, 30 min) reported changes of the alpha wave power of electroencephalogram (EEG). They (Croft et al., 2010) further reported that effects differed between 2-G and 3-G cell phone transmission systems (2-G 894.6 MHz 217-Hz modulation, 0.7 W/kg over 10 gm tissue; 1900-MHz 3-G-modulated signal, 1.7 W/kg over 10 gm tissue; 55 min) on resting alpha activity in young adults. They observed effects after exposure to 2G but not 3G cell phone radiation, whereas Leung et al. (2011) (conditions similar to Croft et al. (2010)) found similar EEG effects (delayed ERD/ERS responses of the alpha power) with both 2G and 3G radiations. However, it is difficult to compare the 2-G and 3-G exposure conditions with different specific absorption rate (SAR) and energy distributions. Ghosn et al. (2015) (GSM 900 MHz, peak SAR 0.93 W/kg, 26 min) also reported GSM EMF affected the alpha band of resting human EEG. Lustenberger et al. (2013) (900 MHz RFR pulsed with 500 msec bursts, spatial peak SAR 0.15 W/kg over 10 gm tissue) found increased slow-wave activity in humans during exposure to pulse-modulated RFR toward the end of the sleep period. Vecchio and associates reported that cell phone RFR affected EEG and the spread of neural synchronization conveyed by inter-hemispherical functional coupling of EEG rhythms (Vecchio et al., 2007) (GSM signal at 902.4 MHz, 8.33 and 217 Hz modulations, peak SAR 0.5 W/kg, 45 min) and modulated event related desynchronization of alpha rhythms and enhanced human cortical neural efficiency (Vecchio et al., 2012a) (exposure conditions same as Vecchio et al., 2007). Nazıroğlu and Gümral (2009) (2450 MHz pulsed at 217 Hz, 1.73 W/kg, 60 min/day for 28 days) reported a significant change in cortical EEG spikes in rats after chronic RFR exposure. RFR exposure modulated the spontaneous low frequency fluctuations in some brain regions (Lv et al., 2014a) (2573 MHz, spatial peak SAR 0.9 and 1.07 W/kg over 10 gm tissue, 30 min) and the synchronization patterns of EEG activation across the whole brain (Lv et al., 2014b) (exposure conditions similar to Lv et al., 2014a) in humans. An interesting finding is that RFR could interact with the activity of brain epileptic foci in epileptic patients (Tombini et al., 2013; Vecchio et al., 2012b). Roggeveen et al. (2015a,b) (1929.1–1939.7 MHz, 0.69 W/kg, 15 min) reported significant changes in several bands of human EEG and detection of radiation peaks when exposed to the RFR from a 3G mobile phone. These effects were observed only when the phone was placed on the ear and not on the heart. Yang et al. (2017) reported a reduction in spectral power in the alpha and beta bands in the frontal and temporal cortical regions of humans exposed to Long-Term Evolution (LTE) cell phone radiation. However, no significant effect on human EEG was reported by Perentos et al. (2007) (continuous wave [CW] RFR 15 min, pulsed RFR 15 min) and Trunk et al. (2013) (1947-MHz 3G UMTS, 1.75 W/kg 2 cm from surface of head model, 30 min), Trunk et al. (2014) (1947-MHz 3G UMTS signals, peak SAR 1.75 W/kg, 15 min)), and Kleinlogel et al. (2008a,b) (1950 MHz UMTS (SAR 0.1 and 1 W/kg) and pulsed 900 MHz GSM (1 W/kg), ~30 min) also reported no significant effects on resting EEG and event-related potentials in humans after exposure to cell phone RFR. Furthermore, Krause et al. (2007) (902 MHz CW or pulsed at 217 Hz, pulse width 0.577 msec, averaged SAR 0.738 W/kg over 10 gm of tissue, peak 1.18 W/kg) reported no significant effect of cell phone radiation on brain oscillatory activity, and Inomata-Terada et al. (2007) (800 MHz TDMA, 0.054 W/kg over 10 gm of tissue, 30 min) concluded that cell phone radiation does not affect the electrical activity of the motor cortex.

There are studies on the effects of cell phone radiation on EEG during sleep. Changes in sleep EEG have been reported by Hung et al. (2007) (GSM 900 MHz, SAR over 10 gm of tissue varied from <0.001 to 0.133 W/kg depending the mode the cell phone was in, during sleep), Loughran et al. (2012) (894.6 MHz pulse-modulated at 217 Hz, peak spatial SAR 0.674 W/kg over 10 gm of tissue, 30 min prior to sleep), Lowden et al. (2011) (GSM 884 MHz, spatial peak SAR 1.4 W/kg, 3 hr prior to sleep), Regel et al. (2007) (pulse-modulated GSM 900 MHz signal, 0.2 or 5 W/kg, 30 min prior to sleep), and Schmid et al. (2012a,b) (900 MHz modulated at 2 Hz, 2 W/kg). No significant effect was reported by Fritzer et al. (2007) (GSM 900 with 2, 8, 217, 1733 Hz modulations, peak SAR within head 1 W/kg, during sleep), Mohler et al. (2010, 2012) (no details on exposure conditions), and Nakatani-Enomoto et al. (2013) (W-CDMA-like signal, SAR over 10 gm tissue in the head and brain 1.52 and 0.13 W/kg, respectively, 3 hr). Loughran et al. (2012) provided an interesting conclusion in their paper: "These results confirm previous findings of mobile phone-like emissions affecting the EEG during non-rapid eye movement (REM) sleep. Importantly, this low level effect was also shown to be sensitive to individual variability. Furthermore, this indicates that "previous negative results are not strong evidence for a lack of an effect…". More recently, Lustenberger et al. (2015) (900 MHz, 2 Hz pulse, peak spatial SAR 2 W/kg over 10 gm tissue, 30 min) reported pulsed-RFR-exposure-related increases in delta-theta EEG frequency range in several fronto-central brain areas in humans during non-REM sleep. Increase in REM sleep (Pelletier et al., 2013) (CW 900 MHz, 1 V/m, 0.0001–0.0003 W/kg, 5 weeks) and increases in duration and frequency of slow-wave sleep (Pelletier et al., 2014) (exposure conditions same as Pelletier et al., 2013) have been reported in developing rats after chronic RFR exposure. Mohammed et al. (2013) reported a disturbance in REM sleep EEG in the rat after long term exposure (1 hr/day for 1 month) to a 900-MHz modulated RFR.

Studies on the effects of RFR on the blood-brain barrier continued. Increase in blood-brain barrier permeability in animals after exposure to RFR was first reported in the 1970s. Such change could lead to entry of toxic substances into the brain. On the other hand, the possibility of using RFR to open up the blood-brain barrier to facilitate entry of therapeutic drugs into the brain has also been explored. In the last decade, the Salford group in Sweden continued to confirm their earlier findings on blood-brain barrier permeability and cell death in the brain (Eberhardt et al., 2008; Nittby et al., 2008a, 2009). Effects were observed after a single exposure (2 hr) to RFR at low SAR (0.00012–0.12 W/kg). In the meantime, there are several studies reporting effects of RFR on the blood-brain barrier. Sirav and Seyhan (2009, 2011) reported increased blood-brain barrier permeability in the rat after a 20-min exposure to continuous wave 900 and 1800 MHz RFR. The SARs in the 2011 study were 0.00426 W/kg for 900-MHz and 0.0014 W/kg for 1800 MHz. Interestingly, the effect was observed only in male and not female rats. In a more recent study, Sirav and Seyhan (2016) studied the effects of pulse-modulated (217 Hz, 557 μs) 900-MHz and 1800-MHz RFR at 0.02 W/kg. They reported an increase in blood-brain barrier permeability in male rats after 20 min of exposure to either 900-MHz or 1800-MHz pulsed RFR, whereas an effect was found in female rats only after exposure to the 900-MHz field. Tang et al. (2015) also reported an increase in blood-brain barrier permeability in rats after repeated exposure (14 or 28 days, 3 hr/day) to a 900 MHz field (brain SAR 2 W/kg). They suggested the involvement of the mkp-1/extracellular signal regulated kinase (ERK) for the effect. Wang LF et al. (2015), using an *in vitro* model, reported broadening of tight junctions in ECV304 cells and astrocytes. The authors implied the involvement of the vascular endothelial growth factor (VEGF)/Flk-1-ERK pathway in the effect. There is a related series of experiments on human subjects by Söderqvist et al. (2009a,b,c). The authors reported a leakage of the blood-cerebrospinal fluid barrier and not the brain-brain barrier in subjects exposed to cell phone or cordless phone radiation. There are studies that reported no significant effect of RFR exposure on the blood-brain barrier. Kumlin et al. (2007) reported no neuronal cell death and significant change in the blood-brain barrier in juvenile rats after exposure to RFR (900 MHz, 0.3–3 W/kg, 2 hr/day, 5 days/week, 5 weeks). de Gannes et al. (2009) reported no significant effect on blood-brain barrier permeability and apoptosis of brain cells in rats after a 2 hr exposure to GSM 900 MHz at brain SAR of 0.14 and 20 W/kg. Finnie et al. (2009a,b) also reported no significant effects on the blood-brain barrier (based on expression of the water channel protein AQP-4 in the brain) in mice after exposure to RFR (900 MHz, 4 W/kg, 60 min or 60 min/day, 5 days/week for 104 weeks). More recently, Poulletier de Gannes et al. (2017) reported no significant changes in blood-brain barrier and neuronal degeneration in rats after a single (2 hr) or repeated (2 h/day, 5 days/week for 4 weeks) exposure to GSM-1800 and UMTS-1950 signals up to a brain average SAR of 13 W/kg. However, an increase in albumin leakage was observed at 50 days after exposure in the brain of rats repeatedly exposed to both RF signals at 13 W/kg. Regarding "dark neurons" in the brain of rats exposed to RFR reported by Salford et al. (2003), which is apparently related to change in the blood-brain barrier, there are five reports showing an increase in dark neurons (Eberhardt et al., 2008; Jorge-Mora et al., 2013; Kerimoğlu et al., 2016a; Köktürk et al., 2013; Odacı et al., 2016), whereas de Gannes et al. (2009), Grafström et al. (2008), and Masuda et al. (2009) did not observe such an effect in the brain of RFR-exposed animals.

Related to the blood-brain barrier is a group of studies on astrocyte and microglia. These are cells in the blood-brain barrier that support the endothelial cells that form the barrier. Effects of RFR on these cells could conceivably affect the function of the blood-brain barrier. RFR-induced effects of astrocytes have been reported by

Ammari et al. (2008a, 2010), Brillaud et al. (2007), Choi and Choi (2016), Liu et al. (2012), Lu et al. (2014), Maskey et al. (2010b, 2012), and Zhao et al. (2007), whereas no significant effect was reported by Bouji et al. (2012), Chen et al. (2014), Kumari et al. (2017) and Watilliaux et al. (2011). In studies on microglia, Hao et al. (2010), He et al. (2016), Lu et al. (2014) and Yang et al. (2010) reported effects of RFR exposure, whereas no significant effect was reported by Finnie et al. (2010), Hirose et al. (2010), and Watilliaux et al. (2011).

There are studies on the effects of cell phone radiation and the auditory system. Most research (Bhagat et al., 2016; Gupta et al., 2015; Kwon 2009, 2010a,b; Parazzini et al., 2009; Stefanics et al., 2007, 2008) reported no effects, which seems to agree with the pre-2007 studies in this area. However, there are two reports by Kaprana et al. (2011) and Khullar et al. (2013) showing effects on auditory brainstem response, two papers by Panda et al. (2010, 2011) that concluded: "Long-term and intensive GSM and Code-Division Multiple Access (CDMA) mobile phone use may cause damage to cochlea as well as the auditory cortex.," and a paper (Mandalà et al., 2014) reporting an effect on auditory-evoked cochlear nerve response. Maskey and Kim (2014) reported a decrease in neurotrophins that are important in the regulation of neuron survival in the superior olivary complex, a neural component of the auditory system, in mice after chronic exposure to RFR. Velayutham et al. (2014) reported hearing loss in cell phone users and Sudan et al. (2013) observed weak associations between cell phone use and hearing loss in children at age 7. These effects may not be caused by the radiation. However, there is a study (Seckin et al., 2014) showing structural damage in the cochlea of the rat after prenatal exposure to RFR. And Özgür et al. (2015) reported neuronal degeneration in the cochlear nucleus of the auditory system in the rat after chronic exposure to RFR. Kwon et al. (2010b) reported that short-term exposure to cell phone radiation did not significantly affect the transmission of sensory stimuli from the cochlea to the midbrain along the auditory nerve and brainstem auditory pathways, and (Kwon et al., 2010a) no significant effect on auditory sensory memory in children. More recently, Çeliker et al. (2017) also reported no significant change in auditory brainstem responses, but increases in neuronal degeneration and apoptosis in the cochlear nucleus in rats exposed to a 2100-MHz field for 30 days.

There are several studies that showed neurological changes in humans after use of wireless devices, but those changes apparently were not caused by exposure to the radiation. Abramson et al. (2009) reported changes in cognitive functions in young adolescents. ("The accuracy of working memory was poorer, reaction time for a simple learning task shorter, associative learning response time shorter and accuracy poorer in children reporting more mobile phone voice calls."). Arns et al. (2007) observed more focused attention in frequent cell phone users, which was probably a "cognitive training effect." Yuan et al. (2011) reported morphological changes in the brain of adolescents with "internet addiction disorder."

There are several studies showing differential effects of different waveforms. This is an important consideration in understanding how EMF interacts with living organisms. Croft et al. (2010) reported that 2G, but not 3G, cell phone radiation affected resting EEG. Hung et al. (2007) showed that 2, 8, 217 Hz-modulated RFR differentially affected sleep. López-Martín et al. (2009) reported that modulated and nonmodulated RFR had different effects on gene expression in the brain. Nylund et al. (2010) found that different carrier frequencies (900 MHz verses 1800 MHz) had different effects on protein expression. Schmid et al. (2012a) concluded that "modulation frequency components (of an RFR) within a physiological range may be sufficient to induce changes in sleep EEG." Mohammed et al. (2013) reported that EEG power spectrum during REM sleep is more susceptible to modulated RFR than the slow wave sleep (SWS). Schneider and Stangassinger (2014) reported different effects of 900-MHz and 1.966-GHz EMFs on social memory functions in the rat. Zhang et al. (2008) reported that an intermittent exposure to RFR had a more potent effect on gene expression in the brain than continuous exposure. Apparently, extremely low frequency (ELF) modulation plays a role in determining the biological effects of RFR. One can find many studies showing the same neurological effects of RFR described above in animals exposed to extremely low frequency electromagnetic field (ELF EMF) (e.g., Carrubba et al., 2007, 2010; Cook et al., 2009; Cui et al., 2012; Perentos et al., 2008). This is of considerable importance, since all cell phone signals are modulated by low frequency components. Furthermore, effects can also depend on the modulation frequency. Bawin et al. (1975) reported an increase in efflux of calcium ions from chick brain tissue after 20 min of exposure to a 147-MHz RFR (1–2 mW/cm^2). The effect occurred when the radiation was sinusoidally amplitude modulated at 6, 9, 11, 16, or 20 Hz, but not at modulation frequencies of 0, 0.5, 3, 25, or 35 Hz. Blackman et al. (1979) also reported a "modulation-frequency window" in RFR-induced calcium ion efflux from brain tissue.

On the neurological effects of RFR, there are many papers published in the last decade indicating that oxidative stress played a role in the effects observed: Akbari et al. (2014), Bodera et al. (2015), Cetin et al. (2014), Dasdag et al. (2009, 2012), Del Vecchio et al. (2009a,b), Deshmukh et al. (2013), Dragicevic et al. (2011), Eser et al. (2013), Gao et al. (2013), Ghazizadeh and Naziroğlu (2014), Hidisoglu et al. (2016), Hu S et al. (2014), Hu (2016), İkinci et al. (2016), Imge et al. (2010), Jing et al. (2012), Kerimoğlu et al. (2016a,b), Kesari et al. (2011), Kim JY et al. (2017), Liu et al. (2011), Maaroufi et al. (2014), Megha et al. (2012), Meral et al. (2007), Motawi et al. (2014), Narayanan et al. (2014), Nazıroğlu and Gümral (2009), Nazıroğlu et al. (2012), Nirwane et al. (2016), Othman et al. (2017), Qin et al. (2014), Saikhedkar et al. (2014), Sharma et al. (2017), Shehu et al. (2016), Sokolovic et al. (2009), Varghese et al. (2017), Xu et al. (2010), Yang et al. (2010), Dragicevic et al. (2011) reported a decrease in mitochondrial free radical production in the hippocampus and cerebral cortex of the mouse after RFR exposure.) There was one study (Poulletier de Gannes et al., 2011) that found no significant oxidative stress in brain cells after exposure to Enhanced Data rate for GSM Evolution (EDGE) signal. Kang et al. (2014) reported that "neither combined RF radiation alone nor combined RF radiation with menadione or H_2O_2 influences the intracellular reactive oxygen species (ROS) level in neuronal cells." The mediating roles of cellular free radicals and oxidative status on the biological effects of EMF are worth looking into. Interestingly, there is a study (Cao et al., 2015) showing that RFR interacts with circadian rhythmicity on antioxidative processes in the rat.

An important issue that has been extensively debated in the media is whether children are more vulnerable to the effect of cell phone radiation than adults. The claim that children have thinner skulls and thus absorb more energy is not valid. And the claim that a child's head absorbs more energy from a cell phone is also debatable. It is quite possible that the pattern of energy distribution of cell phone energy absorption in the head is significantly different between a child and an adult (cf. Christ and Kuster, 2005; Christ et al., 2010; Gandhi et al., 2012). Scientific data on whether a child is biologically more vulnerable to cell phone radiation is sparse. There are several studies that indicate that animals (including humans) of different ages respond differently to cell phone radiation. Bouji et al. (2012) reported differences in neuro-immunity, stress, and behavioral responses to GSM signals between "young adult" (6 weeks old) and "middle age" (12-month old) rats. Croft et al. (2010) showed that GSM signals affected certain electrical activities of the brain in young human adults (19–40 years old), but not in adolescents (13–15 years old) or elderly (55–70 years old) subjects. Leung et al. (2011) reported that performance in a cognitive test was affected by GSM signal in adolescents, but not in young or old human subjects. Noor et al. (2011) reported differences in neurochemical responses to 900-MHz RFR between adult and young rats. And Vecchio et al. (2010) found differences in brain electric activities between young and elderly human subjects responding to GSM signals. It must be pointed out that although these studies reported an age-dependent effect of cell phone radiation, they do not necessarily imply that children are more vulnerable to cell phone radiation than adults. There are several papers showing effects of exposure to RFR during perinatal periods on the development and functions of the nervous system (Aldad et al., 2012; Bas et al., 2013; Cetin et al., 2014; Daniels et al. 2009; Divan et al., 2008, 2011, 2012; Erdem Koç et al., 2016; Gao et al., 2013; Haghani et al., 2013; İkinci et al., 2013; Jing et al., 2012; Köktürk et al., 2013; Lee and Yang, 2014; Odacı et al., 2008, 2013, 2016; Othman et al., 2017; Rağbetli et al., 2009, 2010; Razavinasab et al., 2014; Zareen et al., 2009; Zhang et al., 2015). These studies point to the vulnerability of the development nervous system to RFR. The cerebellum seems to be a structure especially vulnerable to the exposure (Eser et al. 2013; Haghani et al., 2013; Köktürk et al., 2013; Odacı et al., 2016; Rağbetli et al., 2010). Chen et al. (2014) reported that exposure to an 1800-MHz RFR impaired neurite outgrowth of embryonic neural stem cells, which play a critical role in brain development. More recently, Xu et al. (2017) reported that the effect of exposure to an 1800-MHz field on stem and progenitor cell proliferation in the hippocampus of mouse depended on the age of the animal. Stem cells play an important role in embryonic development. And it turns out that they are very sensitive to electric current, particularly in their migration in the body during organogenesis. It has been suggested that electric current can be used as a guidance of migration of stem cells for the treatment of neurodegenerative diseases (Feng et al., 2017). On the other hand, disturbance of stem cells by induced electric currents of electromagnetic fields can cause defects in pre- and postnatal development. This can occur at low intensities of the field. Indeed, there are reports on effects of extremely low frequency (ELF) magnetic and electric fields on stem cells (Bai et al., 2013; Choi et al., 2014; Cho et al., 2012; Kim et al., 2013; Takahashi et al., 2017). ELF EMF is more effective in generating induced electric currents.

With these physiological changes in the brain, what behavioral effects have been reported? Data are summarized in Table 8.1.

TABLE 8.1
Behavioral Effects of Radiofrequency Radiation

	Behavior Studied/Results	Experimental Conditions
	Human studies that showed behavioral effects	
Danker-Hopfe et al. (2015)	Sleep of individuals affected differently- showing both improvements and deteriorations.	GSM 900 MHz and Wideband Code Division Multiple Access (WCDMA)/UMTS, during sleep
de Tommaso et al. (2009)	Reduction in behavioral arousal	GSM 900 MHz, 10 min
Deniz et al. (2017)	Poorer attention in high exposure group	Low (<30 min/day) vs high (>90 min/day) cell phone radiation exposure
Hung et al. (2007)	Sleep latency	GSM 900 MHz with 2, 8, or 217-Hz modulations, 30 min
Leung et al. (2011)	Cognitive functions	2G and 3G cell phone radiation, 10 min
Luria et al. (2009)	Spatial working memory (In a subsequent study (Hareuveny et al., 2011), the authors indicated that some of the effects observed may not be related to RFR exposure.)	GSM phone, 60 min
Lustenberger et al. (2013)	Sleep dependent motor task performance improvement	0.25–0.8 Hz pulsed 900 MHz RFR, all night
Mortazavi et al. (2012)	Decreased reaction time	Cell phone radiation, 10 min
Mortazavi et al. (2013)	Decreased reaction time; poorer short-term memory performance	Occupational exposure to military radar radiation
Movvahedi et al. (2014)	Better short-term memory in elementary school students	Cell phone radiation, 10 min
Redmayne et al. (2013)	Well-being	Use of cellphone and cordless phone
Regel et al. (2007)	Cognitive functions	Pulse modulated GSM 900 MHz signal, 0.2 or 5 W/kg, 30 min
Schoeni et al. (2015)	A change in memory performance	Based on cumulative duration of wireless phone use and RF-EMF dose over one year (GSM and UMTS)
Thomas et al. (2010)	Overall behavioral problems in adolescents	RFR measured by a personal dosimeter over 24 hr

(Continued)

TABLE 8.1 (*Continued*)
Behavioral Effects of Radiofrequency Radiation

	Behavior Studied/Results	Experimental Conditions
Vecchio et al. (2012a)	Better performance in a cognitive motor test	GSM signal at 902.4 MHz, 8.33 and 217 Hz modulations, peak SAR 0.5 W/kg, 45 min
Vecchio et al. (2012b)	Enhanced cognitive motor processes in epileptic patients	GSM phone radiation, 45 min
Vecsei et al. (2013)	Decreased thermal pain perception	UMTS phone-like radiation, 1.75 W/kg, 30 min
Wiholm et al. (2009)	"Virtual" spatial navigation task	884 MHz, peak head SAR 1.4 W/kg, 150 min
Yogesh et al. (2014)	Sleep disturbance, latency, and day dysfunction especially in females	>2 hr/day of mobile phone use
Zheng et al. (2014)	Inattention in adolescents	Use of cell phone >60 min per day
	Human studies that showed no significant behavioral effects	
Calvente et al. (2016)	No definite conclusion can be drawn on cognitive and behavioral functions of 10-year old boys	Environmental RFR 100 kHz to 6 GHz; root mean square 0.286 mW/cm^2; maximum power density 2.76 mW/cm^2
Cinel et al. (2007)	Order threshold task	GSM or unmodulated carrier frequency wave to head, 40 min
Cinel et al. (2008)	Subjective symptoms	GSM or unmodulated carrier frequency wave to head, 40 min
Curcio et al. (2008)	Reaction time task, sequential figure tapping task	GSM (902.4 MHz, 217 Hz modulation, 0.5 W/kg), 3 × 15 min
Curcio et al. (2009)	Objective and subjective vigilance	GSM (902.4 MHz, 8.33 Hz and 217-Hz modulation, 0.5 W/kg), 40 min
Curcio et al. (2012)	Somatosensory task	GSM (902.4 MHz, 8.33 Hz and 217-Hz modulation, 0.5 W/kg), 40 min
Danker-Hopfe et al. (2011)	Effect on sleep	GSM 900 or WCDMA/UMTS, during sleep
Eltiti et al. (2009)	Cognitive functions	GSM 900 or UMTS, 0.001 mW/cm^2, 50 min
Fritzer et al. (2007)	Sleep and cognitive functions	GSM 900 with 2, 8, 217, 1733 Hz modulations, peak SAR within head 1 W/kg, during sleep
Haarala et al. (2007)	Cognitive functions	902 MHz, continuous wave or pulsed (27 Hz, 0.577 ms), head peak SAR 1.18 W/kg, 90 min

(*Continued*)

TABLE 8.1 (*Continued*)
Behavioral Effects of Radiofrequency Radiation

	Behavior Studied/Results	Experimental Conditions
Irlenbusch et al. (2007)	Visual discrimination threshold	GSM 902.4 MHz 217 Hz pulses, 0.1 mW/cm^2, 30 min
Kleinlogel et al. (2008a)	Well-being	1950 MHz UMTS (0.1 and 1 W/kg) or 900 MHz GSM (1 W/kg), 30 min
Kleinlogel et al. (2008b)	Continuous performance test measuring reaction time and false reaction	1950 MHz UMTS (0.1 and 1 W/kg) or 900 MHz GSM (1 W/kg), exposed during measurements
Krause et al. (2007)	Auditory memory task	902 MHz CW or pulsed at 217 Hz, pulse width 0.577 msec, averaged SAR 0.738 W/kg over 10 gm tissue, peak 1.18 W/kg
Kwon et al. (2010a)	Auditory sensory memory in children	GSM 902 MHz pulsed at 217 Hz, temporal lobe peak SAR 1.21 W/kg, average 0.82 W/kg over 10 gm tissue
Loughran et al. (2013)	Cognitive effects and EEG in 11–13 years old adolescents	Modulated GSM 900 (peak SAR 1.4 W/kg or 0.35 W/kg), 30–60 min
Malek et al. (2015)	Cognitive functions in sensitive humans	Pulse-modulated GSM (945 MHZ and 1840 MHz, 28 mW/cm^2) and UMTS (2140 MHz, 38 mW/cm^2), 1 V/m, whole body exposure, Short-term
Mohler et al. (2010, 2012)	Effect on sleep	Environmental far-field RFR and cell and cordless phone radiation
Nakatani-Enomoto et al. (2013)	Effect on sleep	WCDMA, 3 hr
Redmayne et al. (2016)	Cognitive functions in 8–11 years old children	Use of cellular and cordless phone
Riddervold et al. (2008)	Trail making B test	2140 MHz continuous wave and 2140 MHz modulated as UMTS, 45 min
Roser et al. (2016)	No change behavioral problem and concentration capacity	Self-reported and operator-recorded wireless communication device use
Sauter et al. (2011)	Cognitive functions	GSM 900 and WCDMA, 7 hr 15 min in two episodes
Sauter et al. (2015)	Cognitive functions and well-being	Terrestrial Trunked Radio (TETRA) (385 MHz) signals, 2.5 hr
Schmid et al. (2012a)	Cognitive functions	900 MHz pulse modulated at 14 and 217 Hz, peak spatial SAR 2 W/kg, 30 min
Schmid et al. (2012b)	Cognitive functions	900 MHz pulse modulated at 2 Hz, 2 W/kg, 30 min

(*Continued*)

TABLE 8.1 (*Continued*)
Behavioral Effects of Radiofrequency Radiation

	Behavior Studied/Results	Experimental Conditions
Trunk et al. (2013)	Automatic deviance detection processes	1947-MHz 3G UMTS, 1.75 W/kg 2 cm from surface of head model, 30 min
Trunk et al. (2014)	Reaction time to a stimulus	1947-MHz 3G UMTS signals, peak SAR 1.75 W/kg, 15 min
Trunk et al. (2015)	Reaction time to a visual target detection task	1947-MHz UMTS signals, peak SAR 1.75 W/kg, 15 min
Unterlechner et al. (2008)	Attention	UMTS signals, peak SAR 0.63 W/kg at cortex of temporal lobe, 90 min
Wallace et al. (2012)	Cognitive functions	420 MHz TETRA, 0.001 mW/cm^2, 10–50 min, whole body exposure
	Animal studies that showed behavioral effects	
Aldad et al. (2012)	Hyperactive, impaired memory (mouse)	800 and 1900 MHz cell phone radiation, gestation days 1–17 (24 hr/day), tested at 8, 12, and 16 weeks old
Arendash et al. (2010, 2012)	Improved cognitive behavior in mouse model of Alzheimer's disease	918 MHz pulse modulated at 217 Hz, 0.25–1.05 W/kg, 2–6 months or 12 days, 2 hr/day
Banaceur et al. (2013)	Improved cognitive functions in mouse model of Alzheimer's disease	2409 MHz, 1.6 W/kg, 2 hr/day for a month
Barthélémy et al. (2016)	Memory, emotionality, and locomotion in plus maze and open field (rat)	900 MHz modulated at 217 MHz, 15 min (1.5 or 6 W/kg) or 45 min (6 W/kg)
Bouji et al. (2012)	Contextual emotional behavior deficit (rat) (age-dependent effect observed)	900 MHz, 6 W/kg, 15 min
Cammaerts et al. (2012)	Olfactory and/or visual memory deficit in ants	GSM 900 MHz (GSMK modulated), 0.77 V/m, in several periods 1.5–6 days
Cammaerts et al. (2013)	Deterioration of food collection behavior in ants	GSM 900 MHz (GSMK modulated), 0.77 V/m, 180 hr
Cammaerts et al. (2014)	Changes in locomotor and general behaviors in ants	940 MHz pulse-modulated 577 μs width, 0.5–1.5 V/m, 10 min exposure before behavioral observation
Choi and Choi (2016)	Delayed hyperactivity-like behavior (mouse)	Smartphone, 10 min/day, 9–11 weeks
Daniels et al. (2009)	Decreased motor activity and increased grooming (rat)	840 MHz, 6 × 10^{-6} mW/cm^2, pups exposed 3 hr/day from postnatal day 2 to day 14, tested at postnatal day 58

(Continued)

TABLE 8.1 (*Continued*)
Behavioral Effects of Radiofrequency Radiation

	Behavior Studied/Results	Experimental Conditions
Deshmukh et al. (2013)	Impaired cognitive functions (plus maze and water maze) (rat)	900 MHz, 8.47×10^{-5} W/kg, 2 hr/day, 30 days
Deshmukh et al. (2015)	Impaired cognitive functions (plus maze and water maze) (rat)	900 MHz (5.953×10^{-4} W/kg), 1800 MHz (5.835×10^{-4} W/kg), 2450 MHz (6.672×10^{-4} W/kg), 2 hr/day, 180 days
Deshmukh et al. (2016)	Impaired cognitive functions (plus maze and water maze) (rat)	900 MHz (5.953×10^{-4} W/kg), 1800 MHz (5.835×10^{-4} W/kg), 2450 MHz (6.672×10^{-4} W/kg), 2 hr/day, 90 days
Favre (2011)	Induced piping behavior in honeybee workers	Cell phone put close to bee hive
Fragopoulou et al. (2010)	Spatial memory deficit (mouse)	GSM 900 MHz, 0.41–0.98 W/kg, 2 hr/day, 4 days
Hao et al. (2013)	Learning and memory deficit (rat)	916 MHz, 1 mW/cm^2, 6 hr/day, 5 days/week, 10 weeks
Hassanshahi et al. (2017)	Impaired object recognition (rat)	2400 MHz, 12 hr/day, 30 days
Hu et al. (2014)	Spatial memory deficit (rat)	High power microwave, 30 mW/cm^2, average brain SAR 21 W/kg, 15 min/day, 14 days
İkinci et al. (2013)	Learning and memory deficit (rat)	900 MHz, 13th to 21st day of pregnancy, 1 hr/day, offspring tested at 26 days old
Júnior et al. (2014)	Observed stress behavioral patterns (rat)	GSM 180 MHz, 2 V/m, 25 sec every 2 min for 3 days
Kim JH et al. (2017a)	Hyperactivity-like behavior (mouse)	835 MHz, 4 W/kg, 5 hr/day for 12 weeks
Kumar et al. (2009)	Hypoactivity, anxiety behavior (rat)	GSM 900 MHz and 1800 MHz, 50 missed call/day, 4 weeks
Kumari et al. (2017)	Spatial learning deficit and impairment of memory measured by passive avoidance test (mouse)	7.5 KHz magnetic field, 12 or 120 μT, 5 weeks
Kumlin et al. (2007)	Improved spatial learning and memory (rat)	90 MHz, 0.3 or 3 W/kg, 2 hr/day, 5 days/week, 5 weeks
Lee et al. (2015)	Locomotor activity after feeding (fish *Poecilia reticulata* and *Danio rerio*)	RFR from an 1800 MHz cell phone
Li et al. (2015)	Spatial learning and memory deficits (rat)	2.856 MHz 5, 10, 20, or 30 mW/cm^2, 6 min 3 times a week up to 6 weeks
Li et al. (2012)	Spatial learning and memory deficits (rat)	GSM 900 phone, 2 hr/day for 1 month, 0.52–1.08 W/kg

(Continued)

TABLE 8.1 (*Continued*)
Behavioral Effects of Radiofrequency Radiation

	Behavior Studied/Results	Experimental Conditions
Lu et al. (2012)	Spatial memory deficit (rat)	2450 MHz pulsed, 1 mW/cm^2, 3 hr/day, 30 days
Maaroufi et al. (2014)	Spatial learning and memory deficit (rat)	900 MHz, 0.05–0.18 W/cm^2, 1 hr/day, 21 days
Mathur (2008)	Analgesic effect (rat)	73.5 MHz, amplitude modulated at 16 Hz, 0.4 W/kg, 2 hr/day, 45 days
Megha et al. (2012)	Cognitive functions (plus maze and water maze) (rat)	900 MHz (5.953 × 10^{-4} W/kg) or 1800 MHz (5.845 × 10^{-4} W/kg), 2 hr/day, 30 days
Mohammed et al. (2013)	Increased latency of REM sleep (rat)	900 MHz continuous wave, 900 MHz modulated at 8 and 16 Hz, spatial peak SAR 0.245 W/kg, 1 hr/day for 1 month
Narayanan et al. (2009)	Spatial learning and memory deficit (rat)	GSM 900/1800 MHz, 50 missed call/day, 4 weeks
Narayanan et al. (2010)	Passive avoidance deficit (rat)	GSM 900/1800 MHz, 50 missed call/day, 4 weeks
Narayanan et al. (2013)	Elevated plus maze emotionality test deficit (rat)	GSM 900 MHz phone, peak power density 0.1466 mW/cm^2, 1 hr/day for 28 days
Narayanan et al. (2015)	Spatial memory deficit (rat)	GSH 90 MHz phone, peak power density 0.1466 mW/cm^2, 1.15 W/kg, 1 hr/day for 28 days
Nirwane et al. (2016)	Change in social behavior, anxiety behavior, learning impairment (zebrafish)	GSM 900 MHz phone, 1.34 W/kg, 1 hr/day for 14 days
Nittby et al. (2008b)	Reduced memory functions (rat)	GSM 900 MHz, 0.0006 and 0.06 W/kg, 2 hr/week, 55 weeks
Ntzouni et al. (2011)	Non-spatial memory deficit (mouse)	GSM 1800-MHz phone, 022 W/kg, 90 min/day, 17 days
Ntzouni et al. (2013)	Spatial and non-spatial memory deficit (mouse)	GSM 1800-MHz phone, 011 W/kg, 90 min/day, 66–148 days
Odacı et al. (2013)	Motor function (rat)	900 MHz, 10 V/m, exposed 1 hr/day from day 13 to day 21 of pregnancy, offspring tested at 21 days of age
Othman et al. (2017)	Anxiety and deficits in neuromotor maturation mainly in male offspring (rat)	2450 MHz, 2 hr/day from conception to parturition, offspring tested at 28, 30 and 31 days of age
Pelletier et al. (2013)	Food intake increase; changes in sleep parameters; increased food intake (rat)	900 MHz, 1 V/m, 0.3–0.1 W/kg depending on age, 23.5 hr/day, 5 weeks

(*Continued*)

TABLE 8.1 (*Continued*)
Behavioral Effects of Radiofrequency Radiation

	Behavior Studied/Results	Experimental Conditions
Pelletier et al. (2014)	Preferred to sleep in a different temperature environment than controls; sleep parameters (rat)	900 MHz, 1 V/m, 0.3–0.1 W/kg depending on age, 23.5 hr/day, 5 weeks
Qiao et al. (2014)	Spatial memory deficit (rat)	2856 MHz, 30 mW/cm^2, 14 W/kg, 5 min
Qin et al. (2014)	Learning and memory deficits (mouse)	1800 MHz, 0.208 mW/cm^2, 2 hr/day, 30 days
Razavinasab et al. (2014)	Passive avoidance and spatial learning and memory deficits (rat)	900 MHz pulsed RFR, 0.3–0.9 W/kg, 6 hr/day from conception to birth, tested at 30 days of age
Saikhedkar et al. (2014)	Learning and memory deficits (rat)	900 MHz phone, 0.9 W/kg, 4 hr/day, 15 days
Sarapultseva et al. (2014)	Motor activity (protozoa *Spirostomum ambiguum*)	1000 MHz or 10,000 MHz, 0.005–0.05 mW/cm^2, 0.05–10 hr
Schneider and Stangassinger (2014)	Social memory effect (rat)	GSM 900 MHz and UMTS 1966 MHz, 0.4 W/kg, up to 6 months
Sharma et al. (2014)	Spatial learning memory deficit (mouse)	10,000 MHz, 0.25 mW/cm^2, 0.179 W/kg, 2 hr/day, 30 days
Sharma et al. (2017)	Spatial learning and memory deficit (mouse)	10,000 MHz, 0.25 mW/cm^2, 0.179 W/kg, 2 hr/day, 15 days
Shehu et al. (2016)	Anxiety-like behavior (rat)	GSM 900/1800 phones, 10 min call per day for 4 weeks
Sokolovic et al. (2012)	Anxiety-related behavior (rat)	GSM 900 phone, 9.88–13.356 V/m, 0.43–0.135 W/kg, 4 hr/day for 20, 40, 60 days
Tang et al. (2015)	Spatial long term memory deficit (rat)	900 MHz, 1 mW/cm^2, 0.016 W/kg, 3 hr/day for 14–28 days
Vácha et al. (2009)	Magnetoreception disruption (cockroach)	Onset of disruption: 1.2 MHz 12–18 nT; 2.4 MHz 18–44 nT
Varghese et al. (2017)	Learning and memory deficits and expression of anxiety behavior (rat)	2450 MHz, 4 hr/day for 45 days; at power density of 0.778 mW/cm^2, calculated power absorption in the body = 0.04728 W
Wang H et al. (2013)	Spatial memory deficit (rat)	Pulsed 2856 MHz RFR, 5, 10, and 50 mW/cm^2, 6 min
Wang H et al. (2015)	Spatial learning and memory deficits (rat)	Pulsed 2856 MHz RFR, 50 mW/cm^2, 6 min
Wang H et al. (2017)	Spatial learning and memory deficits (rat)	2856 MHz (1.75, 3.5, or 7 W/kg), 6 min/day, 5 days/week, 6 weeks
Wang K et al. (2017)	Increased recognition memory (mouse)	1800 MHz, >2.2 W/kg, 30 min

(*Continued*)

TABLE 8.1 (*Continued*)
Behavioral Effects of Radiofrequency Radiation

	Behavior Studied/Results	Experimental Conditions
Wang LF et al. (2016)	Spatial memory impairment (rat)	GSM 1800 MHz, 30 mW/cm^2, 5 min/day, 5 days /week, 2 months
Zhang et al. (2015)	Increased anxiety-related behavior; spatial memory and learning deficits in male offspring (mouse)	9417 MHz, 200 V/m, 2 W/kg, 12 hr/day on gestation days 3.5–18, offspring tested at 5 weeks of age
Zhang et al. (2017)	Increased anxiety-related behavior (mouse)	1800 MHz, 6 hr/day for 28 days, whole body and brain SAR at 2.7 W/kg and 2.2 W/kg, respectively
	Animal studies that showed no significant behavioral effects	
Ammari et al. (2008b)	Spatial memory (rat)	GSM 900, brain SRR 1.5 W/kg 45 min/day or 6 W/kg 15 min/day, 8 or 24 weeks
Fasseas et al. (2015)	Chemotaxis, short term memory (*Caenorhabditis elegans*)	GSM 1800 MHz (15.4 V/m), WiFi router (9.7 V/m), Digital Enhanced Cordless Telecommunication (DECT) phone (11.3 V/m); various lengths of time (30 min to 24 hr)
Haghani et al. (2013)	Motor function (rat)	Pulsed 900 MHz RFR, SAR 0.5–0.9 W/kg; 6 hr/day during gestation period
Klose et al. (2014)	Learning skills and motor behavior (rat)	GSM-modulated 900 MHz RFR, head only exposure 2 hr/day, 5 days/week from 14 days to 19 months old, 0.7, 2.5 or 10 W/kg
Shirai et al. (2014)	Spatial memory and motor function on F_1, F_2, and F_3 offspring (rat)	2140 MHz WCDMA 20 hr/day from gestation Day 7 to weaning with dam, and offspring alone to 6 weeks old, 3-generations; 0.067–0.14 for a fetus, 0.12–0.36 W/kg for offspring before weaning, 0.12–0.24 W/kg for offspring after weaning
Salunke et al. (2015)	Anxiety, obsessive compulsive disorder (OCD) and depression-like behavior (mouse)	Bluetooth device, 2450 MHz, 60 min/day for 7, 30, 60, 90, or 120 days
Son et al. (2016)	Spatial and nonspatial memory functions (mouse)	1950 MHz; 2 h/day, 5 days/ week, 3 months; 5 W/kg

A majority of the animal studies reported effects, whereas more human studies reported no significant effects. This may be caused by several possible factors: (a) Humans are less susceptible to RFR than are animals. (b) It may be more difficult to do human than animal experiments, since it is, in general, easier to control the variables and confounding factors in an animal experiment. (c) In the animal studies, the cumulative exposure duration was generally longer and studies were carried out after exposure, whereas in the human studies, the exposure was generally one time and testing measurements were carried out mostly during exposure. This raises the question of whether the effects of RFR are cumulative. This consideration could have very important implications on real life human exposure to EMF. However, it must be pointed out that neurophysiological and behavioral changes have been reported in both animals and humans after acute (one time) exposure to RFR, and most of the human EEG studies mentioned above are acute exposure experiments. (d) Most of the human studies are head exposure experiments whereas most of the animal studies involved whole body exposure. Could this have made a difference? Does it mean that effects of RFR on other parts of the body can also affect the nervous system? (e) The nervous system has the capability to adapt to perturbations. Physiological changes in the nervous system do not always manifest as behavioral effects, for example, see Haghani et al. (2013) (changes in electrophysiology of cerebellar Purkinje cells after RFR exposure without behavioral effect in rats) and Schmid et al. (2012a) (RFR exposure induced EEG change but did not affect cognitive test performance in human subjects). It may be that the human brain has higher capability to tolerate and adapt to perturbations than other animals. (f) In the animal studies, the effects studies were mostly learning and memory functions. The hippocampus in the brain, particularly the cholinergic system, plays a major role in learning and memory functions. Various studies indicated that RFR affected electrical activities/morphology/chemistry of the hippocampus in animals (Aboul Ezz et al., 2013; Ammari et al., 2008a,c, 2010; Barcal and Vozeh, 2007; Barthélémy et al., 2016; Bas et al., 2009; Baş et al., 2013; Carballo-Quintás et al., 2011; Choi and Choi, 2016; Erdem Koç et al., 2016; Fragopoulous et al., 2012; Gevrek, 2017; Gökçek-Saraç et al., 2017; Hao et al., 2013; Hassanshahi et al., 2017; Hu et al., 2014; İkinci et al., 2013; Kerimoğlu et al., 2016b; Kesari et al., 2011; Kim JH et al., 2017b; Kim JY et al., 2017; Kumari et al., 2017; Li Y et al., 2012; Li H et al., 2015; López-Martín et al., 2009; Lu et al., 2012; Maskey et al., 2010a,b, 2012; Megha et al., 2015; Mugunthan et al., 2016; Narayanan et al., 2010, 2014, 2015; Ning et al., 2007; Nittby et al., 2008a; Odacı et al., 2008; Rağbetli et al., 2009; Razavinasab et al., 2014; Şahin et al., 2015; Saikhedkar et al., 2014; Sharma et al., 2017; Tang et al., 2015; Tong et al., 2013; Wang H et al., 2013, 2015, 2017; Wang K et al., 2017; Wang LF et al., 2016; Xiong et al., 2015; Xu et al., 2017; Yang et al., 2012; Zhang et al., 2017). As early as 1987, we (Lai et al., 1987) have reported that RFR affected the cholinergic system in the hippocampus of the rat leading to spatial learning and memory deficits. Interestingly, the effect of RFR on the hippocampus apparently involves a sequence of neurological responses in the brain, including activation of endogenous opioids and release of the stress hormone corticotropin releasing factor (Lai, 1994). Thus, it is not surprising that "learning and memory" functions are affected in the rodents by RFR since in most of the studies, the Morris water maze was used to study learning and memory functions. The water maze measures spatial memory, a function that specifically involves the hippocampus. In the human studies listed above, the most common effect studied was cognitive functions. Since the exposure in most of these human studies was localized in the brain, particularly in the temporal cortical area, it is questionable whether the psychological tests used were appropriate.

8.3 DISCUSSION

1. A major concern is that in some of the studies, details of the exposure setup and dosimetry are not provided. This is important since details of the independent variables are very important in interpreting the validity of the experimental results, that is, dependent variables. In many of these studies, a cell phone was used in the exposure of animals and humans. But information on how the cell phone was activated, in many instances, was not provided. Thus, the amount of energy deposited in the body was not known. Some studies used the phone in "stand-by" mode. Mild et al. (2012) reported that when a stationary cell phone is on "stand-by" mode, it actually infrequently emits a very small amount of energy. It is very surprising that in all papers on the effects of RFR on EEG mentioned at the beginning of this paper, only two provided significant information on the exposure parameters. This is alarming. It may indicate that the researchers did not understand the properties of the entity that they were studying. It is good that competent researchers from other disciplines are contributing to the advancement of bioelectromagnetics. But I sincerely think that EMF researchers should get acquainted with the physics of nonionizing electromagnetic fields.
2. Most of the studies were carried out with relatively high levels of RFR compared to environmental levels. However, if you look through the narratives, there are studies that reported effects at very low level, for example, Bak et al., (2010). Indeed, biological/health effects of RFR at levels much lower than most international RFR-exposure guidelines, for example, International Commission on Non-ionizing Radiation Protection (ICNIRP), have been reported (see table 1 in Levitt and Lai, 2010). This raises the question on whether the guidelines used in most countries nowadays are actually obsolete and new exposure guidelines have to be set.
3. Thus, there is ample evidence that RFR exposure affects the nervous system from both acute and long-term exposure experiments. Brain electric activities, nerve cell functions and chemistry, and behavior can be affected. Some explanatory mechanisms for these effects have emerged. One consistent finding is that animals exposed to RFR suffered from memory and learning deficits. These effects can be explained by the results of numerous reports that showed RFR affected the hippocampus, a brain region involved in memory and learning. However, the location and configuration of the human hippocampus are quite different from those of a rodent. There have not been many studies on the effect of RFR on the human hippocampus. Several studies did report deficits in memory in human subjects exposed to RFR, particularly on short-term memory, a function specifically related to

the hippocampus. One recent study (Deniz et al., 2017) showed that chronic cell phone use did not significantly affect the volume of the hippocampus in human subjects. But, the subjects showed poorer attention which is probably not related to the hippocampus. An interesting fact is that learning and memory deficits have also been reported in insects that do not have a hippocampus. Another related aspect is that several papers (Adrendash et al., 2010, 2012; Banaceur et al., 2013; Dragicevic et al., 2011) have indicated that RFR exposure could reverse some of the defects in an animal model of Alzheimer's disease, a neurological disorder involving degeneration of cholinergic innervations in the hippocampus. Interestingly, a similar claim has been reported (Hu et al., 2016) with exposure to extremely low frequency magnetic field.

4. Another very consistent finding is that RFR affects free radical metabolism in the brain. This may explain some of the cellular and physiological effects of RFR on the nervous system. As a matter of fact, oxidative changes in cells and tissues after exposure to RFR is a very common phenomenon (cf. Yakymenko et al., 2016). This happens in many organs of the body and can provide explanation of many reported biological effects of RFR.
5. Many of the effects of RFR on the nervous system, for example, on the hippocampus, oxidative effects, and behavioral effects are also observed with exposure to extremely low frequency electromagnetic field (cf. my section on the neurological effects of ELF EMF in the Bioinitiative Report, www.bioinitiative.info/bioInitiativeReport2012.pdf). There has been speculation whether biological effects observed with low frequency modulated RFR were actually caused by the modulation. There are two reports published in the last decade that seemed to refute this hypothesis. Perentos et al. (2013) reported in human EEG "...a suppression of the global alpha band activity was observed under the pulsed modulated RF exposure, and this did not differ from the continuous RF exposure. No effect was seen in the extremely low frequency condition." This means that pulsing is not essential for the effect observed. Schmid et al. (2012b) compared the effects of a 2-Hz modulated 900-MHz field with a 2-Hz magnetic field on human sleep EEG. Both fields affect sleep EEG, but not identically. The authors concluded that "the study does not support the hypothesis that effects of radio frequency exposure are based on demodulation of the signal only." However, in another study, Schmid et al. (2012a) concluded in a study on sleep EEG "...that modulation frequency components within a physiological range may be sufficient to induce these effects." In our earlier studies (e.g., Lai and Singh, 1995), we found that continuous wave and pulsed RFR produced different effects. Indeed, different effects produced by continuous wave and modulated RFR with the same frequency, exposure conditions, and SAR is a strong indication of the existence of "nonthermal" effects. Another question is whether one type of modulation is different from another in causing biological effects. Cell phone technology advances from one generation to another. Do the research data of a 3G phone apply to 4G or 5G phone radiation? RFR is a complex entity. Its biological effects depend

on many of its physical properties, for example, frequency, direction of the incident waves relative to the object exposed, dielectric properties, size and shape of the exposed object, polarization of the waves, and so on. Thus, it is unlikely that one can easily extrapolate the effects from one form of RFR to another. An assumption that 3G radiation is safe does not necessary imply that 5G radiation is safe. Each one of them has to be investigated separately.

6. An important area of research is on how RFR in the environment affects humans and wildlife. Environmental RFR level has become higher and higher over the past decades due to the employment of RFR wireless devices. Take the example of Bak et al. (2010) mentioned above, an effect on human event-related brain potential was reported after 20 min of exposure to a GSM signal at a power density of 0.0052 mW/cm^2. This is very close to the levels found in some cities. The highest power density of ambient RFR measured near schools and hospitals in Chandigarh, India, was reported to be 0.001148 mW/cm^2 in 2012 (Dhami, 2012). The maximum total RFR power density emitted by FM and TV broadcasting stations and mobile phone base stations in centers of the major cities in the West Bank-Palestine was 0.00386 mW/cm^2 (Lahham and Hammash, 2012). One also has to take into consideration that exposure in the Bak et al. (2010) study was acute (20 min), whereas environmental exposure is chronic. Related to the neurological effect is the magnetic sense possessed by many species of animals. It is essential for their survival. Interference by RFR of magnetic compass orientation in animals has been reported (e.g., Landler et al., 2015; Malkemper et al., 2015; Pakhomov et al., 2017; Schwarze et al., 2016; Vácha et al., 2009). Understanding the effects could help in preserving the ecosystem and ensure survival of the species on this earth.

REFERENCES

Aboul Ezz HS, Khadrawy YA, Ahmed NA, Radwan NM, El Bakry MM. The effect of pulsed electromagnetic radiation from mobile phone on the levels of monoamine neurotransmitters in four different areas of rat brain. *Eur Rev Med Pharmacol Sci.* 17:1782–1788, 2013.

Abramson MJ, Benke GP, Dimitriadis C, Inyang IO, Sim MR, Wolfe RS, Croft RJ. Mobile telephone use is associated with changes in cognitive function in young adolescents. *Bioelectromagnetics.* 30:678–686, 2009.

Akbari A, Jelodar G, Nazifi S. Vitamin C protects rat cerebellum and encephalon from oxidative stress following exposure to radiofrequency wave generated by a BTS antenna model. *Toxicol Mech Methods.* 24:347–352, 2014.

Aldad TS, Gan G, Gao XB, Taylor HS. Fetal radiofrequency radiation exposure from 800–1900 MHz-rated cellular telephones affects neurodevelopment and behavior in mice. *Sci Rep.* 2:312, 2012.

Ammari M, Brillaud E, Gamez C, Lecomte A, Sakly M, Abdelmelek H, de Seze R. Effect of a chronic GSM 900 MHz exposure on glia in the rat brain. *Biomed Pharmacother.* 62:273–281, 2008a.

Ammari M, Gamez C, Lecomte A, Sakly M, Abdelmelek H, De Seze R. GFAP expression in the rat brain following sub-chronic exposure to a 900 MHz electromagnetic field signal. *Int J Radiat Biol.* 86:367–375, 2010.

Ammari M, Jacquet A, Lecomte A, Sakly M, Abdelmelek H, de Seze R. Effect of head-only sub-chronic and chronic exposure to 900-MHz GSM electromagnetic fields on spatial memory in rats. *Brain Inj.* 22:1021–1029, 2008b.

Ammari M, Lecomte A, Sakly M, Abdelmelek H, de-Seze R. Exposure to GSM 900 MHz electromagnetic fields affects cerebral cytochrome c oxidase activity. *Toxicol.* 250:70–74, 2008c.

Arendash GW, Mori T, Dorsey M, Gonzalez R, Tajiri N, Borlongan C. Electromagnetic treatment to old Alzheimer's mice reverses β-amyloid deposition, modifies cerebral blood flow, and provides selected cognitive benefit. *PLoS One.* 7:e35751, 2012.

Arendash GW, Sanchez-Ramos J, Mori T, Mamcarz M, Lin X, Runfeldt M, Wang L et al. Electromagnetic field treatment protects against and reverses cognitive impairment in Alzheimer's disease mice. *J Alzheimers Dis.* 19:191–210, 2010.

Arns M, Van Luijtelaar G, Sumich A, Hamilton R, Gordon E. Electroencephalographic, personality, and executive function measures associated with frequent mobile phone use. *Int J Neurosci.* 117:1341–1360, 2007.

Bai WF, Xu WC, Feng Y, Huang H, Li XP, Deng CY, Zhang MS. Fifty-Hertz electromagnetic fields facilitate the induction of rat bone mesenchymal stromal cells to differentiate into functional neurons. *Cytotherapy.* 15:961–970, 2013.

Bak M, Dudarewicz A, Zmyślony M, Sliwinska-Kowalska M. Effects of GSM signals during exposure to event related potentials (ERPs). *Int J Occup Med Environ Health.* 23:191–199, 2010.

Banaceur S, Banasr S, Sakly M, Abdelmelek H. Whole body exposure to 2.4 GHz WIFI signals: Effects on cognitive impairment in adult triple transgenic mouse models of Alzheimer's disease (3xTg-AD). *Behav Brain Res.* 240:197–201, 2013.

Barcal J, Vozeh F. Effect of whole-body exposure to high-frequency electromagnetic field on the brain cortical and hippocampal activity in mouse experimental model. *NeuroQuantology.* 5:292–302, 2007.

Barthélémy A, Mouchard A, Bouji M, Blazy K, Puigsegur R, Villégier AS. Glial markers and emotional memory in rats following acute cerebral radiofrequency exposures. *Environ Sci Pollut Res Int.* 23:25342–25355, 2016.

Bas O, Odacı E, Kaplan S, Acer N, Ucok K, Colakoglu S. 900 MHz electromagnetic field exposure affects qualitative and quantitative features of hippocampal pyramidal cells in the adult female rat. *Brain Res.* 1265:178–185, 2009.

Baş O, Sönmez OF, Aslan A, İkinci A, Hancı H, Yıldırım M, Kaya H, Akça M, Odacı E. Pyramidal cell loss in the cornu ammonis of 32-day-old female rats following exposure to a 900 megahertz electromagnetic field during prenatal days 13–21. *NeuroQuantology.* 11:591–599, 2013.

Bawin SM, Kaczmarek LK, Adey WR. Effects of modulated VHF fields on the central nervous system. *Annals NY Acad Sci.* 247:74–81, 1975.

Bhagat S, Varshney S, Bist SS, Goel D, Mishra S, Jha VK. Effects on auditory function of chronic exposure to electromagnetic fields from mobile phones. *Ear Nose Throat J.* 95:E18–E22, 2016.

Blackman CF, Elder JA, Weil CM, Benane SG, Eichinger DC, House DE. Induction of calcium-ion efflux from brain tissue by radio-frequency radiation: Effects of modulation frequency and field strength. *Radio Sci.* 14(6S):93–98, 1979.

Bodera P, Stankiewicz W, Antkowiak B, Paluch M, Kieliszek J, Sobiech J, Niemcewicz M. Influence of electromagnetic field (1800 MHz) on lipid peroxidation in brain, blood, liver and kidney in rats. *Int J Occup Med Environ Health.* 28:751–759, 2015.

Bouji M, Lecomte A, Hode Y, de Seze R, Villégier AS. Effects of 900 MHz radiofrequency on corticosterone, emotional memory and neuroinflammation in middle-aged rats. *Exp Gerontol.* 47:444–451, 2012.

Brillaud E, Piotrowski A, de Seze R. Effect of an acute 900 MHz GSM exposure on glia in the rat brain: A time-dependent study. *Toxicology*. 238:23–33, 2007.

Calvente I, Pérez-Lobato R, Núñez MI, Ramos R, Guxens M, Villalba J, Olea N, Fernández MF. Does exposure to environmental radiofrequency electromagnetic fields cause cognitive and behavioral effects in 10-year-old boys? *Bioelectromagnetics*. 37:25–36, 2016.

Cammaerts MC, De Doncker P, Patris X, Bellens F, Rachidi Z, Cammaerts D. GSM 900 MHz radiation inhibits ants' association between food sites and encountered cues. *Electromagn Biol Med*. 31:151–165, 2012.

Cammaerts MC, Rachidi Z, Bellens F, De Doncker P. Food collection and response to pheromones in an ant species exposed to electromagnetic radiation. *Electromagn Biol Med*. 32:315–332, 2013.

Cammaerts M-C, Vandenbosch GAE, Volski V. Effect of short-term GSM radiation at representative levels in society on a biological model: The ant Myrmica sabuleti. *J Insect Beh*. 27:514–526, 2014.

Cao H, Qin F, Liu X, Wang J, Cao Y, Tong J, Zhao H. Circadian rhythmicity of antioxidant markers in rats exposed to 1.8 GHz radiofrequency fields. *Int J Environ Res Public Health*. 12:2071–2087, 2015.

Carballo-Quintás M, Martínez-Silva I, Cadarso-Suárez C, Alvarez-Figueiras M, Ares-Pena FJ, López-Martín E. A study of neurotoxic biomarkers, c-fos and GFAP after acute exposure to GSM radiation at 900 MHz in the picrotoxin model of rat brains. *Neurotoxicology*. 32:478–494, 2011.

Carrubba S, Frilot C, Chesson AL, Marino AA. Nonlinear EEG activation evoked by low-strength low-frequency magnetic fields. *Neurosci Lett*. 417:212–216, 2007.

Carrubba S, Frilot C 2nd, Chesson AL Jr, Marino AA. Mobile-phone pulse triggers evoked potentials. *Neurosci Lett*. 469:164–168, 2010.

Çeliker M, Özgür A, Tümkaya L, Terzi S, Yılmaz M, Kalkan Y, Erdoğan E. Effects of exposure to 2100 MHz GSM-like radiofrequency electromagnetic field on auditory system of rats. *Braz J Otorhinolaryngol*. 83:691–696, 2017.

Cetin H, Nazıroğlu M, Celik O, Yüksel M, Pastacı N, Ozkaya MO. Liver antioxidant stores protect the brain from electromagnetic radiation (900 and 1800 MHz)-induced oxidative stress in rats during pregnancy and the development of offspring. *J Matern Fetal Neonatal Med*. 27:1915–1921, 2014.

Chen C, Ma Q, Liu C, Deng P, Zhu G, Zhang L, He M et al. Exposure to 1800 MHz radiofrequency radiation impairs neurite outgrowth of embryonic neural stem cells. *Sci Rep*. 4:5103, 2014.

Cho H, Seo YK, Yoon HH, Kim SC, Kim SM, Song KY, Park JK. Neural stimulation on human bone marrow-derived mesenchymal stem cells by extremely low frequency electromagnetic fields (ELF-EMFs). *Biotechnol Prog*. 28:1329–1335, 2012.

Choi Y-J, Choi Y-S. Effects of electromagnetic radiation from smartphones on learning ability and hippocampal progenitor cell proliferation in mice. *Osong Pub Health Res Persp*. 7:12–17, 2016.

Choi YK, Lee DH, Seo YK, Jung H, Park JK, Cho H. Stimulation of neural differentiation in human bone marrow mesenchymal stem cells by extremely low-frequency electromagnetic fields incorporated with MNPs. *Appl Biochem Biotechnol*. 174:1233–1245, 2014.

Christ A, Gosselin MC, Christopoulou M, Kühn S, Kuster N. Age-dependent tissue-specific exposure of cell phone users. *Phys Med Biol*. 55:1767–1783, 2010.

Christ A, Kuster N. Differences in RF energy absorption in the heads of adults and children. *Bioelectromagnetics*. (Suppl 7):S31–S44, 2005.

Cinel C, Boldini A, Russo R, Fox E. Effects of mobile phone electromagnetic fields on an auditory order threshold task. *Bioelectromagnetics*. 28:493–496, 2007.

Cinel C, Russo R, Boldini A, Fox E. Exposure to mobile phone electromagnetic fields and subjective symptoms: A double-blind study. *Psychosom Med.* 70:345–348, 2008.

Cook CM, Saucier DM, Thomas AW, Prato FS. Changes in human EEG alpha activity following exposure to two different pulsed magnetic field sequences. *Bioelectromagnetics.* 30:9–20, 2009.

Croft RJ, Hamblin DL, Spong J, Wood AW, McKenzie RJ, Stough C. The effect of mobile phone electromagnetic fields on the alpha rhythm of human electroencephalogram. *Bioelectromagnetics.* 29:1–10, 2008.

Croft RJ, Leung S, McKenzie RJ, Loughran SP, Iskra S, Hamblin DL, Cooper NR. Effects of 2G and 3G mobile phones on human alpha rhythms: Resting EEG in adolescents, young adults, and the elderly. *Bioelectromagnetics.* 31:434–444, 2010.

Cui Y, Ge Z, Rizak JD, Zhai C, Zhou Z, Gong S, Che Y. Deficits in water maze performance and oxidative stress in the hippocampus and striatum induced by extremely low frequency magnetic field exposure. *PLoS One.* 7:e32196, 2012.

Curcio G, Ferrara M, Limongi T, Tempesta D, Di Sante G, De Gennaro L, Quaresima V, Ferrari M. Acute mobile phones exposure affects frontal cortex hemodynamics as evidenced by functional near-infrared spectroscopy. *J Cereb Blood Flow Metab.* 29:903–910, 2009.

Curcio G, Nardo D, Perrucci MG, Pasqualetti P, Chen TL, Del Gratta C, Romani GL, Rossini PM. Effects of mobile phone signals over BOLD response while performing a cognitive task. *Clin Neurophysiol.* 123:129–136, 2012.

Curcio G, Valentini E, Moroni F, Ferrara M, De Gennaro L, Bertini M. Psychomotor performance is not influenced by brief repeated exposures to mobile phones. *Bioelectromagnetics.* 29:237–241, 2008.

Daniels WM, Pitout IL, Afullo TJ, Mabandla MV. The effect of electromagnetic radiation in the mobile phone range on the behaviour of the rat. *Metab Brain Dis.* 24:629–641, 2009.

Danker-Hopfe H, Dorn H, Bahr A, Anderer P, Sauter C. Effects of electromagnetic fields emitted by mobile phones (GSM 900 and WCDMA/UMTS) on the macrostructure of sleep. *J Sleep Res.* 20(1 Pt 1):73–81, 2011.

Danker-Hopfe H, Dorn H, Bolz T, Peter A, Hansen ML, Eggert T, Sauter C. Effects of mobile phone exposure (GSM 900 and WCDMA/UMTS) on polysomnography based sleep quality: An intra- and inter-individual perspective. *Environ Res.* 145:50–60, 2015.

Dasdag S, Akdag MZ, Kizil G, Kizil M, Cakir DU, Yokus B. Effect of 900 MHz radio frequency radiation on beta amyloid protein, protein carbonyl, and malondialdehyde in the brain. *Electromagn Biol Med.* 31:67–74, 2012.

Dasdag S, Akdag MZ, Ulukaya E, Uzunlar AK, Ocak AR. Effect of mobile phone exposure on apoptotic glial cells and status of oxidative stress in rat brain. *Electromagn Biol Med.* 28:342–354, 2009.

de Gannes FP, Billaudel B, Taxile M, Haro E, Ruffié G, Lévêque P, Veyret B, Lagroye I. Effects of head-only exposure of rats to GSM-900 on blood-brain barrier permeability and neuronal degeneration. *Radiat Res.* 172:359–367, 2009.

de Tommaso M, Rossi P, Falsaperla R, Francesco Vde V, Santoro R, Federici A. Mobile phones exposure induces changes of contingent negative variation in humans. *Neurosci Lett.* 464:79–83, 2009.

Del Vecchio G, Giuliani A, Fernandez M, Mesirca P, Bersani F, Pinto R, Ardoino L, Lovisolo GA, Giardino L, Calzà L. Effect of radiofrequency electromagnetic field exposure on *in vitro* models of neurodegenerative disease. *Bioelectromagnetics.* 30:564–572, 2009a.

Del Vecchio G, Giuliani A, Fernandez M, Mesirca P, Bersani F, Pinto R, Ardoino L, Lovisolo GA, Giardino L, Calzà L. Continuous exposure to 900 MHz GSM-modulated EMF alters morphological maturation of neural cells. *Neurosci Lett.* 455:173–177, 2009b.

Deniz OG, Kaplan S, Selcuk MB, Terzi M, Altun, Yurt KK, Aslan K, Davis D. Effects of short and long term electromagnetic fields exposure on the human hippocampus. *J Micros Ultrastru.* 5:191–197, 2017.

Deshmukh PS, Banerjee BD, Abegaonkar MP, Megha K, Ahmed RS, Tripathi AK, Mediratta PK. Effect of low level microwave radiation exposure on cognitive function and oxidative stress in rats. *Indian J Biochem Biophys.* 50:114–119, 2013.

Deshmukh PS, Megha K, Nasare N, Banerjee BD, Ahmed RS, Abegaonkar MP, Tripathi AK, Mediratta PK. Effect of low level subchronic microwave radiation on rat brain. *Biomed Environ Sci.* 29:858–867, 2016.

Deshmukh PS, Nasare N, Megha K, Banerjee BD, Ahmed RS, Singh D, Abegaonkar MP, Tripathi AK, Mediratta PK. Cognitive impairment and neurogenotoxic effects in rats exposed to low-intensity microwave radiation. *Int J Toxicol.* 34:284–290, 2015.

Dhami AK. Study of electromagnetic radiation pollution in an Indian city. *Environ Monit Assess.* 184:6507–6512, 2012.

Divan HA, Kheifets L, Obel C, Olsen J. Prenatal and postnatal exposure to cell phone use and behavioral problems in children. *Epidemiology.* 19:523–529, 2008.

Divan HA, Kheifets L, Obel C, Olsen J. Cell phone use and behavioural problems in young children. *J Epidemiol Community Health.* 66:524–529, 2012.

Divan HA, Kheifets L, Olsen J. Prenatal cell phone use and developmental milestone delays among infants. *Scand J Work Environ Health.* 37:341–348, 2011.

Dragicevic N, Bradshaw PC, Mamcarz M, Lin X, Wang L, Cao C, Arendash GW. Long-term electromagnetic field treatment enhances brain mitochondrial function of both Alzheimer's transgenic mice and normal mice: A mechanism for electromagnetic field-induced cognitive benefit? *Neuroscience.* 185:135–149, 2011.

Eberhardt JL, Persson BR, Brun AE, Salford LG, Malmgren LO. Blood-brain barrier permeability and nerve cell damage in rat brain 14 and 28 days after exposure to microwaves from GSM mobile phones. *Electromagn Biol Med.* 27:215–229, 2008.

Eltiti S, Wallace D, Ridgewell A, Zougkou K, Russo R, Sepulveda F, Fox E. Short-term exposure to mobile phone base station signals does not affect cognitive functioning or physiological measures in individuals who report sensitivity to electromagnetic fields and controls. *Bioelectromagnetics.* 30:556–563, 2009.

Erdem Koç G, Kaplan S, Altun G, Gümüş H, Gülsüm Deniz Ö, Aydin I, Emin Onger M, Altunkaynak Z. Neuroprotective effects of melatonin and omega-3 on hippocampal cells prenatally exposed to 900 MHz electromagnetic fields. *Int J Radiat Biol.* 92:590–595, 2016.

Eser O, Songur A, Aktas C, Karavelioglu E, Caglar V, Aylak F, Ozguner F, Kanter M. The effect of electromagnetic radiation on the rat brain: An experimental study. *Turk Neurosurg.* 23:707–715, 2013.

Fasseas MK, Fragopoulou AF, Manta AK, Skouroliakou A, Vekrellis K, Margaritis LH, Syntichaki P. Response of Caenorhabditis elegans to wireless devices radiation exposure. *Int J Radiat Biol.* 91:286–293, 2015.

Favre D. Mobile phone-induced honeybee worker piping. *Apidologie.* 42:270–279, 2011.

Feng JF, Liu J, Zhang L, Jiang JY, Russell M, Lyeth BG, Nolta JA, Zhao M. Electrical guidance of human stem cells in the rat brain. *Stem Cell Reports.* 9:177–189, 2017.

Finnie JW, Blumbergs PC, Cai Z, Manavis J. Expression of the water channel protein, aquaporin-4, in mouse brains exposed to mobile telephone radiofrequency fields. *Pathology.* 41:473–475, 2009a.

Finnie JW, Cai Z, Manavis J, Helps S, Blumbergs PC. Microglial activation as a measure of stress in mouse brains exposed acutely (60 minutes) and long-term (2 years) to mobile telephone radiofrequency fields. *Pathology.* 42:151–154, 2010.

Finnie JW, Chidlow G, Blumbergs PC, Manavis J, Cai Z. Heat shock protein induction in fetal mouse brain as a measure of stress after whole of gestation exposure to mobile telephony radiofrequency fields. *Pathology*. 41:276–279, 2009b.

Fragopoulou AF, Miltiadous P, Stamatakis A, Stylianopoulou F, Koussoulakos SL, Margaritis LH. Whole body exposure with GSM 900-MHz affects spatial memory in mice. *Pathophysiology*. 17:179–187, 2010.

Fragopoulou AF, Samara A, Antonelou MH, Xanthopoulou A, Papadopoulou A, Vougas K, Koutsogiannopoulou E et al. Brain proteome response following whole body exposure of mice to mobile phone or wireless DECT base radiation. *Electromagn Biol Med*. 31:250–274, 2012.

Fritzer G, Göder R, Friege L, Wachter J, Hansen V, Hinze-Selch D, Aldenhoff JB. Effects of short- and long-term pulsed radiofrequency electromagnetic fields on night sleep and cognitive functions in healthy subjects. *Bioelectromagnetics*. 28:316–325, 2007.

Gandhi OP, Morgan LL, de Salles AA, Han YY, Herberman RB, Davis DL. Exposure limits: The underestimation of absorbed cell phone radiation, especially in children. *Electromagn Biol Med*. 31:34–51, 2012.

Gao X, Luo R, Ma B, Wang H, Liu T, Zhang J, Lian Z, Cui X. [Interference of vitamin E on the brain tissue damage by electromagnetic radiation of cell phone in pregnant and fetal rats]. *Wei Sheng Yan Jiu*. 42:642–646, 2013 (Article in Chinese).

Gevrek F. Histopathological, immunohistochemical, and stereological analysis of the effect of Gingko biloba (Egb761) on the hippocampus of rats exposed to long-term cellphone radiation. *Histol Histopathol*. 11943, 2017 Nov 9.

Ghazizadeh V, Nazıroğlu M. Electromagnetic radiation (Wi-Fi) and epilepsy induce calcium entry and apoptosis through activation of TRPV1 channel in hippocampus and dorsal root ganglion of rats. *Metab Brain Dis*. 29:787–799, 2014.

Ghosn R, Yahia-Cherif L, Hugueville L, Ducorps A, Lemaréchal JD, Thuróczy G, de Seze R, Selmaoui B. Radiofrequency signal affects alpha band in resting electroencephalogram. *J Neurophysiol*. 113:2753–2759, 2015.

Gökçek-Saraç Ç, Er H, Kencebay Manas C, Kantar Gok D, Özen Ş, Derin N. Effects of acute and chronic exposure to both 900 and 2100 MHz electromagnetic radiation on glutamate receptor signaling pathway. *Int J Radiat Biol*. 93:980–989, 2017.

Grafström G, Nittby H, Brun A, Malmgren L, Persson BR, Salford LG, Eberhardt J. Histopathological examinations of rat brains after long-term exposure to GSM-900 mobile phone radiation. *Brain Res Bull*. 77:257–263, 2008.

Gupta N, Goyal D, Sharma R, Arora KS. Effect of prolonged use of mobile phone on brainstem auditory evoked potentials. *J Clin Diagn Res*. 9:CC07–9, 2015.

Haarala C, Takio F, Rintee T, Laine M, Koivisto M, Revonsuo A, Hämäläinen H. Pulsed and continuous wave mobile phone exposure over left versus right hemisphere: Effects on human cognitive function. *Bioelectromagnetics*. 28:289–295, 2007.

Haghani M, Shabani M, Moazzami K. Maternal mobile phone exposure adversely affects the electrophysiological properties of Purkinje neurons in rat offspring. *Neuroscience*. 250:588–598, 2013.

Hao D, Yang L, Chen S, Tong J, Tian Y, Su B, Wu S, Zeng Y. Effects of long-term electromagnetic field exposure on spatial learning and memory in rats. *Neurol Sci*. 34:157–164, 2013.

Hao Y, Yang X, Chen C, Yuan-Wang, Wang X, Li M, Yu Z. STAT3 signalling pathway is involved in the activation of microglia induced by 2.45 GHz electromagnetic fields. *Int J Radiat Biol*. 86:27–36, 2010.

Hareuveny R, Eliyahu I, Luria R, Meiran N, Margaliot M. Cognitive effects of cellular phones: A possible role of non-radiofrequency radiation factors. *Bioelectromagnetics*. 32:585–588, 2011.

Hassanshahi A, Shafeie SA, Fatemi I, Hassanshahi E, Allahtavakoli M, Shabani M, Roohbakhsh A, Shamsizadeh A. The effect of Wi-Fi electromagnetic waves in unimodal and multimodal object recognition tasks in male rats. *Neurol Sci.* 38:1069–1076, 2017.

He GL, Luo Z, Shen TT, Li P, Yang J, Luo X, Chen CH, Gao P, Yang XS. Inhibition of STAT3- and MAPK-dependent PGE2 synthesis ameliorates phagocytosis of fibrillar β-amyloid peptide (1–42) via EP2 receptor in EMF-stimulated N9 microglial cells. *J Neuroinflammation.* 13:296, 2016.

Hidisoglu E, Kantar Gok D, Er H, Akpinar D, Uysal F, Akkoyunlu G, Ozen S, Agar A, Yargicoglu P. 2100-MHz electromagnetic fields have different effects on visual evoked potentials and oxidant/antioxidant status depending on exposure duration. *Brain Res.* 1635:1–11, 2016.

Hirose H, Sasaki A, Ishii N, Sekijima M, Iyama T, Nojima T, Ugawa Y. 1950 MHz IMT-2000 field does not activate microglial cells *in vitro*. *Bioelectromagnetics.* 31:104–112, 2010.

Hountala CD, Maganioti AE, Papageorgiou CC, Nanou ED, Kyprianou MA, Tsiafakis VG, Rabavilas AD, Capsalis CN. The spectral power coherence of the EEG under different EMF conditions. *Neurosci Lett.* 441:188–192, 2008.

Hu S, Peng R, Wang C, Wang S, Gao Y, Dong J, Zhou H et al. Neuroprotective effects of dietary supplement Kang-fu-ling against high-power microwave through antioxidant action. *Food Funct.* 5:2243–2251, 2014.

Hu Y, Lai J, Wan B, Liu X, Zhang Y, Zhang J, Sun D et al. Long-term exposure to ELF-MF ameliorates cognitive deficits and attenuates tau hyperphosphorylation in 3xTg AD mice. *Neurotoxicology.* 53:290–300, 2016.

Hung CS, Anderson C, Horne JA, McEvoy P. Mobile phone "talk-mode" signal delays EEG-determined sleep onset. *Neurosci Lett.* 421:82–86, 2007.

İkinci A, Mercantepe T, Unal D, Erol HS, Şahin A, Aslan A, Baş O et al. Morphological and antioxidant impairments in the spinal cord of male offspring rats following exposure to a continuous 900 MHz electromagnetic field during early and mid-adolescence. *J Chem Neuroanat.* 75(Pt B):99–104, 2016.

İkinci A, Odacı E, Yıldırım M, Kaya H, Akça M, Hancı H, Aslan A, Sönmez OF, Baş O. The effects of prenatal exposure to a 900 megahertz electromagnetic field on hippocampus morphology and learning rehavior in rat pups. *NeuroQuantology.* 11:582–590, 2013.

Imge EB, Kiliçoğlu B, Devrim E, Cetin R, Durak I. Effects of mobile phone use on brain tissue from the rat and a possible protective role of vitamin C—A preliminary study. *Int J Radiat Biol.* 86:1044–1049, 2010.

Inomata-Terada S, Okabe S, Arai N, Hanajima R, Terao Y, Frubayashi T, Ugawa Y. Effects of high frequency electromagnetic field (EMF) emitted by mobile phones on the human motor cortex. *Bioelectromagnetics.* 28:553–561, 2007.

Irlenbusch L, Bartsch B, Cooper J, Herget I, Marx B, Raczek J, Thoss F. Influence of a 902.4 MHz GSM signal on the human visual system: Investigation of the discrimination threshold. *Bioelectromagnetics.* 28:648–654, 2007.

Jing J, Yuhua Z, Xiao-qian Y, Rongping J, Dong-mei G, Xi C. The influence of microwave radiation from cellular phone on fetal rat brain. *Electromagn Biol Med.* 31:57–66, 2012.

Jorge-Mora T, Köktürk S, Yardimoglu M, Celikozlu SD, Dolanbay EG, Cimbiz A. Effect of Lycopersicon esculentum extract on apoptosis in the rat cerebellum, following prenatal and postnatal exposure to an electromagnetic field. *Exp Ther Med.* 6:52–56, 2013.

Júnior LC, Guimarães ED, Musso CM, Stabler CT, Garcia RM, Mourão-Júnior CA, Andreazzi AE. Behavior and memory evaluation of Wistar rats exposed to 1 · 8 GHz radiofrequency electromagnetic radiation. *Neurol Res.* 36:800–803, 2014.

Kang KA, Lee HC, Lee JJ, Hong MN, Park MJ, Lee YS, Choi HD, Kim N, Ko YK, Lee JS. Effects of combined radiofrequency radiation exposure on levels of reactive oxygen species in neuronal cells. *J Radiat Res.* 55:265–276, 2014.

Kaprana AE, Chimona TS, Papadakis CE, Velegrakis SG, Vardiambasis IO, Adamidis G, Velegrakis GA. Auditory brainstem response changes during exposure to GSM-900 radiation: An experimental study. *Audiol Neurootol.* 16:270–276, 2011.

Kerimoğlu G, Aslan A, Baş O, Çolakoğlu S, Odacı E. Adverse effects in lumbar spinal cord morphology and tissue biochemistry in Sprague Dawley male rats following exposure to a continuous 1-h a day 900-MHz electromagnetic field throughout adolescence. *J Chem Neuroanat.* 78:125–130, 2016a.

Kerimoğlu G, Hancı H, Baş O, Aslan A, Erol HS, Turgut A, Kaya H, Çankaya S, Sönmez OF, Odacı E. Pernicious effects of long-term, continuous 900-MHz electromagnetic field throughout adolescence on hippocampus morphology, biochemistry and pyramidal neuron numbers in 60-day-old Sprague Dawley male rats. *J Chem Neuroanat.* 77:169–175, 2016b.

Kesari KK, Kumar S, Behari J. 900-MHz microwave radiation promotes oxidation in rat brain. *Electromagn Biol Med.* 30:219–234, 2011.

Khullar S, Sood A, Sood S. Auditory brainstem responses and EMFs generated by mobile phones. *Indian J Otolaryngol Head Neck Surg.* 65(Suppl 3):645–649, 2013.

Kim HJ, Jung J, Park JH, Kim JH, Ko KN, Kim CW. Extremely low-frequency electromagnetic fields induce neural differentiation in bone marrow derived mesenchymal stem cells. *Exp Biol Med (Maywood).* 238:923–931, 2013.

Kim JH, Yu DH, Huh YH, Lee EH, Kim HG, Kim HR. Long-term exposure to 835 MHz RF-EMF induces hyperactivity, autophagy and demyelination in the cortical neurons of mice. *Sci Rep.* 7:41129, 2017a.

Kim JH, Yu DH, Kim HJ, Huh YH, Cho SW, Lee JK, Kim HG, Kim HR. Exposure to 835 MHz radiofrequency electromagnetic field induces autophagy in hippocampus but not in brain stem of mice. *Toxicol Ind Health.* 34(1):23–35, 2017b Jan 1:748233717740066. doi: 10.1177/0748233717740066.

Kim JY, Kim HJ, Kim N, Kwon JH, Park MJ. Effects of radiofrequency field exposure on glutamate-induced oxidative stress in mouse hippocampal HT22 cells. *Int J Radiat Biol.* 93:249–256, 2017.

Kleinlogel H, Dierks T, Koenig T, Lehmann H, Minder A, Berz R. Effects of weak mobile phone—Electromagnetic fields (GSM, UMTS) on well-being and resting EEG. *Bioelectromagnetics.* 29:479–487, 2008a.

Kleinlogel H, Dierks T, Koenig T, Lehmann H, Minder A, Berz R. Effects of weak mobile phone—Electromagnetic fields (GSM, UMTS) on event related potentials and cognitive functions. *Bioelectromagnetics.* 29:488–497, 2008b.

Klose M, Grote K, Spathmann O, Streckert J, Clemens M, Hansen VW, Lerchl A. Effects of early-onset radiofrequency electromagnetic field exposure (GSM 900 MHz) on behavior and memory in rats. *Radiat Res.* 182:435–447, 2014.

Köktürk S, Yardimoglu M, Celikozlu SD, Dolanbay EG, Cimbiz A. Effect of Lycopersicon esculentum extract on apoptosis in the rat cerebellum, following prenatal and postnatal exposure to an electromagnetic field. *Exp Ther Med.* 6:52–56, 2013.

Krause CM, Pesonen M, Haarala Björnberg C, Hämäläinen H. Effects of pulsed and continuous wave 902 MHz mobile phone exposure on brain oscillatory activity during cognitive processing. *Bioelectromagnetics.* 28:296–308, 2007.

Kumar RS, Sareesh NN, Nayak S, Mailankot M. Hypoactivity of Wistar rats exposed to mobile phone on elevated plus maze. *Indian J Physiol Pharmacol.* 53:283–286, 2009.

Kumari K, Koivisto H, Viluksela M, Paldanius KMA, Marttinen M, Hiltunen M, Naarala J, Tanila H, Juutilainen J. Behavioral testing of mice exposed to intermediate frequency magnetic fields indicates mild memory impairment. *PLoS One.* 12(12):e0188880, 2017 Dec 4.

Kumlin T, Iivonen H, Miettinen P, Juvonen A, van Groen T, Puranen L, Pitkäaho R, Juutilainen J, Tanila H. Mobile phone radiation and the developing brain: Behavioral and morphological effects in juvenile rats. *Radiat Res.* 168:471–479, 2007.

Kwon MS, Huotilainen M, Shestakova A, Kujala T, Näätänen R, Hämäläinen H. No effects of mobile phone use on cortical auditory change-detection in children: An ERP study. *Bioelectromagnetics*. 31:191–199, 2010a.

Kwon MS, Jääskeläinen SK, Toivo T, Hämäläinen H. No effects of mobile phone electromagnetic field on auditory brainstem response. *Bioelectromagnetics*. 31:48–55, 2010b.

Kwon MS, Kujala T, Huotilainen M, Shestakova A, Näätänen R, Hämäläinen H. Preattentive auditory information processing under exposure to the 902 MHz GSM mobile phone electromagnetic field: A mismatch negativity (MMN) study. *Bioelectromagnetics*. 30:241–248, 2009.

Lahham A, Hammash A. Outdoor radiofrequency radiation levels in the West Bank-Palestine. *Radiat Prot Dosimetry*. 149:399–402, 2012.

Lai H, Horita A, Chou CK, Guy AW. Low-level microwave irradiation affects central cholinergic activity in the rat. *J Neurochem*. 48:40–45, 1987.

Lai H, Singh NP. Acute low-intensity microwave exposure increases DNA single-strand breaks in rat brain cells. *Bioelectromagnetics*. 16:207–210, 1995.

Lai H. Neurological effects of microwave irradiation. In *Advances in Electromagnetic Fields in Living Systems, Vol. 1*, Lin JC (ed.), Plenum Press, New York, 1994, pp. 27–80.

Landler L, Painter MS, Youmans PW, Hopkins WA, Phillips JB. Spontaneous magnetic alignment by yearling snapping turtles: Rapid association of radio frequency dependent pattern of magnetic input with novel surroundings. *PLoS One*. 10(5):e0124728, 2015.

Lee D, Lee J, Lee I. Cell phone generated radio frequency electromagnetic field effects on the locomotor behaviors of the fishes Poecilia reticulata and Danio rerio. *Int J Radiat Biol*. 91:845–850, 2015.

Lee W, Yang K-L. Using medaka embryos as a model system to study biological effects of the electromagnetic fields on development and behavior. *Ecotoxicol Environ Safety*. 108:187–194, 2014.

Leung S, Croft RJ, McKenzie RJ, Iskra S, Silber B, Cooper NR, O'Neill B et al. Effects of 2G and 3G mobile phones on performance and electrophysiology in adolescents, young adults and older adults. *Clin Neurophysiol*. 122:2203–2216, 2011.

Levitt BB, Lai H. Biological effects from exposure to electromagnetic radiation emitted by cell tower base stations and other antenna arrays. *Environ Rev*. 18:369–395, 2010.

Li H, Peng R, Wang C, Qiao S, Yong Z, Gao Y, Xu X et al. Alterations of cognitive function and 5-HT system in rats after long term microwave exposure. *Physiol Behav*. 40:236–246, 2015.

Li Y, Shi C, Lu G, Xu Q, Liu S. Effects of electromagnetic radiation on spatial memory and synapses in rat hippocampal CA1. *Neural Regen Res*. 7:1248–1255, 2012.

Liu ML, Wen JQ, Fan YB. Potential protection of green tea polyphenols against 1800 MHz electromagnetic radiation-induced injury on rat cortical neurons. *Neurotox Res*. 20:270–276, 2011.

Liu YX, Tai JL, Li GQ, Zhang ZW, Xue JH, Liu HS, Zhu H et al. Exposure to 1950-MHz TD-SCDMA electromagnetic fields affects the apoptosis of astrocytes via caspase-3-dependent pathway. *PLoS One*. 7:e42332, 2012.

López-Martín E, Bregains J, Relova-Quinteiro JL, Cadarso-Suárez C, Jorge-Barreiro FJ, Ares-Pena FJ. The action of pulse-modulated GSM radiation increases regional changes in brain activity and c-Fos expression in cortical and subcortical areas in a rat model of picrotoxin-induced seizure proneness. *J Neurosci Res*. 87:1484–1499, 2009.

Loughran SP, Benz DC, Schmid MR, Murbach M, Kuster N, Achermann P. No increased sensitivity in brain activity of adolescents exposed to mobile phone-like emissions. *Clin Neurophysiol*. 124:1303–1308, 2013.

Loughran SP, McKenzie RJ, Jackson ML, Howard ME, Croft RJ. Individual differences in the effects of mobile phone exposure on human sleep: Rethinking the problem. *Bioelectromagnetics*. 33:86–93, 2012.

Lowden A, Akerstedt T, Ingre M, Wiholm C, Hillert L, Kuster N, Nilsson JP, Arnetz B. Sleep after mobile phone exposure in subjects with mobile phone-related symptoms. *Bioelectromagnetics*. 32:4–14, 2011.

Lu Y, He M, Zhang Y, Xu S, Zhang L, He Y, Chen C et al. Differential pro-inflammatory responses of astrocytes and microglia involve STAT3 activation in response to 1800 MHz radiofrequency fields. *PLoS One*. 9:e108318, 2014.

Lu Y, Xu S, He M, Chen C, Zhang L, Liu C, Chu F, Yu Z, Zhou Z, Zhong M. Glucose administration attenuates spatial memory deficits induced by chronic low-power-density microwave exposure. *Physiol Behav*. 106:631–637, 2012.

Luria R, Eliyahu I, Hareuveny R, Margaliot M, Meiran N. Cognitive effects of radiation emitted by cellular phones: The influence of exposure side and time. *Bioelectromagnetics*. 30:198–204, 2009.

Lustenberger C, Murbach M, Durr R, Schmid MR, Kuster N, Achermann P, Huber R. Stimulation of the brain with radiofrequency electromagnetic field pulses affects sleep-dependent performance improvement. *Brain Stimul*. 6:805–811, 2013.

Lustenberger C, Murbach M, Tüshaus L, Wehrle F, Kuster N, Achermann P, Huber R. Inter-individual and intra-individual variation of the effects of pulsed RF EMF exposure on the human sleep EEG. *Bioelectromagnetics*. 36:169–177, 2015.

Lv B, Chen Z, Wu T, Shao Q, Yan D, Ma L, Lu K, Xie Y. The alteration of spontaneous low frequency oscillations caused by acute electromagnetic fields exposure. *Clin Neurophysiol*. 125:277–286, 2014a.

Lv B, Su C, Yang L, Xie Y, Wu T. Whole brain EEG synchronization likelihood modulated by long term evolution electromagnetic fields exposure. *Conf Proc IEEE Eng Med Biol Soc*. 2014:986–989, 2014b.

Maaroufi K, Had-Aissouni L, Melon C, Sakly M, Abdelmelek H, Poucet B, Save E. Spatial learning, monoamines and oxidative stress in rats exposed to 900 MHz electromagnetic field in combination with iron overload. *Behav Brain Res*. 258:80–89, 2014.

Maganioti AE, Hountala CD, Papageorgiou CC, Kyprianou MA, Rabavilas AD, Capsalis CN. Principal component analysis of the P600 waveform: RF and gender effects. *Neurosci Lett*. 478:19–23, 2010.

Malek F, Rani KA, Rahim HA, Omar MH. Effect of short-term mobile phone base station exposure on cognitive performance, body temperature, heart rate and blood pressure of Malaysians. *Sci Rep*. 5:13206, 2015.

Malkemper EP, Eder SH, Begall S, Phillips JB, Winklhofer M, Hart V, Burda H. Magnetoreception in the wood mouse (Apodemus sylvaticus): Influence of weak frequency-modulated radio frequency fields. *Sci Rep*. 29(4):9917, 2015.

Mandalà M, Colletti V, Sacchetto L, Manganotti P, Ramat S, Marcocci A, Colletti L. Effect of Bluetooth headset and mobile phone electromagnetic fields on the human auditory nerve. *Laryngoscope*. 124:255–259, 2014.

Maskey D, Kim HJ, Kim HG, Kim MJ. Calcium-binding proteins and GFAP immunoreactivity alterations in murine hippocampus after 1 month of exposure to 835 MHz radiofrequency at SAR values of 1.6 and 4.0 W/kg. *Neurosci Lett*. 506:292–296, 2012.

Maskey D, Kim M, Aryal B, Pradhan J, Choi IY, Park KS, Son T et al. Effect of 835 MHz radiofrequency radiation exposure on calcium binding proteins in the hippocampus of the mouse brain. *Brain Res*. 1313:232–241, 2010a.

Maskey D, Kim MJ. Immunohistochemical localization of brain-derived neurotrophic factor and glial cell line-derived neurotrophic factor in the superior olivary complex of mice after radiofrequency exposure. *Neurosci Lett*. 564:78–82, 2014.

Maskey D, Pradhan J, Aryal B, Lee CM, Choi IY, Park KS, Kim SB, Kim HG, Kim MJ. Chronic 835-MHz radiofrequency exposure to mice hippocampus alters the distribution of calbindin and GFAP immunoreactivity. *Brain Res.* 1346:237–246, 2010b.

Masuda H, Ushiyama A, Takahashi M, Wang J, Fujiwara O, Hikage T, Nojima T, Fujita K, Kudo M, Ohkubo C. Effects of 915 MHz electromagnetic-field radiation in TEM cell on the blood-brain barrier and neurons in the rat brain. *Radiat Res.* 172:66–73, 2009.

Mathur R. Effect of chronic intermittent exposure to AM radiofrequency field on responses to various types of noxious stimuli in growing rats. *Electromagn Biol Med.* 27:266–276, 2008.

Megha K, Deshmukh PS, Banerjee BD, Tripathi AK, Abegaonkar MP. Microwave radiation induced oxidative stress, cognitive impairment and inflammation in brain of Fischer rats. *Indian J Exp Biol.* 50:889–896, 2012.

Megha K, Deshmukh PS, Ravi AK, Tripathi AK, Abegaonkar MP, Banerjee BD. Effect of low-intensity microwave radiation on monoamine neurotransmitters and their key regulating enzymes in rat brain. *Cell Biochem Biophys.* 73:93–100, 2015.

Meral I, Mert H, Mert N, Deger Y, Yoruk I, Yetkin A, Keskin S. Effects of 900-MHz electromagnetic field emitted from cellular phone on brain oxidative stress and some vitamin levels of guinea pigs. *Brain Res.* 1169:120–124, 2007.

Mild KH, Andersen JB, Pedersen GF. Is there any exposure from a mobile phone in stand-by mode? *Electromagn Biol Med.* 31:52–56, 2012.

Mohammed HS, Fahmy HM, Radwah NM, Elsayed AA. Non-thermal continuous and modulated electromagnetic radiation fields effects on sleep EEG of rats. *J Adv Res.* 4:81–187, 2013.

Mohler E, Frei P, Braun-Fahrländer C, Fröhlich J, Neubauer G, Röösli M; Qualifex Team. Effects of everyday radiofrequency electromagnetic-field exposure on sleep quality: A cross-sectional study. *Radiat Res.* 174:347–356, 2010.

Mohler E, Frei P, Fröhlich J, Braun-Fahrländer C, Röösli M; QUALIFEX-team. Exposure to radiofrequency electromagnetic fields and sleep quality: A prospective cohort study. *PLoS One.* 7:e37455, 2012.

Mortazavi SM, Rouintan MS, Taeb S, Dehghan N, Ghaffarpanah AA, Sadeghi Z, Ghafouri F. Human short-term exposure to electromagnetic fields emitted by mobile phones decreases computer-assisted visual reaction time. *Acta Neurol Belg.* 112:171–175, 2012.

Mortazavi SM, Taeb S, Dehghan N. Alterations of visual reaction time and short term memory in military radar personnel. *Iran J Public Health.* 42:428–435, 2013.

Motawi TK, Darwish HA, Moustafa YM, Labib MM. Biochemical modifications and neuronal damage in brain of young and adult rats after long-term exposure to mobile phone radiations. *Cell Biochem Biophys.* 70:845–855, 2014.

Movvahedi MM, Tavakkoli-Golpayegani A, Mortazavi SA, Haghani M, Razi Z, Shojaie-Fard MB, Zare M et al. Does exposure to GSM 900 MHz mobile phone radiation affect short-term memory of elementary school students? *J Pediatr Neurosci.* 9:121–124, 2014.

Mugunthan N, Shanmugasamy K, Anbalagan J, Rajanarayanan S, Meenachi S. Effects of long term exposure of 900–1800 MHz radiation emitted from 2G mobile phone on mice hippocampus- A histomorphometric study. *J Clin Diagn Res.* 10:AF01–6, 2016.

Nakatani-Enomoto S, Furubayashi T, Ushiyama A, Groiss SJ, Ueshima K, Sokejima S, Simba AY et al. Effects of electromagnetic fields emitted from W-CDMA-like mobile phones on sleep in humans. *Bioelectromagnetics.* 34:589–598, 2013.

Narayanan SN, Kumar RS, Karun KM, Nayak SB, Bhat PG. Possible cause for altered spatial cognition of prepubescent rats exposed to chronic radiofrequency electromagnetic radiation. *Metab Brain Dis.* 30:1193–1206, 2015.

Narayanan SN, Kumar RS, Kedage V, Nalini K, Nayak S, Bhat PG. Evaluation of oxidant stress and antioxidant defense in discrete brain regions of rats exposed to 900 MHz radiation. *Bratisl Lek Listy*. 115:260–266, 2014.

Narayanan SN, Kumar RS, Paval J, Kedage V, Bhat MS, Nayak S, Bhat PG. Analysis of emotionality and locomotion in radio-frequency electromagnetic radiation exposed rats. *Neurol Sci*. 34:1117–1124, 2013.

Narayanan SN, Kumar RS, Potu BK, Nayak S, Bhat PG, Mailankot M. Effect of radio-frequency electromagnetic radiations (RF-EMR) on passive avoidance behaviour and hippocampal morphology in Wistar rats. *Ups J Med Sci*. 115:91–96, 2010.

Narayanan SN, Kumar RS, Potu BK, Nayak S, Mailankot M. Spatial memory performance of Wistar rats exposed to mobile phone. *Clinics (Sao Paulo)*. 64:231–234, 2009.

Nazıroğlu M, Çelik Ö, Özgül C, Çiğ B, Doğan S, Bal R, Gümral N, Rodríguez AB, Pariente JA. Melatonin modulates wireless (2.45 GHz)-induced oxidative injury through TRPM2 and voltage gated Ca(2+) channels in brain and dorsal root ganglion in rat. *Physiol Behav*. 105:683–692, 2012.

Naziroğlu M, Gümral N. Modulator effects of L-carnitine and selenium on wireless devices (2.45 GHz)-induced oxidative stress and electroencephalography records in brain of rat. *Int J Radiat Biol*. 85:680–689, 2009.

Ning W, Xu SJ, Chiang H, Xu ZP, Zhou SY, Yang W, Luo JH. Effects of GSM 1800 MHz on dendritic development of cultured hippocampal neurons. *Acta Pharmacol Sin*. 28:1873–1880, 2007.

Nirwane A, Sridhar V, Majumdar A. Neurobehavioural changes and brain oxidative stress induced by acute exposure to GSM 900 mobile phone radiations in Zebrafish (Danio rerio). *Toxicol Res*. 32:123–132, 2016.

Nittby H, Brun A, Eberhardt J, Malmgren L, Persson BR, Salford LG. Increased blood-brain barrier permeability in mammalian brain 7 days after exposure to the radiation from a GSM-900 mobile phone. *Pathophysiology*. 16:103–112, 2009.

Nittby H, Grafström G, Tian DP, Malmgren L, Brun A, Persson BR, Salford LG, Eberhardt J. Cognitive impairment in rats after long-term exposure to GSM-900 mobile phone radiation. *Bioelectromagnetics*. 29:219–232, 2008a.

Nittby H, Widegren B, Krogh M, Grafström G, Berlin H, Rehn G, Eberhardt JL, Malmgren L, Persson BRR, Salford L. Exposure to radiation from global system for mobile communications at 1,800 MHz significantly changes gene expression in rat hippocampus and cortex. *Environmentalist*. 28:458–465, 2008b.

Noor NA, Mohammed HS, Ahmed NA, Radwan NM. Variations in amino acid neurotransmitters in some brain areas of adult and young male albino rats due to exposure to mobile phone radiation. *Eur Rev Med Pharmacol Sci*. 15:729–742, 2011.

Ntzouni MP, Skouroliakou A, Kostomitsopoulos N, Margaritis LH. Transient and cumulative memory impairments induced by GSM 1.8 GHz cell phone signal in a mouse model. *Electromagn Biol Med*. 32:95–120, 2013.

Ntzouni MP, Stamatakis A, Stylianopoulou F, Margaritis LH. Short-term memory in mice is affected by mobile phone radiation. *Pathophysiology*. 18:193–199, 2011.

Nylund R, Kuster N, Leszczynski D. Analysis of proteome response to the mobile phone radiation in two types of human primary endothelial cells. *Proteome Sci*. 8:52, 2010.

Odacı E, Bas O, Kaplan S. Effects of prenatal exposure to a 900 MHz electromagnetic field on the dentate gyrus of rats: A stereological and histopathological study. *Brain Res*. 1238:224–229, 2008.

Odacı E, Hancı H, İkinci A, Sönmez OF, Aslan A, Şahin A, Kaya H, Çolakoğlu S, Baş O. Maternal exposure to a continuous 900-MHz electromagnetic field provokes neuronal loss and pathological changes in cerebellum of 32-day-old female rat offspring. *J Chem Neuroanat*. 75(Pt B):105–110, 2016.

Odacı E, İkinci A, Yıldırım M, Kaya H, Akça M, Hancı H, Sönmez OF, Aslan A, Okuyan M, Baş O. The effects of 900 megahertz electromagnetic field applied in the prenatal period on spinal cord morphology and motor behavior in female rat pups. *NeuroQuantology*. 11:573–581, 2013.

Othman H, Ammari M, Sakly M, Abdelmelek H. Effects of prenatal exposure to WIFI signal (2.45 GHz) on postnatal development and behavior in rat: Influence of maternal restraint. *Behav Brain Res*. 326:291–302, 2017.

Özgür A, Tümkaya L, Terzi S, Kalkan Y, Erdivanlı ÖÇ, Dursun E. Effects of chronic exposure to electromagnetic waves on the auditory system. *Acta Otolaryngol*. 135:765–770, 2015.

Pakhomov A, Bojarinova J, Cherbunin R, Chetverikova R, Grigoryev PS, Kavokin K, Kobylkov D, Lubkovskaja R, Chernetsov N. Very weak oscillating magnetic field disrupts the magnetic compass of songbird migrants. *J R Soc Interface*. 14(133), 2017 Aug. pii: 20170364. doi: 10.1098/rsif.2017.0364.

Panda NK, Jain R, Bakshi J, Munjal S. Audiologic disturbances in long-term mobile phone users. *J Otolaryngol Head Neck Surg*. 39:5–11, 2010.

Panda NK, Modi R, Munjal S, Virk RS. Auditory changes in mobile users: Is evidence forthcoming? *Otolaryngol Head Neck Surg*. 144:581–585, 2011.

Parazzini M, Sibella F, Lutman ME, Mishra S, Moulin A, Sliwinska-Kowalska M, Woznicka E et al. Effects of UMTS cellular phones on human hearing: Results of the European project EMFnEAR. *Radiat Res*. 172:244–251, 2009.

Pelletier A, Delanaud S, de Seze R, Bach V, Libert JP, Loos N. Does exposure to a radiofrequency electromagnetic field modify thermal preference in juvenile rats? *PLoS One*. 9:e99007, 2014.

Pelletier A, Delanaud S, Décima P, Thuroczy G, de Seze R, Cerri M, Bach V, Libert JP, Loos N. Effects of chronic exposure to radiofrequency electromagnetic fields on energy balance in developing rats. *Environ Sci Pollut Res Int*. 20:2735–2746, 2013.

Perentos N, Croft RJ, McKenzie RJ, Cosic I. The alpha band of the resting electroencephalogram under pulsed and continuous radio frequency exposures. *IEEE Trans Biomed Eng*. 60:1702–1710, 2013.

Perentos N, Croft RJ, McKenzie RJ, Cvetkovic D, Cosic I. Comparison of the effects of continuous and pulsed mobile phone like RF exposure on the human EEG. *Australas Phys Eng Sci Med*. 30:274–280, 2007.

Perentos N, Croft RJ, McKenzie RJ, Cvetkovic D, Cosic I. The effect of GSM-like ELF radiation on the alpha band of the human resting EEG. *Conf Proc IEEE Eng Med Biol Soc*. 2008:5680–5683, 2008.

Poulletier de Gannes F, Haro E, Hurtier A, Taxile M, Ruffié G, Billaudel B, Veyret B, Lagroye I. Effect of exposure to the edge signal on oxidative stress in brain cell models. *Radiat Res*. 175:225–230, 2011.

Poulletier de Gannes F, Masuda H, Billaudel B, Poque-Haro E, Hurtier A, Lévêque P, Ruffié G, Taxile M, Veyret B, Lagroye I. Effects of GSM and UMTS mobile telephony signals on neuron degeneration and blood-brain barrier permeation in the rat brain. *Sci Rep*. 7(1):15496, 2017 Nov 14. doi: 10.1038/s41598-017-15690-1.

Qiao S, Peng R, Yan H, Gao Y, Wang C, Wang S, Zou Y et al. Reduction of Phosphorylated Synapsin I (Ser-553) Leads to spatial memory impairment by attenuating GABA release after microwave exposure in Wistar Rats. *PLoS One*. 9:e95503, 2014.

Qin F, Yuan H, Nie J, Cao Y, Tong J. [Effects of nano-selenium on cognition performance of mice exposed in 1800 MHz radiofrequency fields]. *Wei Sheng Yan Jiu*. 43:16–21, 2014 (Article in Chinese).

Rağbetli MC, Aydinlioğlu A, Koyun N, Rağbetli C, Bektas S, Ozdemir S. The effect of mobile phone on the number of Purkinje cells: A stereological study. *Int J Radiat Biol*. 86:548–554, 2010.

Rağbetli MC, Aydinlioğlu A, Koyun N, Rağbetli C, Karayel M. Effect of prenatal exposure to mobile phone on pyramidal cell numbers in the mouse hippocampus: A stereological study. *Int J Neurosci*. 119:1031–1041, 2009.

Razavinasab M, Moazzami K, Shabani M. Maternal mobile phone exposure alters intrinsic electrophysiological properties of CA1 pyramidal neurons in rat offspring. *Toxicol Ind Health*. 32:968–979, 2014.

Redmayne M, Smith CL, Benke G, Croft RJ, Dalecki A, Dimitriadis C, Kaufman J et al. Use of mobile and cordless phones and cognition in Australian primary school children: A prospective cohort study. *Environ Health*. 15:26, 2016.

Redmayne M, Smith E, Abramson MJ. The relationship between adolescents' well-being and their wireless phone use: A cross-sectional study. *Environ Health*. 12:90, 2013.

Regel SJ, Tinguely G, Schuderer J, Adam M, Kuster N, Landolt HP, Achermann P. Pulsed radio-frequency electromagnetic fields: Dose-dependent effects on sleep, the sleep EEG and cognitive performance. *J Sleep Res*. 16:253–258, 2007.

Riddervold IS, Pedersen GF, Andersen NT, Pedersen AD, Andersen JB, Zachariae R, Mølhave L, Sigsgaard T, Kjaergaard SK. Cognitive function and symptoms in adults and adolescents in relation to rf radiation from UMTS base stations. *Bioelectromagnetics*. 29:257–267, 2008.

Roggeveen S, van Os J, Lousberg R. Does the brain detect 3G mobile phone radiation peaks? An explorative in-depth analysis of an experimental study. *PLoS One*. 10:e0125390, 2015a.

Roggeveen S, van Os J, Viechtbauer W, Lousberg R. EEG changes due to experimentally induced 3G mobile phone radiation. *PLoS One*. 10:e0129496, 2015b.

Roser K, Schoeni A, Röösli M. Mobile phone use, behavioural problems and concentration capacity in adolescents: A prospective study. *Int J Hyg Environ Health*. 219:759–769, 2016.

Şahin A, Aslan A, Baş O, İkinci A, Özyılmaz C, Fikret Sönmez O, Çolakoğlu S, Odacı E. Deleterious impacts of a 900 MHz electromagnetic field on hippocampal pyramidal neurons of 8-week-old Sprague Dawley male rats. *Brain Res*. 1624:232–238, 2015.

Saikhedkar N, Bhatnagar M, Jain A, Sukhwal P, Sharma C, Jaiswal N. Effects of mobile phone radiation (900 MHz radiofrequency) on structure and functions of rat brain. *Neurol Res*. 36:1072–1076, 2014.

Salford LG, Brun AE, Eberhardt JL, Malmgren L, Persson BR. Nerve cell damage in mammalian brain after exposure to microwaves from GSM mobile phones. *Environ Health Perspect*. 111:881–883, 2003.

Salunke BP, Umathe SN, Chavan JG. Behavioral in-effectiveness of high frequency electromagnetic field in mice. *Physiol Behav*. 140:32–37, 2015.

Sarapultseva EI, Igolkina JV, Tikhonov VN, Dubrova YE. The *in vivo* effects of low-intensity radiofrequency fields on the motor activity of protozoa. *Int J Radiat Biol*. 90:262–267, 2014.

Sauter C, Dorn H, Bahr A, Hansen ML, Peter A, Bajbouj M, Danker-Hopfe H. Effects of exposure to electromagnetic fields emitted by GSM 900 and WCDMA mobile phones on cognitive function in young male subjects. *Bioelectromagnetics*. 32:179–190, 2011.

Sauter C, Eggert T, Dorn H, Schmid G, Bolz T, Marasanov A, Hansen ML, Peter A, Danker-Hopfe H. Do signals of a hand-held TETRA transmitter affect cognitive performance, well-being, mood or somatic complaints in healthy young men? Results of a randomized double-blind cross-over provocation study. *Environ Res*. 140:85–94, 2015.

Schmid MR, Loughran SP, Regel SJ, Murbach M, Bratic Grunauer A, Rusterholz T, Bersagliere A, Kuster N, Achermann P. Sleep EEG alterations: Effects of different pulse-modulated radio frequency electromagnetic fields. *J Sleep Res*. 21:50–58, 2012a.

Schmid MR, Murbach M, Lustenberger C, Maire M, Kuster N, Achermann P, Loughran SP. Sleep EEG alterations: Effects of pulsed magnetic fields versus pulse-modulated radio frequency electromagnetic fields. *J Sleep Res*. 21:620–629, 2012b.

Schneider J, Stangassinger M. Nonthermal effects of lifelong high-frequency electromagnetic field exposure on social memory performance in rats. *Behav Neurosci.* 128:633–637, 2014.

Schoeni A, Roser K, Röösli M. Memory performance, wireless communication and exposure to radiofrequency electromagnetic fields: A prospective cohort study in adolescents. *Environ Int.* 85:343–351, 2015.

Schwarze S, Schneider NL, Reichl T, Dreyer D, Lefeldt N, Engels S, Baker N, Hore PJ, Mouritsen H. Weak broadband electromagnetic fields are more disruptive to magnetic compass orientation in a night-migratory songbird (Erithacus rubecula) than strong narrow-band fields. *Front Behav Neurosci.* 10:55, 2016.

Seckin E, Suren Basar F, Atmaca S, Kaymaz FF, Suzer A, Akar A, Sunan E, Koyuncu M. The effect of radiofrequency radiation generated by a Global System for Mobile Communications source on cochlear development in a rat model. *J Laryngol Otol.* 128:400–405, 2014.

Sharma A, Kesari KK, Saxena VK, Sisodia R. Ten gigahertz microwave radiation impairs spatial memory, enzymes activity, and histopathology of developing mice brain. *Mol Cell Biochem.* 435:1–13, 2017.

Sharma A, Sisodia R, Bhatnagar D, Saxena VK. Spatial memory and learning performance and its relationship to protein synthesis of Swiss albino mice exposed to 10 GHz microwaves. *Int J Radiat Biol.* 90:29–35, 2014.

Shehu A, Mohammed A, Magaji RA, Muhammad MS. Exposure to mobile phone electromagnetic field radiation, ringtone and vibration affects anxiety-like behaviour and oxidative stress biomarkers in albino Wistar rats. *Metab Brain Dis.* 31:355–362, 2016.

Shirai T, Imai N, Wang J, Takahashi S, Kawabe M, Wake K, Kawai H, Watanabe S-I, Furukawa F, Fujiwara O. Multigenerational effects of whole body exposure to 2.14 GHz W-CDMA cellular phone signals on brain function in rats. *Bioelectromagnetics.* 35:497–511, 2014.

Sirav B, Seyhan N. Blood-brain barrier disruption by continuous-wave radio frequency radiation. *Electromagn Biol Med.* 28:215–222, 2009.

Sirav B, Seyhan N. Effects of radiofrequency radiation exposure on blood-brain barrier permeability in male and female rats. *Electromagn Biol Med.* 30:253–260, 2011.

Sırav B, Seyhan N. Effects of GSM modulated radio-frequency electromagnetic radiation on permeability of blood-brain barrier in male & female rats. *J Chem Neuroanat.* 75(Pt B):123–127, 2016.

Söderqvist F, Carlberg M, Hansson Mild K, Hardell L. Exposure to an 890-MHz mobile phone-like signal and serum levels of S100B and transthyretin in volunteers. *Toxicol Lett.* 189:63–66, 2009a.

Söderqvist F, Carlberg M, Hardell L. Mobile and cordless telephones, serum transthyretin and the blood-cerebrospinal fluid barrier: A cross-sectional study. *Environ Health.* 21(8):19, 2009b.

Söderqvist F, Carlberg M, Hardell L. Use of wireless telephones and serum S100B levels: A descriptive cross-sectional study among healthy Swedish adults aged 18-65 years. *Sci Total Environ.* 407:798–805, 2009c.

Sokolovic D, Djindjic B, Nikolic J, Bjelakovic G, Pavlovic D, Kocic G, Krstic D, Cvetkovic T, Pavlovic V. Melatonin reduces oxidative stress induced by chronic exposure of microwave radiation from mobile phones in rat brain. *J Radiat Res.* 49:579–586, 2009.

Sokolovic D, Djordjevic B, Kocic G, Babovic P, Ristic G, Stanojkovic Z, Sokolovic DM, Veljkovic A, Jankovic A, Radovanovic Z. The effect of melatonin on body mass and behaviour of rats during an exposure to microwave radiation from mobile phone. *Bratisl Lek Listy.* 113:265–269, 2012.

Son Y, Jeong YJ, Kwon JH, Choi HD, Pack JK, Kim N, Lee YS, Lee HJ. 1950 MHz radiofrequency electromagnetic fields do not aggravate memory deficits in 5xFAD mice. *Bioelectromagnetics.* 37(6):391–399, 2016.

Stefanics G, Kellényi L, Molnár F, Kubinyi G, Thuróczy G, Hernádi I. Short GSM mobile phone exposure does not alter human auditory brainstem response. *BMC Public Health*. 7:325, 2007.

Stefanics G, Thuróczy G, Kellényi L, Hernádi I. Effects of twenty-minute 3G mobile phone irradiation on event related potential components and early gamma synchronization in auditory oddball paradigm. *Neuroscience*. 157:453–462, 2008.

Sudan M, Kheifets L, Arah OA, Olsen J. Cell phone exposures and hearing loss in children in the Danish National Birth Cohort. *Paediatr Perinat Epidemiol*. 27:247–257, 2013.

Takahashi M, Saito A, Jimbo Y, Nakasono S. Evaluation of the effects of power-frequency magnetic fields on the electrical activity of cardiomyocytes differentiated from human induced pluripotent stem cells. *J Toxicol Sci*. 42:223–231, 2017.

Tang J, Zhang Y, Yang L, Chen Q, Tan L, Zuo S, Feng H, Chen Z, Zhu G. Exposure to 900 MHz electromagnetic fields activates the mkp-1/ERK pathway and causes blood-brain barrier damage and cognitive impairment in rats. *Brain Res*. 1601:92–101, 2015.

Thomas S, Heinrich S, von Kries R, Radon K. Exposure to radio-frequency electromagnetic fields and behavioural problems in Bavarian children and adolescents. *Eur J Epidemiol*. 25:135–141, 2010.

Tombini M, Pellegrino G, Pasqualetti P, Assenza G, Benvenga A, Fabrizio E, Rossini PM. Mobile phone emissions modulate brain excitability in patients with focal epilepsy. *Brain Stimul*. 6:448–454, 2013.

Tong J, Chen S, Liu XM, Hao DM. [Effect of electromagnetic radiation on discharge activity of neurons in the hippocampus CA1 in rats]. *Zhongguo Ying Yong Sheng Li Xue Za Zhi*. 29:423–427, 2013 (Article in Chinese).

Trunk A, Stefanics G, Zentai N, Bacskay I, Felinger A, Thuróczy G, Hernádi I. Lack of interaction between concurrent caffeine and mobile phone exposure on visual target detection: An ERP study. *Pharmacol Biochem Behav*. 124:412–420, 2014.

Trunk A, Stefanics G, Zentai N, Bacskay I, Felinger A, Thuróczy G, Hernádi I. Effects of concurrent caffeine and mobile phone exposure on local target probability processing in the human brain. *Sci Rep*. 5:14434, 2015.

Trunk A, Stefanics G, Zentai N, Kovács-Bálint Z, Thuróczy G, Hernádi I. No effects of a single 3G UMTS mobile phone exposure on spontaneous EEG activity, ERP correlates, and automatic deviance detection. *Bioelectromagnetics*. 34:31–42, 2013.

Unterlechner M, Sauter C, Schmid G, Zeitlhofer J. No effect of an UMTS mobile phone-like electromagnetic field of 1.97 GHz on human attention and reaction time. *Bioelectromagnetics*. 29:145–153, 2008.

Vácha M, Puzová T, Kvícalová M. Radio frequency magnetic fields disrupt magnetoreception in American cockroach. *J Exp Biol*. 212(Pt 21):3473–3477, 2009.

Varghese R, Majumdar A, Kumar G, Shukla A. Rats exposed to 2.45 GHz of non-ionizing radiation exhibit behavioral changes with increased brain expression of apoptotic caspase 3. *Pathophysiology*. 25(1):19–30, 2017 Nov 14. pii: S0928-4680(17)30052-4. doi: 10.1016/j.pathophys.2017.11.001.

Vecchio F, Babiloni C, Ferreri F, Buffo P, Cibelli G, Curcio G, van Dijkman S, Melgari JM, Giambattistelli F, Rossini PM. Mobile phone emission modulates inter-hemispheric functional coupling of EEG alpha rhythms in elderly compared to young subjects. *Clin Neurophysiol*. 121:163–171, 2010.

Vecchio F, Babiloni C, Ferreri F, Curcio G, Fini R, Del Percio C, Rossini PM. Mobile phone emission modulates interhemispheric functional coupling of EEG alpha rhythms. *Eur J Neurosci*. 25:1908–1913, 2007.

Vecchio F, Buffo P, Sergio S, Iacoviello D, Rossini PM, Babiloni C. Mobile phone emission modulates event-related desynchronization of α rhythms and cognitive-motor performance in healthy humans. *Clin Neurophysiol*. 123:121–128, 2012a.

Vecchio F, Tombini M, Buffo P, Assenza G, Pellegrino G, Benvenga A, Babiloni C, Rossini PM. Mobile phone emission increases inter-hemispheric functional coupling of electroencephalographic alpha rhythms in epileptic patients. *Int J Psychophysiol.* 84:164–171, 2012b.

Vecsei Z, Csathó A, Thuróczy G, Hernádi I. Effect of a single 30 min UMTS mobile phone-like exposure on the thermal pain threshold of young healthy volunteers. *Bioelectromagnetics.* 34:530–541, 2013.

Velayutham P, Govindasamy GK, Raman R, Prepageran N, Ng KH. High-frequency hearing loss among mobile phone users. *Indian J Otolaryngol Head Neck Surg.* 66(Suppl 1):169–172, 2014.

Wallace D, Eltiti S, Ridgewell A, Garner K, Russo R, Sepulveda F, Walker S et al. Cognitive and physiological responses in humans exposed to a TETRA base station signal in relation to perceived electromagnetic hypersensitivity. *Bioelectromagnetics.* 33:23–39, 2012.

Wang H, Peng R, Zhao L, Wang S, Gao Y, Wang L, Zuo H et al. The relationship between NMDA receptors and microwave induced learning and memory impairment: A long-term observation on Wistar rats. *Int J Radiat Biol.* 91:262–269, 2015.

Wang H, Peng R, Zhou H, Wang S, Gao Y, Wang L, Yong Z et al. Impairment of long-term potentiation induction is essential for the disruption of spatial memory after microwave exposure. *Int J Radiat Biol.* 89:1100–1107, 2013.

Wang H, Tan S, Xu X, Zhao L, Zhang J, Yao B, Gao Y, Zhou H, Peng R. Long term impairment of cognitive functions and alterations of NMDAR subunits after continuous microwave exposure. *Physiol Behav.* 181:1–9, 2017.

Wang LF, Tian DW, Li HJ, Gao YB, Wang CZ, Zhao L, Zuo HY et al. Identification of a novel rat NR2B subunit gene promoter region variant and its association with microwave-induced neuron impairment. *Mol Neurobiol.* 53:2100–2111, 2016.

Wang K, Lu JM, Xing ZH, Zhao QR, Hu LQ, Xue L, Zhang J, Mei YA. Effect of 1.8 GHz radiofrequency electromagnetic radiation on novel object associative recognition memory in mice. *Sci Rep.* 7:44521, 2017.

Wang LF, Li X, Gao YB, Wang SM, Zhao L, Dong J, Yao BW et al. Activation of VEGF/Flk-1-ERK pathway induced blood-brain barrier injury after microwave exposure. *Mol Neurobiol.* 52:478–491, 2015.

Wang LF, Tian DW, Li HJ, Gao YB, Wang CZ, Zhao L, Zuo HY et al. Identification of a Novel Rat NR2B Subunit Gene Promoter Region Variant and Its Association with Microwave-Induced Neuron Impairment. *Mol Neurobiol.* 53:2100–2111, 2016.

Watilliaux A, Edeline JM, Lévêque P, Jay TM, Mallat M. Effect of exposure to 1,800 MHz electromagnetic fields on heat shock proteins and glial cells in the brain of developing rats. *Neurotox Res.* 20:109–119, 2011.

Wiholm C, Lowden A, Kuster N, Hillert L, Arnetz BB, Akerstedt T, Moffat SD. Mobile phone exposure and spatial memory. *Bioelectromagnetics.* 30:59–65, 2009.

Xiong L, Sun CF, Zhang J, Gao YB, Wang LF, Zuo HY, Wang SM et al. Microwave exposure impairs synaptic plasticity in the rat hippocampus and PC12 cells through over-activation of the NMDA receptor signaling pathway. *Biomed Environ Sci.* 28:13–24, 2015.

Xu F, Bai Q, Zhou K, Ma L, Duan J, Zhuang F, Xie C, Li W, Zou P, Zhu C. Age-dependent acute interference with stem and progenitor cell proliferation in the hippocampus after exposure to 1800 MHz electromagnetic radiation. *Electromagn Biol Med.* 36:158–166, 2017.

Xu S, Zhou Z, Zhang L, Yu Z, Zhang W, Wang Y, Wang X et al. Exposure to 1800 MHz radiofrequency radiation induces oxidative damage to mitochondrial DNA in primary cultured neurons. *Brain Res.* 1311:189–196, 2010.

Yakymenko I, Tsybulin O, Sidorik E, Henshel D, Kyrylenko O, Kyrylenko S. Oxidative mechanisms of biological activity of low-intensity radiofrequency radiation. *Electromagn Biol Med.* 35:186–202, 2016.

Yang L, Chen Q, Lv B, Wu T. Long-term evolution electromagnetic fields exposure modulates the resting state EEG on alpha and beta bands. *Clin EEG Neurosci.* 48:168–175, 2017.

Yang X, He G, Hao Y, Chen C, Li M, Wang Y, Zhang G, Yu Z. The role of the JAK2-STAT3 pathway in pro-inflammatory responses of EMF-stimulated N9 microglial cells. *J Neuroinflammation.* 7:54, 2010.

Yang XS, He GL, Hao YT, Xiao Y, Chen CH, Zhang GB, Yu ZP. Exposure to 2.45 GHz electromagnetic fields elicits an HSP-related stress response in rat hippocampus. *Brain Res Bull.* 88:371–378, 2012.

Yogesh S, Abha S, Priyanka S. Mobile usage and sleep patterns among medical students. *Indian J Physiol Pharmacol.* 58:100–103, 2014.

Yuan K, Qin W, Wang G, Zeng F, Zhao L, Yang X, Liu P et al. Microstructure abnormalities in adolescents with internet addiction disorder. *PLoS One.* 6:e20708, 2011.

Zareen N, Khan MY, Ali Minhas L. Derangement of chick embryo retinal differentiation caused by radiofrequency electromagnetic fields. *Congenit Anom (Kyoto).* 49:15–19, 2009.

Zhang JP, Zhang KY, Guo L, Chen QL, Gao P, Wang T, Li J, Guo GZ, Ding GR. Effects of 1.8 GHz radiofrequency fields on the emotional behavior and spatial memory of adolescent mice. *Int J Environ Res Public Health.* 14(11), 2017. pii: E1344. doi: 10.3390/ijerph14111344.

Zhang SZ, Yao GD, Lu DQ, Chiang H, Xu ZP. [Effect of 1.8 GHz radiofrequency electromagnetic fields on gene expression of rat neurons]. *Zhonghua Lao Dong Wei Sheng Zhi Ye Bing Za Zhi.* 26:449–452, 2008 (Article in Chinese).

Zhang Y, Li Z, Gao Y, Zhang C. Effects of fetal microwave radiation exposure on offspring behavior in mice. *J Radiat Res.* 56:261–268, 2015.

Zheng F, Gao P, He M, Li M, Wang C, Zeng Q, Zhou Z, Yu Z, Zhang L. Association between mobile phone use and inattention in 7102 Chinese adolescents: A population-based cross-sectional study. *BMC Public Health.* 14:1022, 2014.

Zhao TY, Zou SP, Knapp PE. Exposure to cell phone radiation up-regulates apoptosis genes in primary cultures of neurons and astrocytes. *Neurosci Lett.* 412:34–38, 2007.

9 Radiobiological Arguments for Assessing the Electromagnetic Hazard to Public Health for the Beginning of the Twenty-First Century

The Opinion of the Russian Scientist

Yury G. Grigoriev

CONTENTS

9.1 CARESSING ELECTROMAGNETIC SMOG IN THE PAST, AND NOW: UNCONTROLLED ELECTROMAGNETIC CHAOS IN THE HUMAN ENVIRONMENT

The author of this chapter began his journey in science as a radiobiologist from the first difficult steps in the implementation of the State Program for nuclear energy in Russia—in 1949. There were high requirements for the implementation of scientific programs, the shortness of time, the clarity of tasks, strict implementation of the schedule, and a complete absence of meaningless discussions. A special role was given to experimental studies on both large (dogs) and small (rats and mice) animals. Strict protocol conditions were created for general and local irradiation of animals, mainly with gamma radiation, with the assessment of applied and absorbed doses, and with dosimetry monitoring. It was important to create a clinical picture of various forms of radiation sickness to develop methods for the prevention and treatment of this serious disease. The Institute of Biophysics has a clinic for treatment of patients who received acute radiation in emergency situations in industry (both in terms of the area of the irradiated body and the amount of absorbed dose).

Working daily in this specific scientific and at the same time practical atmosphere, I was able to cope 37 years later with the problems that occurred in the first days after the Chernobyl accident (April 26, 1986). It was my duty to receive patients from the Chernobyl nuclear power plant, to organize their sanitation and hospitalization, to prevent additional radiation exposure from other patients because of their very strong "contamination" with radioactive substances, and to ensure subsequent treatment.

A total of 259 patients and 23 donors were hospitalized. On May 15, 1986, I was included in the Government Commission for the liquidation of the accident at the Chernobyl nuclear power plant and on the same day flew to the Chernobyl nuclear power plant. The situation changed dramatically when I immersed myself in assessing the health risks of non-ionizing electromagnetic radiation, which received at that time the harmless name "electromagnetic smog," and began to be constantly present in the human habitat. Initially, these were different broadcasting stations, emissions from space objects, power lines, and household appliances, and special attention was paid to radar stations. The population living near airports was sometimes irradiated with EMF exceeding the permissible levels, but this was tolerated.

In the 1960s, with the development of the television and radio network in the USSR, there arose a practical need to ensure the safety of the population in conditions when relatively large sources of RF EMF were located on the border or on the territory of residential buildings. The Kiev Institute of Communal Hygiene was leader of this program. Under the leadership of M.G. Shandala, the State Program on the Justification of permissible levels of Non-Ionizing Radiation of the Radio Frequency Range for the population was launched. Unique experiments were conducted, lasting up to several months, using low nonthermal levels of exposure. We received very valuable results which have been published in numerous peer-reviewed journals of the USSR (Shandala and Vinogradov, 1982; Vinogradov and Dumansky, 1974, 1975).

In 1997, we reanalyzed all early publications and once again confirmed that the results obtained were correctly chosen for the basis for the standardization of RF EMF exposure for the population in the USSR. The reader can find the results of this generalization in the International Science and Technology Center (ISTC) report in Russian and English (ISTC, 2003).

However, even before the era of mobile communication, in the United States, doubt was expressed about the reliability of the results of these experiments. At the same time, western authors proceeded from the elementary postulate that the human body can not react to nonthermal exposure, claiming that there are no known mechanisms for nonthermal exposure and therefore our results were not correct.

There was a very complicated situation with EMF standards. The differences in the standards between the USSR and the USA were significant; their magnitudes differed by three orders of magnitude. Considering this, a Soviet-American group of well-known specialists was established. The head of the Soviet group was M.G. Shandala. From the US side, very well-known experts were included (professors Guy, Fry, Lai, McRae), and others. I was able to take part in the working meeting of this group three times. However, we were unable to reach a common opinion for standard recommendation.

Various joint commissions were created, numerous international meetings, round tables, and informal forums were held which claimed only thermal effects. This view was actively supported by industry. Promoting this concept, the WHO Advisory Committee, ICNIRP, IEEE, ANSI have defended only one concept—thermal effects. Based on these positions, the WHO Advisory Committee, ICNIRP, and IEEE became completely scientifically bankrupt (Decision of the Parliamentary Assembly of the Council of Europe May 2011 with a demand to revise the standards. More than 25 countries adopted stricter standards—Belgium, Brazil, Spain, Israel, Italy, Canada, United Kingdom, etc.).

With the increasing use of mobile communications among the population, many specialists have neglected radiobiological concepts, for example, the concept of a critical organ or critical system, the possibility of accumulating bioeffects, the degree of residual damage, and long-term effects. The novelty of the almost daily life-long exposure to RF EMF of the human brain did not receive attention, and the precautionary principle proposed by WHO, that children are at risk, was completely disregarded. It was the first time in human civilization to include children into a risk group (Grigoriev, 2014; Markov and Grigoriev, 2015).

Until now, isolated studies have been carried out without taking into account the basic radiobiological arguments to assess the dangers of mobile communication for public health. This occurs against the backdrop of periodically appearing publications that mobile communication is not dangerous to the health of the population, which is outrageous. Attempts are still being made to assert that mobile communication does not have a negative impact on children. Naturally, the increase in the geometric proportion of the general anthropogenic background of RF EMF comes primarily because of the increase in the number of base stations (BS). However, the transition to the 5G standard will lead to a further sharp increase in the number of base stations and additional irradiation. The standard 5G will use low frequencies (6–3.7 Hz), medium frequencies (3.7–24 Hz), and high frequencies (24–26 GHz and higher). The antennas of the millimeter signals are planned to be installed on any residential house and in schools. According to information from the US, in California, up to 50,000 new millimeter base stations should be installed (Moskowitz, 2017). A declaration of the world scientific community has already been signed with a recommendation to officials in the European Union to introduce a moratorium on the deployment of 5G telecommunication networks until the potential risks to human health and the environment are fully investigated by scientists independent of the industry (EU 5G Appeal, 10 August, 2017).

Really, today there is round-the-clock exposure of the population to different carrier frequencies and with different modulations.

Mobile phones (MT) are open sources of electromagnetic radiation which are accessible to all population groups. They can be purchased in almost any store without the availability of guidance materials. With the use of MT, local irradiation of the brain and nervous receptive structures of the inner ear predominantly occurs. For the first time in the whole period of civilization, the brain became a critical organ. The variety of mobile phones and other gadgets expands the geography of their uncontrolled use. The proposed tariffs increase the duration of the conversation and thus increase the total absorbed dose by the brain.

The most basic principles of protection are not brought to the consciousness of the population in an accessible form: **protection by time and distance.** And this means that one needs to talk less on the mobile phone, the conversation should be short and business oriented, and, if possible, keep the phone away from the ear or use a speakerphone or an appropriate headset.

Sometimes we see a substitution in the significance of the results. For example, an attempt is made to study the unfavorable effects from the electromagnetic radiation of the BS. The intensity of the RF EMF of BS is extremely low and additionally there are a lot of other factors affecting the test population. In fact, there is a substitution of concepts! At the same time, some authors try to introduce these "effective instruments of protection" into schools, accompanied by the words that with these instruments make it safe to use mobile phones without restrictions. In this electromagnetic chaos, an attempt is made to profit from the sale of many so-called local means of protection (covers, stickers, etc.).

Thus, in just 25 years, there was a global breakthrough in the use of wireless communication by the population which significantly changed the situation of man-made electromagnetic pollution of the external environment and the methodology for assessing the health risks for the all population groups.

Twenty-five years ago, when the era of mobile communication had only begun, the steps and technogenic pollution of the environment was well predicted, there were normative documents, and the concept of the thermal effect of RF EMF was accepted as an axiom. This situation was characterized as an innocuous "electromagnetic smog."

Now, 25 years later, this situation can be characterized as "electromagnetic chaos," which is beginning to be realized by the main scientific community and government circles. In fact, this is the era of "electromagnetic" lawlessness of electromagnetic pollution of the environment.

It is clear that the scientific community and public health services were not prepared for an epochal change in communication among the population, which is directly related to the constant additional impact of RF EMF on the body of the population.

We observe the complete confusion of both scientists and governmental officials in many countries that take opposite sides or simply ignore a situation that can be characterized as "electromagnetic chaos" in the habitat of the population. We can characterize this situation as a global uncontrolled experiment (Markov and Grigoriev, 2013).

9.2 STUDY OF THE BIOLOGICAL EFFECT OF NON-IONIZING ELECTROMAGNETIC RADIATION OF NONTHERMAL INTENSITY IN THE REGIME OF ACUTE EXPERIMENTS

The first experiments with biological model systems were held in our laboratory of the Institute of Biophysics of the USSR Ministry of Health in 1977, primarily to confirm the hypothesis of a possible biological effect of the electromagnetic field of a nonthermal intensity.

We selected the basic models based on participation in the central nervous system (CNS) response. This choice was influenced by earlier studies of Yu. Kholodov published in 1975–1992, in which he showed the high radiosensitivity of the CNS to various types of permanent, alternating magnetic fields and electromagnetic fields of various frequencies.

Back in 1996, we pointed to the necessity of evaluation of the biological effects of complex EMF generation regimes and of various types of modulation (Grigoriev et al., 1995). A number of experiments in our laboratory were carried out using various modes of modulation and a structurally complicated electromagnetic signal. There were reasons to suppose that the complication from the electromagnetic signals due to modulation or changes in other parameters would lead to a "forced" response of the organism when the RF EMF is exposed to a very low nonthermal intensity.

As a deputy director, I succeeded in attracting a large team of researchers, including specialists in various fields: radiobiologists, biophysicists, physiologists, electrophysiologists, morphologists, physicists, and engineers. A unique irradiator base was created. Several anechoic chambers were built; a number of EMF generators were purchased. Serious attention was paid to the importance of dosimetry of EMF.

A large series of studies was performed on the characteristic of changes in the total bioelectrical activity of the brain under conditions of acute single and repeated effects of RF EMF with various regimes, including modulation and a more complex structure of the electromagnetic signal. The research was conducted on volunteers (mobile phone users), on rabbits, small laboratory animals (rats), and brain sections (Lukyanova, 2015).

In our laboratory, beginning in 1983, studies were carried out on the effect of memory formation during irradiation with RF EMF of chickens used as an imprinting model (Grigorev et al., 1984, Grigoriev and Stepanov, 1998; 2000). Previously, this model was not used to study the biological effect of RF EMF. The purpose of this study was to evaluate the formation of memory in chickens after preliminary exposure to electromagnetic fields of low nonthermal levels, and establish the so-called dose relationship between different levels of RF EMF and functional changes (substitutions) in the most sensitive system—in the brain in accordance with the criterion of memory disorder. Experiments showed the direct effect of RF EMF on the brain with nonthermal intensity (Grigoriev and Stepanov, 1998; 2000).

Another study was carried out with 10 volunteers—users of mobile phones under short-term EMF exposure of the head (Grigoriev et al., 1999). The standard MNT-50, GSM-900, and GSM-180, output power 1.0, 0.25 and 0.12 W, respectively, were applied. There were repeated exposures with single times of 5, 10, and 20 minutes. Prior to, during, and after the exposure, the EEG was recorded for 2 hours; the condition of the cardiovascular system was checked, muscle tone was assessed, psychological tests were performed, and blood from the vein was used to characterize possible changes in hormonal status. Changes in the bioelectrical activity of the brain were observed–an increase in the power of the alpha rhythm. These changes were not permanent and persisted for the first 60–120 minutes after the completion of RF EMF exposure.

It was shown that 300 μW/cm^2, with a complex mode of modulation (pulse repetition frequency 0.16 Hz, pulse duration 16 ms, rectangular shape, 100% modulation depth) and bioelectric activity in the parietal-occipital and antero-central regions induced more significant changes than after exposure to only one carrier frequency (1.5 GHz) in continuous mode (Lukyanova, 2002). Based on numerous experiments, we came to the conclusion that the burst-pulse mode is more efficient than the continuous mode without modulation.

Lukyanova (1999) registered pre-convulsive electroencephalography activity in rabbits after exposure to EMF 1.2 GHz in pulsed mode, meander, 100 Hz, 400 μW/cm^2 in impulse. Based on the results of our studies, as well as the results obtained by other authors, we came to the conclusion that RF EMF of low intensity can have a synchronizing effect on the bioelectric processes in the brain, which can lead to the development of convulsive syndrome.

In our laboratory, it was shown that the influence of a certain form of modulation of the carrier electromagnetic field or complex regimes of the active EMF leads to the possibility of developing a convulsive syndrome in rabbits (Grigoriev and Sidorenko, 2010).

It is necessary to pay attention to the statement about the renewal of nerve cells in the hippocampus. In the adult hippocampus, neurogenesis is carried out continuously, and this process serves as the neurobiological basis for the formation of new memory (Van Praag et al., 2002). It is established that the hippocampus, which retains the ability of neurogenesis, plays a key role in the formation of long-term memory, information, and its distribution in the higher parts of the brain. From these results follows the assumption of a possible increased sensitivity of nerves.

Unfortunately, acute experiments with short-term exposure to RF do not allow to draw conclusions about the degree of danger of cellular communication for public health due to the impossibility of assessing the classical radiobiological criterion–the process of accumulation of adverse consequences and the development of long-term consequences. However, the results presented in this chapter allow us to affirm that RF EMF of low intensity, nonthermal level causes a biological response, which was taken into account when assessing standards for chronic exposure conditions.

9.3 CHRONIC EFFECTS OF RF EMF WITH NON-THERMAL INTENSITY

The mobile communication user subjects his brain every day to a local electromagnetic exposure, and his whole body is irradiated around the clock and for life. In this regard, the evaluation of the development of the body's response in the process of chronic long-term exposure acquires special significance (Gigoriev, 1997, 1999; Belyev and Grigoriev, 2007; Markov and Grigoriev, 2013; Markov, 2015; Grigoriev and Grigoriev, 2016).

The deterioration in the health of the population is difficult to connect with the impact of EMF from base stations, since the population is faced with numerous other factors of the environment. With this in mind, experiments simulating the chronic impact of RF EMF are gaining importance.

Earlier in this paper, we pointed out that a special program in the Institute of Communal Hygiene in Kiev produced unique results in experiments on the chronic effect of RF EMF with nonthermal intensity. On the basis of these data it was concluded that RF EMF of nonthermal intensity in conditions of chronic long-term RF EMF action can lead to the development of adverse reactions.

However, in the West, probably because of neglecting publications in Russian language, the notion that nonthermal RF EMF intensities can not cause any biological effect was introduced. With a persistence worthy of imitation, experts did not get acquainted with these results and did not use the results obtained in the USSR when developing international regulatory documents for RF EMF. A single point of view was promoted that only thermal effects are possible with the subsequent conclusion that the existing technogenic levels of the electromagnetic field in the habitat of the population do not pose a danger to general health. US scientists visited our laboratory under the sign "Show all your data." We showed the data, but after many days of discussions, they still had only one hypothesis: only the thermal effect of RF EMF (Figure 9.1).

This one-sided interpretation of the thermal effect steadily persisted during the years. It is time to break this monotonous trend. The first to do this were the scientists of Austria. G. Oberfeld in 2010 organized a round table with the participation of American scientists S. Sage and C. Blockman, scholars of other countries, and the author of the article. A proposal was made to reduce the allowable level to 1 μW/cm^2.

The author of this article in 2014 proposed to WHO to reproduce experiments using the nonthermal level of high-frequency EMF, performed by M.G. Shandala and

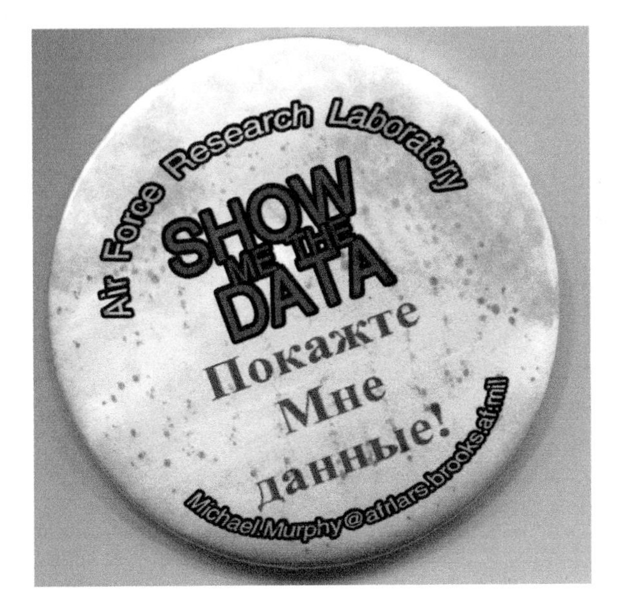

FIGURE 9.1 A badge of the US delegation member M. Murphy in Russia with a request (in Russian): "Show me the data."

his colleagues. We suggested that this experiment be carried out under the auspices of WHO and the Scientific International Monitoring Committee. In 2005, our offer was accepted.

Two previously conducted experiments with low levels of RF EMF on immunological effects were chosen, the results of which were mentioned earlier in this chapter (Vinogradov and Dumansky 1974, 1975; Shandala and Vinogradov, 1982).

The previously used protocol was implemented and in addition, the modern conditions of RF EMF exposure and dosimetry methods were created. In addition, more correct planning of all stages of the study using a blind method was carried out. The program and protocol of the experiment, with a detailed description of all stages of the study, were coordinated with WHO and approved by an independent Scientific Review Committee, which included scientists from the United States, Italy, and Germany.

In coordination with WHO, the leading institution was chosen to be our laboratory of the Institute of Biophysics. The irradiation of animals and dosimetry was performed with the participation of French specialists. The conditions of EMF action guaranteed a uniform irradiation of all groups of experimental animals in equal absorbed doses.

The work with animals during the quarantine period (14 days) and the whole period of exposure (30 days) was performed by a "neutral" (not interested in the results) radiobiological laboratory of ionizing radiation of the Institute of Biophysics. The employees of this laboratory were not familiar with the tasks of the experiment, which ensured the implementation of the blind method in the entire experiment and in subsequent work with experimental encrypted material by other performers.

The experiment started in October 2006. The entire cycle of the experiment, including the processing of the samples, analysis of the results, and the preparation of the conclusion were carried out with the active participation of the Scientific Supervisory Committee–external observers representing scientists from Germany (J. Bushmann), Italy (C. Pioli), and the United States (R. Sypnewski), and also with the active all round assistance of the former head of the WHO International Program, "EMF and Health," M. Repacholi.

The experiment was entirely implemented by the WHO protocol and the framework of the international program required three years of work (2005–2007). The report on the results of the experiment and the general conclusion were submitted to WHO and to the Committee on Scientific Observations. The main results of this experiment are published in Grigoriev et al. (2010a).

"This study was conducted using the methodology of the original experiments conducted in the USSR (Vinogradov and Dumansky, 1974, 1975; Shandala and Vinogradov, 1982). Autoimmunity was evaluated using the original methodology developed in the USSR (Vinogradov and Dumansky, 1974, 1975; Shandala and Vinogradov, 1982). The original methodology was a CFT, however, our study was expanded to include the ELISA test. The Russian study was conducted in accordance with WHO recommendations on RF biological research and Good Laboratory Practice (GLP) principles. The results of our immunology study using the CFT and ELISA tests partly confirmed the results of the Soviet research groups on the possible induction of autoimmune responses (formation of antibodies to brain tissues) and stress reactions from RF EMF exposure (30-day exposure for 7 h/day for 5 days/week at a power density of 5 W/m^2), that is, long-term non-thermal RF exposure. The results of our study on prenatal development of offspring suggested possible adverse effects of the blood serum from exposed rats (30-day exposure for 7 h/day for 5 days/week at a power density of 5 W/m^2) on pregnancy and embryo–fetal development in rats, in agreement with the earlier results of Shandala and Vinogradov (1982), although the model used by Shandala and Vinogradov (1982), which was intentionally replicated here, is not considered an appropriate one for assessing human health effects from RF exposure."

The main results of this experiment were published in the journal Radiation Biology, Radioecology RAS in 2010 in five reports in Russian (Grigoriev et al. (2010b), Message 1; Grigoriev et al. (2010c), Message 2; Ivanov et al. (2010) Message 3; Grigoriev et al. (2010d), Message 4; Lyaginskaya et al. (2010), Message 5); as well as in English (Grigoriev et al. Bioelectromagnetics, 2010a).

Consequently, we obtained the results confirming the validity of the database used in 1956 in order to justify the standards for RF EMF in the USSR—10 $\mu W/cm^2$, which have not changed so far in Russia.

These data allow us to conclude that the immune system can be considered as a critical system when evaluating the biological effect of RF EMF of low intensity. The above results, indicating the presence of dose dependency under the influence of low intensity RF EMF, make it possible to use the results in the development of regulatory documents.

Earlier, we analyzed the risk of developing so-called somatic long-term effects under the action of various factors, including the chronic effect of RF EMF of low nonthermal intensities (Grigoriev et al. (2003)). One of the reasons for the development of this type of long-term consequences may be a decrease in the body's compensatory reserves and, as a consequence, acceleration of the aging processes. Previous studies have shown that long-term adverse effects as a result of prolonged exposure to RF EMF can be expressed in an increase in the incidence of morbidity from the main body systems (central nervous, cardiovascular, immune, etc.) and exert additional influence on the deterioration of public health. In a number of other studies with prolonged exposure to RF EMF, an earlier development of age-related disorders in the body and a possible reduction in life expectancy were noted (Tyagin, 1971; Nikitina, 2004). Bondareva and Zolkina (2017) evaluated the thermal effect of electromagnetic radiation from a mobile phone in the area of the auricle. All phones used in the experiment had a significantly lower SAR value than the standard set. In the experiment, 20 people aged 22–71 years, who for half an hour were talking on a mobile phone, participated. The results showed that the tympanic membrane was heated with $2.52 \pm 0.2°C$. Topographically, auditory and vestibular nerve receptor structures are located directly behind the tympanic membrane and cannot escape the heating. Given the daily repeated impact on these structures, we can expect adverse manifestations of hearing and vestibular disorders in "heavy users" of mobile phones.

The population has been using mobile communication for more than 25 years. To date, according to epidemiological studies, a carcinogenic effect is possible in the users of cell phones, which has been identified as a specific adverse manifestation of the effect of RF EMF.

Over the past ten years, there has been an active discussion among the world community about the possibility of developing brain cancer among users of cell phones. At the same time, a number of international organizations have diametrically opposing points of view. For example, the WHO International Agency for Research on Cancer (IARC), published in May 2011 a press release in which RF EMF mobile phones are referred to as the promoters of brain glioma tumors in group 2B. However, at the meetings of the WHO Advisory Committee on the International Program "EMF and Public Health" in 2011 and 2012, an opinion was promoted that there is no confidence in this IARC decision.

Of course, most of the negative opinions on this issue are formed under the influence of industry and financial interests. Unfortunately, many scientists participate in lobbying for their interests. As a result, the world lobbying syndicate was established, with constant financial support, which prevents objectively informing the population about the possible adverse effects of RF EMF on public health.

A group of Swedish scientists led by Hardell L. has been conducting complex epidemiological studies for over 15 years on the analysis of the development of brain tumors in cellular communication users. **The authors pointed out the increased risk of developing brain tumors in mobile phone users with a** "waiting period" of 10 years with a risk from 1.3–1.8. An increased risk of astrocytoma and acoustic neurinoma on the ipsilateral side of the brain has been found. The risk of developing brain tumors increases up to 5 times in people who started using cell phones and portable phones at the age of 8–10 years, and the development of the tumor depends on the duration of the use of the cell phone. Hardell L. and co-authors consider it necessary to classify the promoter activity of EMF cell phones in group 1, "as carcinogenic to humans." (Hardell et al., 2015). Of course, long-term consequences are important radiobiological criteria.

At the beginning of 2016, a statistical report was published on data obtained in the USA on the basis of the materials of the National Cancer Institute (NCI), the National Cancer Registry Program (NPCR), and the United States Agency international development (USAID) epidemiological surveillance program for 2008–2012. Conclusions were drawn about the increase in the development of brain tumors in the US population of different age groups for the period 2000–2010. The authors of these materials believe that the increase in brain tumors was significant and associate this growth with the use of cellular communication (Gittleman et al., 2015; Ostrom et al., 2015).

In May 2016, a report was published on the results of a large-scale experiment conducted in the framework of the US National Toxicology Program (NTP) (Microwave News, May 2016; http://bit.ly/WSJsaferemr). The report is presented by the National Institute of Environmental Health (NIEHS US). For 18 years, since 1999, the Scientific Program of this experiment has been developed, an independent form of financing for this project has been determined, an appropriate experimental base has been created and, finally, a two-year experiment was conducted. This program was financed by the US Government and the cost of this experiment amounted to $25 million.

The rats were exposed to the RF EMF of cell phones every 10 minutes, followed by a 10-minute break for 18 hours, resulting in nine hours per day for two years. Two GSM and CDMA standards were used. The frequency of the signals was 900 MHz.

Four groups were used for each type of cell phone standard: resulting in three experimental groups of 180 rats and a control group—shame exposure (90 rats). The lowest intensity of exposure was SAR 1.5 W/kg, the other two groups were exposed with intensities of SAR 3 and 6 W/kg, which eliminated tissue heating, that is, the "thermal effect."

This study showed a statistically significant increase in the incidence of cancer among rats that were electromagnetically exposed to GSM or CDMA signals for two years. As a result of exposure, tumors were developed in 30 of the 540 rats (5.5%), or in one of the 18 rats exposed to the EMF of the cell phone. In addition, some rats were diagnosed with precancerous hyperplasia. Thus, in 46 of the 540 rats, or in one of the 12 rats exposed to the EMF of the cell phone, cancer or precancerous cell hyperplasia developed. The development of tumors was directly dependent on the intensity of EMF. A significant dose-effect relationship was obtained.

In a group of rats exposed to EMF of a low-intensity cellular phone (1.5 W/kg), 12 of 180 rats, or one of 15 rats developed tumors or pretumor cell hyperplasia. In the group of rats with the highest exposure (6 W/kg), in 24 out of 180 rats, or in one of the 8 male rats, a cancer or premalignant hyperplasia developed. Irradiated rats developed two types of tumors: gliomas and schwannoma. Both types of tumors were previously detected in cell phone users during epidemiological studies. **It is very important that "none of the unirradiated control rats had the development of any type of tumor."**

The results showed that nonthermal levels of RF EMF can cause the development of tumors in the brain. This conclusion contradicts the current INCRIP recommendations, which recommend a permissible level for a cell phone of 2.0 W/kg. Thus, the results of a unique two-year experiment to assess the possible development of brain tumors in cell phone users (US National Toxicology Program—NTP, 1999–2016) have increased the reliability of the global conclusion about possible health risks to the EMF population when using cellular communication and the impact of EMF RF nonthermal intensity.

Concerned about the hesitancy of WHO and the widespread global adoption of wireless technology, more than 200 EMF scientists from 40 countries submitted a petition in May 2016 to the United Nations, WHO, and world leaders to review EMF safety levels in the light of recent research and warn the public about the risks associated with exposure to RF EMF.

9.4 CONCLUSIONS

At present, there are no unified approaches to assessing the health hazards of the RF EMF of mobile communications. There is a wide variation in the permissible RF EMF levels. The possibility of developing long-term consequences is underestimated. The technical solutions for the creation of new types of wireless communication outrun scientific research to assess the danger to the public. The precautionary principle is ignored when placing base stations. There is a desire to ensure that all schools use Wi-Fi.

The large spread, uncontrolled, use of this connection by all groups of the population, including children, continues although the mobile phone is an open source of radiation, and the critical body is the user's brain.

In conditions of the existing electromagnetic chaos, it is necessary to inform the population that mobile communication in the absence of self-control can be dangerous for health, and as an independent choice for the population, it is necessary to introduce the category of "voluntary risk."

We must finally stop the electromagnetic chaos.

REFERENCES

Belyev I., Grigoriev Y. 2007. Problems in assessment of risk from exposures to microwaves of mobile communication Radiation biology. *Radioecology*. 47(6), p. 727–730.

Bondareva E., Zolkina E. 2017. Evaluation of the thermal effect of electromagnetic radiation of a mobile phone on the brain. *Fundamental and Applied Problems of Technology and Technology*. 2(322), p. 145–150. (In Russian).

Gittleman H. et al. 2015. Trends in central nervous system tumor incidence relative to other common cancers in adults, adolescents, and children in the United States, 2000 to 2010. *Cancer*. 2015, 121(1), p. 102–112.

Grigoriev Y. 1997. Bioelectromagnetics compatibility (Problems of protecting people against electromagnetic radiation. *Electrical Technolgy*. 13, p. 121–130.

Grigoriev Y. 1999. The impact of electromagnetic fields of man-made nature on man (assessment of danger). *Medicine of Extreme Situations*. 2, p. 34–35. (In Russian).

Grigoriev Y. 2014. Mobile phone and adverse effect on the user's brain—risk assessment. Radiation Biology. *Radioecology*. 54(2), p. 215–216. (In Russian).

Grigoriev Y., Beskhlebnova L., Mityaeva Z. 1984. Combined action of microwaves and gamma radiation on imprinting in chickens irradiated in early embryogenesis. *Radiobiology*. 24(c. 2), p. 204–207. (In Russian).

Grigoryev Y., Grigoriev O. 2016. Cellular and Health. Electromagnetic charge. Radiobiological and hygienic problems. *Forecast of Danger. Moscow*. 2016, 574 p. (In Russian).

Grigoriev Y., Grigoriev O., Ivanov A. et al. 2010a. Confirmation studies of Soviet research on immunological effects of microwaves: Russian Immunology results. *Bioelectromagnetics*, 31(8), p. 589–602.

Grigoriev Y., Grigoriev O., Ivanov A., Lyaginskaya A. et al. 2010b. Autoimmune processes after prolonged exposure to low intensity electromagnetic fields (Experimental results). Message 1. Mobile communication and changing the electromagnetic environment of the population. The need for additional justification for existing hygienic standards. *Radiation Biology. Radioecology*. 50(1), p. 5–11. (In Russian).

Grigoryev Y., Grigoriev O., Merkulov A. et al. 2010c. Message 2. General scheme and conditions of the study. Creation of conditions for irradiation with electromagnetic fields in accordance with the tasks of the experiment. The condition of animals during prolonged irradiation. *Radiation Biology. Radioecology*. 50(1), p. 12–16. (In Russian).

Grigoryev Y., Lukyanova S., Grigoriev O. et al. 1999. Human reaction to the electromagnetic radiation of a cellular phone. *Materials of the International Meeting 'Electromagnetic fields. Biological Action and Hygienic Regulation*. Moscow, 1998. Izd. WHO, Geneva, pp. 525–536. (In Russian).

Grigoriev Y., Lukyanova S., Makarov V., Rinskov V. 1995. Motor activity of rabbits in conditions of chronic low-intensity pulse microwave irradiation. *Radiation biology. Radioecology*. 35(1), p. 29–35. (In Russian).

Grigoryev Y., Mikhailov V., Ivanov A. et al. 2010d. Message 4. Manifestation of oxidative intracellular stress reactions after chronic exposure to EMF RF of low intensity in rats. *Radiation Biology. Radioecology*. 50(1), p. 22–27. (In Russian).

Grigoriev Y., Shafirkin A., Niktina V., Vasin A. 2003. The effects of the chronic effect of ionizing radiation and electromagnetic fields on the hygienic regulation are remote. *Radiation Biology. Radioecology*. T.43(5), p. 565–578. (In Russian).

Grigoriev Y., Sidorenko V. 2010. Electromagnetic fields of nonthermal level and evaluation of the possibility of development of convulsive syndrome. *Radiation Biology. Radioecology*. 505, p. 552–559. (In Russian).

Grigoriev Y., Stepanov V. 1998. Formation of memory (imprinting) at chickens after preliminary exposure of electromagnetic fields of low levels. *Radiation biology. Radioecology*. 38(2), p. 223–231. (In Russian).

Grigoriev Y., Stepanov V. 2000. Microwave effect on embryo brain: dose dependence and the effect of modulation. B.J. Klauenberg and D. Miklavic (eds), *Radio Frequency Radiation Dosimetry*, Kluwer Academic Publishers, Dordrecht, p. 31–37.

Hardell L., Carlberg M. et al. 2015. Cell and cordless phone risk for glioma: Analysis of pooled case-control studies in Sweden, 1997–2003 and 2007–2009. *Pathophysiology*. 22:1–13. Available online. http://dx.doi.org/10.10167j.pathophys.2014.10.001

IARC/A/WHO. 2011. Classifies radiofrequency electromagnetic fields as possibly carcinogenic to humans. Press release, No 208, 31 May, 2011, 3 p.

ISTC. 2003. Project No. 2362, Analytical Report 'Biological Effects of Electromagnetic Fields of the Radio Frequency Range Applied to the Problem of Normalization (Results of the Experiments in the Ussr-Russia)', Moscow, IBP, 2003, supervisor Yu. Grigoryev.

Ivanov A., Grigoriev Y., Maltsev V. et al. 2010. Message 3. Effect of EMF RF nonthermal intensity on the level of complementary anti-tumor antibodies. *Radiation Biology. Radioecology*. 50(1), p. 12–16. (In Russian).

Lukyanova S. 1999. Reaction of the central nervous system to low-intensity short-term microwave radiation. *Materials of the International Meeting 'Electromagnetic Fields. Biological Action and Hygienic Regulation*. Moscow, 1998. Izd. WHO, Geneva, p. 401–408. (In Russian).

Lukyanova S. 2015. *Electromagnetic Field Super High Frequency not—Thermal Intensity as a Stimulus to the Central Nervous System*. Moscow, 200 p. (In Russian).

Lukyanova S.N. 2002. Phenomenology and genesis of changes in the total bioelectric activity of the brain on electromagnetic radiation. *Radiation Biology. Radioecology*. T.42(3), p. 308–331. (In Russian).

Lyaginskaya A., Grigoriev Y., Osipov V.A. et al. 2010. Message 5. Study of the influence of serum of irradiated rats with low-intensity electromagnetic fields on the course of pregnancy, fetal development, offspring. *Radiation Biology. Radioecology*. 50(1), p. 28–36. (In Russian).

Markov M. 2015. Benefit and hazard of electromagnetic fields. In: *Electromagnetic Fields in Biology and Medicine*. CRC Press, p. 15–28.

Markov M., Grigoriev Y. 2013. *Wi-Fi Technology an Uncontrolled Experiment*. J. Nexus, 17(1), p. 15–20.

Markov M., Grigoriev Y. 2015. Protect children from EMF. *Electromagnetic Biology and Medicine*. 34(3), p. 251–256.

Moskowitz J. 2017. 5G wireless technology: Millimeter wave health effects. *Electromagnetic Radiation Safety*. No. 3, pp. 3–6.

Nikitna V.N. 2004. Influence of modulated electromagnetic fields on aging processes. *Proceedings of Int. Shipbuilding Confirmation*, Russia, p. 60–66. (In Russian).

Ostrom Q., Gittleman H., Fulop J. et al. 2015. CBTRUS statistical report: Primary brain and central nervous system tumors diagnosed in the United States in 2008–2012. *Neuro-Oncology*. 17(Supplement 4), p. 1–62.

Shandala M., Vinogradov G. 1982. *Autoallergic Effects of Electromagnetic Energy of the MW-Range Exposure and their Influence on a Foetus and Posterity. The Bulletin of the Academy of Medical Sciences of the USSR*. Moscow: Medicina. p. 13–16. (In Russian).

Tyagin N. 1971. Clinical aspects of irradiation of the microwave range. *Leningrad Medicine* 231 p. (In Russian).

Van Praag H., Shinder A., Christa B. et al. 2002. Functional neurogenesis in adult hippocampus. *Netere*. 445(6875), p. 1030–1034.

Vinogradov G., Dumansky Y. 1974. Change of antigenic properties of fabrics and autoallergic processes at influence of MW-energy. *Bulletin of Experimental Biology and Medicine*. 8, p. 76–79. (In Russian).

Vinogradov G., Dumansky Y. 1975. On the sensitization action of ultrahigh frequency electromagnetic fields. *Gigiena i Sanitariya*. 9, p. 31–35. (In Russian).

Wyde M., Cesta M., Blystone C. et al. 2015. Report of Partial findings from the National Toxicology Program Carcinogenesis Studies of Cell Phone Radiofrequency Radiation in Hsd: Sprague Dawley® SD rats (Whole Body Exposure), (US National Toxicology Program—NTP), 1999–2016. https://doi.org/10.1101/055699.

10 A Longitudinal Study of Psychophysiological Indicators in Pupils Users of Mobile Communications in Russia (2006–2017)

Children Are in the Group of Risk

Yury G. Grigoriev and Natalia I. Khorseva

CONTENTS

10.1 INTRODUCTION

We would start this paper by asking several principle questions. **WHY** does mankind allow, for the first time in the history of civilization, the child's brain to be exposed daily to radio frequency electromagnetic fields, **why** are devices that are potential sources of electromagnetic radiation sold in stores and are freely accessible to children, **why** do children use sources of radio frequency electromagnetic fields without control and at their sole discretion (Grigoriev and Khorseva, 2014)? **Why** do the international forums need to return to school cable links and to abandon Wi-Fi (Reykjavik Appeal on wireless technology in schools, 2017)? **Why** has an international group of experts of the European Cancer and Environment Research Institute (ECERI) proposed to create an international group of scientists and lawyers to discuss the possibility that the deliberation of the electromagnetic pollution may be considered by the International Criminal Court (ICC) as a true crime against the health of the population? (ECERI Newsletter. No. 6, June 2017)? **Why** has the lack of real action aimed at reducing electromagnetic effects on the children been replaced by endless years of fruitless discussions? (Grigoriev and Grigoriev, 2013).

10.2 THE REAL SITUATION CAN BE ASSESSED AS THE PERFORMANCE OF A GLOBAL, UNRESTRAINED EXPERIMENT INVOLVING CHILDREN

We should admit the fact that the largest group of users of mobile communication is small children and teens who "must" have a connection almost 24 hours a day. If in 2009 in the work of Khurana and coworkers, the fact that the use of a mobile phone starts at the age of three looked sensational (Khurana et al., 2009), the studies that Kabali and coworkers conducted in the US showed that more than a third of ***babies*** six months old start to use computerized toys, including smartphones and tablets, and by the age of two years, the mobile devices are in use by the vast majority of children (Kabali et al., 2015).

However, there is still no way to evaluate and predict the potential damage to the brain of children by this early exposure to EMF. In this regard, the precautionary principle and WHO IARC classification should apply in discussing the potential dangers for children with the "use today and tomorrow of the cellular communication device."

10.2.1 Sources of Exposure to RF EMF Children

First of all, the base stations represent a constant source of technogenic environmental pollution. They generate RF EMF round the clock almost during the entire life of the human population, including children.

Next is the impact on children's health of the number of sources of WiFi as well as many varieties of gadgets. Even if one considers this irradiation to be of less intensity, we have the case of absorbed radiation energy from different sources acting together and initiating various effects which are difficult to predict and assess.

There are publications that WiFi affects the brain activity of children and can reduce working memory (Maganioti et al., 2010; Papageorgiou et al., 2011). From our view point, the authors' assumption requires additional confirmation.

In 2015, Lukyanova compiled and analyzed studies published during the last 40 years on changes in bioelectrical activity of brain and other reactions of the central

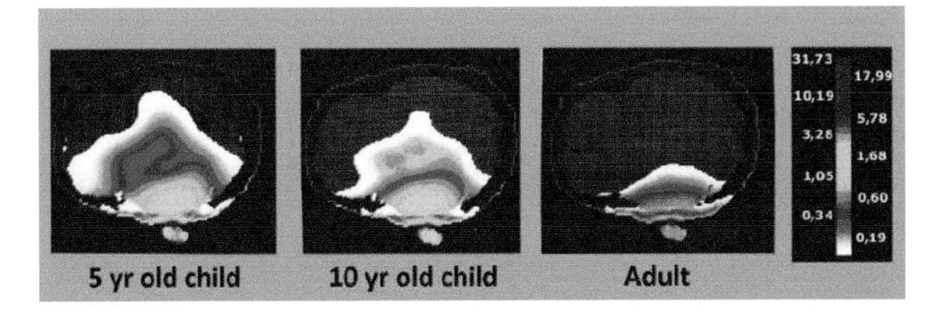

FIGURE 10.1 Distribution of absorbed energy in the brains of adults and children of different ages (5 and 10 years) using mobile phone. (From Gandhi O P et al. 1996. *IEEE Trans Microw Theory Tech.* 44(10): 1884–1897.)

nervous system to RF electromagnetic fields with nonthermal intensity (Lukyanova, 2015). The author came to the conclusion that nonthermal RF EMF at the short-term exposure may be characterized as a weak nonspecific irritant. In addition, WiFi can affect the brain of children in cases where it comes from laptops on their knees (Findlay and Dimbylow, 2010).

The most dangerous source of RF EMF is the mobile phone because the brain of the individual is directly exposed to the microwave radiation: the cerebral cortex, subcortical structures, receptor nerve structures of the vestibular, and auditory and visual analyzers. In 1996, Gandhi showed that the maximum value of the absorbed dose (SAR) in a child's brain is almost 2 times higher than that of an adult and there is a greater depth of penetration into the brain structures (Gandhi, 1996) (Figure 10.1).

This is because the child has a smaller head size, thinner skull, and brain tissue has a larger specific conductivity than that of adults (Ghandhi and Kang, 2002). Moreover, the child holds the phone more tightly to his ear, due to the lack of cartilage in the ear. The domestic measurements showed that during the use of mobile telephone (MT) in adults the heating of the external auditory canal occurs (Berezina, 2015).

During the postnatal development of human tissues, the number and size of cells increase, and the proportion of water content decreases. Such changes generally lead to significant changes in the dielectric properties of tissues. The results show that the maximum SAR levels in the brain tissues of small children (3 months) are 61% and 78% higher than in adults (Mohammed et al., 2017).

It is necessary to remember that children' organisms are in the process of constant development, and no one can predict the problem of remote consequences which may be the result of exposure to RF EMF at an early age.

In 2003, the WHO formulated a conclusion that children are more vulnerable to environmental factors than adults: "Children differ from adults. Children have unique vulnerabilities when they grow and develop; there are 'Windows of susceptibility': periods when their organs and system may acquire a special sensitivity to the effects of certain environmental threats." (WHO, Backgrounder N 3, 2003, 5p.).

This should be considered in the hazard assessment and the availability of a cumulative process in conditions of chronic and repeated impacts.

10.2.2 Radiobiological Evaluation of the Potential Health Effects of RF EMFs on Children

Even before the wide spread use of mobile communication, during the 1970s–1980s in the USSR, experimental studies to characterize the age-related sensitivity to EMFs were carried out. The results of these studies showed that the organisms of young animals are more sensitive to RF radiation (Chernova, 1982; Chernova and Kuzminskya, 1979; Kazarin and Shvaiko, 1983, 1988; Pol'ka, 1989).

Further studies by Russian scientists demonstrated that chronic RF EMF exposure comparable by intensity with the MT irradiation disturbed the creation of conditioned reflexes and consolidation of memory trace, and also revealed changes in neurons in many brain structures, including the cerebral cortex, hippocampus, and basal ganglia (Navakatikyan, 1988, 1992; Pryakhin et al., 2007).

Similar studies outside the USSR have registered in young rats the increase in the permeability of the blood-brain barrier (BBB) to the albumin and as a consequence, histochemical changes in the nerve cells of the brain (Salford et al., 2003a,b).

Recently published data suggests that the cells of the hippocampus of the adult brain maintain the ability to divide, that is, continuing neurogenesis, and this process serves as the neurobiological basis for the formation of new memory. It was also found that the hippocampus, which retains the ability for neurogenesis, plays a key role in the formation of long-term memory, in the integration of the obtained memory by brain information, and its distribution in the higher parts of the brain. As a result, the constantly dividing cells of the hippocampus may have a unique susceptibility to physical factors of the environment, including the radiation from mobile phones (Choi and Choi, 2016; Li et al., 2012; Narayanan et al., 2010; O'Connor et al., 2010), although not all researchers adhere to these conclusions (O'Connor et al., 2010).

The existence of the accumulation of changes/effects during repeated or long-term chronic exposure is one of the most important criteria for assessing the risk of exposure to RF EMF from mobile phones for the population when developing appropriate standards. This was facilitated by the results of a cycle of long-term epidemiological studies of Swedish scientists led by Hardell.

With increasing the time of active use of mobile phones by the population, there is very strong evidence, presented as publications and documents of a number of authoritative agencies and scientific forums, about the possibility of the development of brain tumors among users of MT (Hardell et al., 2004, 2009, 2013; Hardell and Carlberg, 2015; IARC, 2011; Lahkola et al., 2008; US NPCR, 2015). The authors concluded that for the users of cellular phones, the risk of brain tumor development increases with a "waiting period" of 10 years having a risk value of 1.3–1.8. An increased risk of developing astrocytomas and acoustic neuromas on the ipsilateral side of the brain was discovered. The risk of developing brain tumors increases up to 5 times in people who began using cell and portable phones at the age of 8–10 years, and the development of the tumor depends on the duration of cell phone usage.

In 2011, the International Agency for Research on Cancer (IARC) classified radio frequency electromagnetic fields in group 2B as a possible carcinogen based on an increased risk for glioma (IARC WHO. Classifying radio frequency electromagnetic fields as possibly carcinogenic to humans (Press release No. 208, 31 May 2011, 3 p.),

IARC specifically noted that this decision is of great importance for the population, especially for users of mobile phones among young people and children.

In 2015, the results of three national programs of the United States (National Program of Cancer Registries (NPCR), a program of the National Cancer Institute (NCI) and the program for epidemiological observations (SER)) for the assessment of brain cancer in the populations of different age groups for the period 2000–2010 were published (de Salles et al., 2006; Ghandhi and Kang, 2002; Gittleman et al., 2015; Ostrom et al., 2015). A significant increase in the incidence of primary malignant brain tumors and central nervous system (CNS) in American children (0–14 years) was found between 2000 and 2010, with an annual percent change (APC) of 0.6%. In adolescents (15–19 years), there was a significant increase in the incidence of primary malignant brain tumors.

Doubts in the possibility of the development of brain tumors among users of MT forced Swedish scientists to publish two papers in 2017, which reanalysed previously obtained results, with the consideration of many possible methodological errors (Carlberg and Hardell, 2017a,b). It evaluated the power of scientific data to determine whether there is a causal relationship between a risk factor and the associated development of gliomas of the brain and using a wireless phone (Hardell and Carlberg, 2015). The authors present convincing arguments in favor of the conclusion that glioma is caused by RF radiation. The authors strongly recommended a review of current regulatory guidelines for RF exposure in order to protect the population from the effects of low frequency radiation.

Also in 2016, a preliminary report on the results of a two year large-scale experiment on rats conducted under the National Toxicology Program of the United States (NTP) was published (Microwave News, May 2016; http://bit.ly/WSJsaferemr) and performed by the National Institute of Environmental Health United States (US NIEHS). This program was funded by the US Government with the costs amounting to 25 million dollars.

Male rats were exposed to RF EMFs of cell phones every 10 minutes with a subsequent 10-minute break for 18 hours, resulting in nine hours a day for two years. Two standards from GSM and CDMA with a frequency of 900 MHz were used.

For each type of standard cell phone, there were four groups: three experimental groups of 180 rats and the control group for sham exposure (90 rats). The lowest intensity of exposure amounted to SAR 1.5 W/kg, and the remaining two experimental groups were exposed to SAR 3 and 6 W/kg, which excluded the heating of tissue, that is, the "thermal effect."

The study showed a significant increase in cancer rates among rats that were subjected to the electromagnetic influence of GSM or CDMA signals for two years. In the control group, the development of tumors was not found.

These results clearly demonstrate that nonthermal levels of RF EMFs can cause development of tumors in the brain. It should be noted that epidemiological observations are used not only to predict the occurrence of brain tumors when children use MT, but also to investigate the possible development of other somatic disorders. The authors state that there is a correlation between the registered violations and the mode of use of MT. However, these publications raise a lot of questions because their results are not based on the experience of the authors themselves, and the methodology of individual observations was not used (Anttila et al., 2006; Carter et al., 2016; Chernenkov and

Gumenyuk, 2009; George et al., 2015; Huss et al., 2015; Hysing et al., 2015; Inyang et al., 2010a,b; Kheifets and Repacholi, 2005; Sillanpaa and Anttila, 1996; Sudan et al., 2012, 2013; Tomas, 2010; Van den Bulck, 2007; Zheng et al., 2015).

In addition, the research of the influence of the EMF RF mobile phones on the psychophysiological parameters of children and adolescents and the results obtained are highly ambiguous (Calvente et al., 2016; Curcio et al., 2008; Schoeni et al., 2015a,b; Thomas et al., 2010).

We have data from our own experience of the long-term monitoring of children as users of MT, where we were in constant personal contact with children, their parents, and teachers. The results of these studies are presented below.

10.3 PSYCHOPHYSIOLOGICAL INDICATORS AS MARKERS OF THE IMPACT OF EMF RF MOBILE PHONES TO THE CENTRAL NERVOUS SYSTEM OF CHILDREN AND ADOLESCENTS

In our studies, we used psychophysiological indicators, because in this situation, the "critical organ" is the child's brain. Previously, on a large amount of statistical material (more than 3500 children and adolescents), it was shown that psychophysiological indicators, along with other medical indicators, are very sensitive markers in other exposures to a number of unfavorable environmental factors (Khorseva, 2004). The study was conducted in the Lyceum 10 and 17, in the city of Khimki, Moskow region. It is important to note that in addition to the main group of children who used MT (1161), a control group of children and adolescents not using MT (370 people) was formed. ***The presence of a control group is an undeniable advantage of our studies.***

10.3.1 The Main Results of Our Ten-Year Study

The psychophysiological parameters were recorded both with the use of the automated workplace of the psychophysiologist and with the help of a computer program developed by us, LUM (Local Universal Monitoring).

10.3.1.1 Hearing Analyzer

For studying the effect of mobile phone electromagnetic radiation on the auditory system, we used the parameters of a simple audiomotor reaction, since it was established that the determination of the time of simple sensorimotor reactions quite clearly reflects the functional relationships in the cerebral cortex. In our studies, we applied a complex of characteristics of a simple audiomotor reaction. It included recording the change in reaction time and the degree of its instability (variability, in the stereo- and mono-presentation of the audio signal), as well as the level of violations of phonemic perception. The latter parameter was developed by Khorseva. The index is obtained empirically and reflects the wrong perception of similar sounding or similar in articulation speech sounds, manifested in the pass/substitution of letters, the permutation of the syllables, the wrong reading or uttering words, etc. (Khorseva and Zakharova, 2011a,b).

We described for the first time the effects of changing the phonemic perception, the laterality of their changes, the number of missed signals, and the time change of a simple audiomotor reaction in MT child users. The effect of increasing the time of a simple audiomotor reaction in comparison with the age dynamics in both stereo and mono-presentation of the sound signal was manifested only when it achieved a certain total time of use of the child of MT. In our study, this total time is 360 minutes, provided that the child started using a mobile phone at the age of 7. For children older than 9 years, the effect of slowing the age-related dynamics of the audiomotor reaction is observed at a higher total exposure to 750 min (Grigoriev and Khorseva, 2014).

It is shown that for all children, MT users increased the number of violations of phonemic perception. In 79.3% of cases, we registered a contralateral effect, that is, an increase in the number of disorders recorded on the side opposite the impact of EMF RF of the mobile phone.

Next, we traced the age characteristics of this effect. It has been established that with age, the frequency of manifestations of the contralateral effect of changes in the number of violations of phonemic perception as a whole for each age group decreases.

Our results are in good agreement with the work of the otolaryngologists Panda et al. (2007, 2010, 2011), who for several years, conducted a study of the auditory analyzer for mobile phone users. It has been shown that if the MT is used more than one hour a day for more than four years, dysfunction of the auditory analyzer occurs: a decrease in the perception of high-frequency sounds (s, f, h, t, z), which may indicate a violation of the phonemic perception.

10.3.1.2 The Visual Analyzer

Investigations of the effect of electromagnetic radiation from the MT on the visual analyzer were carried out using such indicators as visual acuity in near vision, speed of visual discrimination, and the time of a simple visual-motor reaction (SVMR).

It was found that such indicators as visual acuity and speed of visual discrimination in children users of MT were not different from the control group, that is, apparently these indicators were not sensitive to the radiation of MT.

Further, an analysis was made of the effect of the slowing down of the dynamics of a simple visual-motor reaction with both binocular and monocular presentation of a light signal. In contrast to the parameters of a simple auditory motor reaction (PSRM), for which the effect of slowing dynamics was detected with a total usage time of the mobile phone by the child, 360 min, the total time of use for a simple visual-motor reaction (PZMR) was 730 min. Such effects were found in children aged 7 years.

One more effect, which we observed for both the SSRM and the PZMR, should be especially noted. With short duration of use of MT (up to six months) and intense daily use up to 2 min/day, we noted a decrease in the response time of both auditory and motor-motor reactions, which may be related to the child's central nervous system stress response to a new type of external effect, radiation from an MT. A further increase in the duration of use and the daily load leads to the effects described above. These effects were observed for all age groups.

10.3.1.3 Fatigue and Working Capacity

In our studies, we recorded fatigue indicators (through the index of muscular tension, determined with the help of tremorometry) and working capacity (through

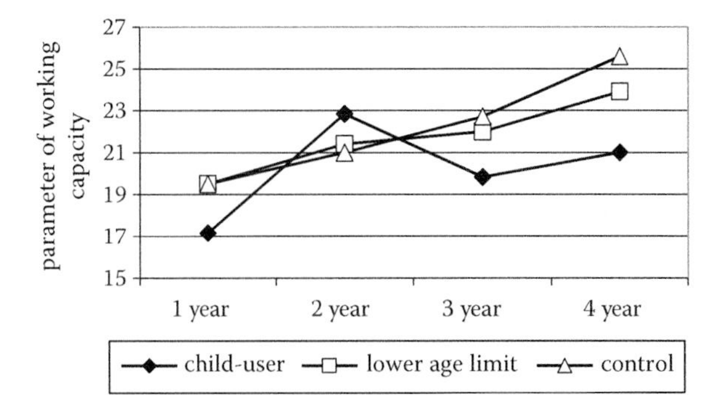

FIGURE 10.2 Comparison of dynamics of individual parameters of working capacity children from the test and control groups (daily time of use: 1 year—2 min; 2 year—5 min; 3 year—15 min; 4 year—10 min).

the parameters of the tapping test), which are objective not subjective methods. In the course of longitudinal studies, it was found that, in comparison with the control group, an increase in fatigue was registered for children in 39.7% of cases, and in 30.3% of cases this increase was significant. Parameters of working capacity for children decreased in 50.7% of cases.

It can be seen that for schoolboy from the test group at the fourth year of observations, an indicator of working capacity has decreased the lower of limit of the age norm, while schoolboy for the control group, parameters of the working capacity are within normal limits (Figure 10.2).

In further studies, we were using the parameters of a ten fingers chaotic tapping test using the computer program LUM (Local Universal Monitoring). This program provides for the registration of more than 20 parameters, including the total number of clicks, and characterizes the level of development of fine motor skills of the hand and working capacity (patent of the Russian Federation No. 2314743). It should be especially emphasized that the data of children and teenage mobile users were processed on the basis of the normative indicators of children and adolescents of the control groups.

In general, only in 8.5% from all data (1364 measurements) is at the level of formation of fine motor skills and working capacity within the limits of the age norm for children and adolescents 7–11 years of age (we examined children and adolescents 7 years old—311 people, 8–348 people, 9–339 people, 10–311 people). This situation already affects the performance of written work, the handwriting of children and adolescents.

Given that the level of motor skills and the formation of cognitive processes are directly dependent, one can expect changes in attention and memory in children and adolescents. In this regard, a special place is occupied by studies of the possible impact on cognitive functions of the RF EMF from mobile phones.

10.3.1.4 Cognitive Functions. Arbitrary Attention and Semantic Memory

Our studies, providing dynamic observations of changes in attention and memory rates, revealed the stress response of a new environmental factor (MT radiation). With a short duration of MT use (up to six months), and daily intensity up to 2 min/day, we recorded an improvement in the parameters of cognitive processes (increasing productivity and accuracy, reducing the time of the task). We recall that similar effects were also revealed for simple audio and visual motor responses.

Nevertheless, with the increase in the duration and total time of MT use by children, it was noted that not only the stability parameters of arbitrary attention decreased (productivity indicators worsened by 14.3% and accuracy indicators by 19.4%), but semantic memory also decreased (decreased the accuracy factor by 19.4%, increased in time by 30.1%). Below is an example of changing individual indicators of arbitrary attention and semantic memory in a schoolchild for 6 years (Figure 10.3).

As can be seen from the presented data, changes in the mode of using MT leads to changes in the indices of cognitive processes. Decreasing the daily use of MT in the second year of observation leads to an increase in the productivity index (Figure 10.3a); greater accuracy and a significant reduction in the execution time of the task (Figure 10.3b).

A small time of use in the period of 2–5 years of observation leads to the following effects. The productivity index is significantly increased (Figure 10.3a), which corresponds to the age dynamics for the control group pupils; the accuracy rate is very high. The parameters of accuracy and time of the task execution fluctuate depending on the change in the daily load regime (Figure 10.3b). During this period of time, the task was carried out quickly with high accuracy. However, for the 6th year of observation, with a sharp increase in the daily use time of up to 25 min/day, all parameters of arbitrary attention deteriorated: decreased accuracy and productivity, and time of task execution increased.

In addition, the analysis of the indices of arbitrary attention and semantic memory obtained by testing students using our programs LUM allowed us to more thoroughly

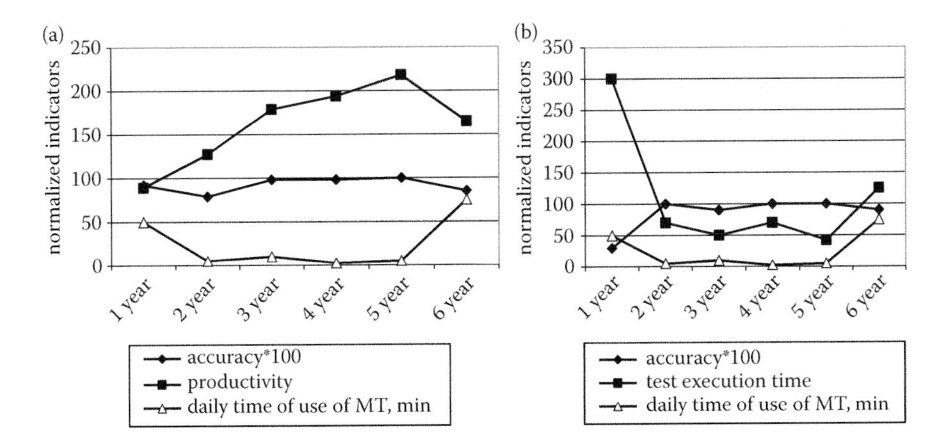

FIGURE 10.3 Example of changing individual performance of arbitary attention (a) and semantic memory (b) (performance and accuracy) during longitudinal observations. The indicators are normalized. Daily load of using MT: 1 year—10 min; 2 year—1 min; 3 year—2 min; 4 year—0.5 min; 5 year—2 min; 6 year—25 min.

assess the change in performance, in particular, semantic memory in groups of 7 years (2012–2014, time observations). It should be noted that, in contrast to the group of first-graders who were under observation in the period 2007–2012, the use of MT in groups of children during the monitoring in 2012–2014 had significantly increased the time use every day and in duration of the use (about 55% of the students started to used MT with 5–6 years).

This immediately influenced the parameters, particularly on the semantic memory: with a duration of MT use for one year with a daily load of no more than 2 minutes/day, a slight change in accuracy was observed, but the task execution time increased by 1.3 compared to the control. However, in the group of users whose daily load exceeded 20 minutes, other patterns were revealed. If the duration of MT use was 0.5 years, the registered accuracy index decreased by 30%, and the time of the task fulfillment increased by 1.4 times. With one year use, there was an increase in the time of the task of 1.69 times and a decrease in the accuracy parameter of 20%. Similar changes were found for school children and other age groups.

10.3.1.4.1 The Statistical Analysis of the Data

The statistical analysis of the data was carried out at the BIOSTASTIKA Center under the leadership of Leonov V.P. The array of data of indicators of voluntary attention and semantic memory on the whole array of data since 2006, which contained 2086 observations, including 25 signs, was analyzed.

Tables 10.1 and 10.2 show the level of formation of arbitrary attention and the semantic memory of children and teenage users of MT at the ages of 5–16.5 years.

From these results, it can be seen that only 41% of measurements can be attributed to a high level of formation of indicators of arbitrary attention (both indicators at the level of high values), while 29.62% of measurements are a combination of medium and high values, 8.3% are at the level of average values, and 21% are a disharmonious combination of indicators (high to average accuracy and lower limit/low/very low productivity and vice versa).

TABLE 10.1
Analysis of the Level of Development of Voluntary Attention in Children of Mobile Users Across the Dataset (2084 Observations)

	Productivity Indicators				
Accuracy's Indicators	Tall	Average	The Lower Limit of Normal	Low	Very Low
Tall	41,03	17,1	4,32	3,41	0,77
Average	12,52	8,3	1,73	1,39	0,58
The lower limit of normal	1,78	1,78	0,67	0,48	0,1
Low	1,01	1,01	0,48	0,58	0,24
Very low	0,1	0,1	0,05	0,4	0,38

Data in %.

TABLE 10.2
Analysis of the Level of the Formation of the Semantic Memory in Children Users by Mobile Communication Throughout the Entire Dataset (2083 Measurements)

	Time Indicators for the Test				
Accuracy's Indicators	**Tall**	**Average**	**The Lower Limit of Normal**	**Low**	**Very Low**
Tall	33,6	11,95	1,92	3,22	1,2
Average	9,22	8,98	1,58	3,89	2,06
The lower limit of normal	4,27	2,88	0,82	2,5	0,96
Low	2,45	2,4	0,96	0,82	1,2
Very low	0,53	0,53	0	0,29	0,77

Data in %.

It is established that only 33.6% of the measurements can be attributed to a high level of the formation of semantic memory indicators (both indicators at the level of high values), 21.17% of measurements are a combination of medium and high values, 8.98% are at the level of average values, and 36.25% are a disharmonious combination of indicators (high/average accuracy and low limit /low/very low time parameters task execution and vice versa).

However, it should be noted that when comparing the level of development of arbitrary attention and semantic memory, there is some imbalance: high levels of development of arbitrary attention were revealed in 41.03% of children and adolescents against 33.6% for increased semantic (semantic memory); the disharmonious level for indices of arbitrary attention is set for 21%, and for semantic memory it is 36.25%. It is possible that this may reflect the fact that the parameters of semantic memory for children users of mobile communication indicators were reduced to a greater extent than the voluntary attention.

Statistical analysis of data using conjugacy tables showed the following: although the strength of the connection of these qualitative characteristics for both parameters of voluntary attention and semantic memory is not very strong, it is statistically significant ($p < 0.0001$).

So, the longitudinal changes in the psychophysiological indicators of children who use mobile phones convincingly show that chronic exposure to electromagnetic radiation from a mobile phone may negatively affect the central nervous system of the child:

1. The reaction time to sound and light stimuli is increased;
2. There is an increase in the number of violations of phonemic perception and the number of missed signals when a sound stimulus is presented;
3. Indicators of arbitrary attention and semantic memory deteriorate;
4. There are increased parameters of fatigue and decreased parameters of working capacity

It should be especially noted that in most cases in children who are active users of mobile communication, changes in psychophysiological indicators either were within the lower limit of the norm or already go beyond it.

We believe that the changes listed above may and in some cases already do affect the success of the training. However, observance of the elementary rules of a safe mode of using MT can significantly reduce the level of negative effects of electromagnetic radiation from mobile phones. And we already have confirmation of this statement.

Over the past three years, a complex of preventive measures was implemented on the basis of the Lyceum 17 with the participation of all participants of the educational process aimed at reducing the negative impact of the RF EMF of the MT (schoolchildren, parents, teachers, and the Lyceum administration). A series of lectures was organized for parents, teachers, and the administration of the educational institution. During this period, using the program Universal Local Monitoring, the levels of cognitive processes (arbitrary attention and semantic memory), parameters of working capacity, and the level of development of fine motor skills were studied. An individual survey of children on the use of MT was conducted.

It was found that the safe mode of use (headphones, speakerphone, use of SMS, MMS) statistically significantly improve ALL psychophysiological indicators.

We believe that the results of our longitudinal observations clearly show that the RF EMF from mobile phones affects psychophysiological indicators of children and adolescents. Based on our results, it can be confidently affirmed that children are located in the group at risk. It should be recognized and the efforts of the scientific community to reduce the risk of adverse effects on the organisms of children should be made. One of the possible ways of reducing the impact of electromagnetic fields on children is an understanding of the dangers by the parents and children, the use of mobile communication, and a voluntary choice of the form of communication, that is, the introduction of the concept of "voluntary risk."

REFERENCES

Anttila P, Metsahonkala L, Sillanpaa M. 2006. Long-term trends in the incidence of headache in Finnish schoolchildren. *Pediatrics*. 117: 1197–201.

Berezina A A. 2015. Assessment of the impact of mobile communication, the change of temperature in the external ear. *Proceedings of the III International Scientific and Technical Internet-Conference "Information Systems and Technologies 2015" FGBOU VPO "State University-Educational Scientific-Industrial Complex"*. Limited Liability Company "Siberian crane" (Orel, April 01–May 31), 8–19 (in Russian).

Calvente I, Pérez-Lobato R, Núñez M I et al. 2016. Does exposure to environmental radiofrequency electromagnetic fields cause cognitive and behavioral effects in 10-year-old boys? *Bioelectromagnetics*. Jan.; 37(1): 25–36. doi: 10.1002/bem.21951

Carlberg M, Hardell L. 2017a. Evaluation of mobile phone and cordless phone use and Glioma risk using the Bradford Hill viewpoints from 1965 on association or causation. *Biomed Res Int*. 2017:9218486. Epub 2017 Mart 16. https://www.ncbi.nlm.nih.gov/pmc/articles/PMC5376454/

Carlberg M, Hardell L. 2017b. New review paper finds that cell phone and cordless phone use causes brain cancer. *Electromagnetic Radiation Safety*, April 13, 2017. http://www.saferemr.com/2017/04/cell-phone-and-cordless-phone-use.html

Carter B, Rees P, Hale L et al. 2016. Association between portable screen-based media device access or use and sleep outcomes: A systematic review and meta-analysis. *JAMA Pediatr.* Dec 1; 170(12): 1202–8, access mode https://www.ncbi.nlm.nih.gov/pmc/articles/PMC5380441

Chernenkov Y V, Gumenyuk O. 2009. Hygienic aspects of studying the effects of mobile phones and personal computers on schoolchildren's health. *Hygiene and Sanitation.* May-Jun; (3): 84–6 (in Russian).

Chernova S A. 1982. Some endocrine and biological aspects of the effects of electromagnetic fields of UHF range on young and senescent rats. *Proc. Dokl. All-Union Symposium. Biological Effects of Electromagnetic Fields.* Pushchino, 30–1 (in Russian).

Chernova S A, Kuzminskya G N. 1979. *Some Indicators Pituitary-Gonadal and Pituitary-Adrenal System Under the Action of Microwave Electromagnetic Field of Low Intensity in KN.: Questions of Hygiene of Labour in the Electronic Industry.* M: Medicine 77–82 (in Russian).

Choi Y-J, Choi Y-S. 2016. Effects of electromagnetic radiation from smartphones on learning ability and hippocampal progenitor cell proliferation in mice. *Osong Public Health Res Perspect.* 7(1): 12–7, access mode https://www.ncbi.nlm.nih.gov/pmc/articles/PMC4776265/

Curcio G, Valentini E, Moroni F et al. 2008. Psychomotor performance is not influenced by brief repeated exposures to mobile phones. *Bioelectromagnetics.* 29(3): 237–41.

de Salles A A, Bulla G, Rodriguez C E. 2006. Electromagnetic absorption in the head of adults and children due to mobile phone operation close to the head. *Electromagn Biol Med.* 25(4): 349–60.

ECERI. Newsletter. No. 6, June 2017, access mode http://www.saferemr.com/2017/06/

Findlay R, Dimbylow P. 2010. SAR in a child vowel phantom from exposure to wireless computer networks (Wi-Fi). *Phys Med Biol.* 55: 405–11.

Gandhi O P. 1996. d'Arsonval medal: address. some bioelectromagnetics research at the University of Utah: Acceptance speech on the occasion of receiving the d'Arsonval Medal. *Bioelectromagnetics.* 17(1): 3–9.

Gandhi O P, Lazzi G, Furse C. 1996. Electromagnetic absorption in the human head and neck for mobile telephones at 835 and 1900MHz. *IEEE Trans Microw Theory Tech.* 44(10): 1884–97.

Ghandhi O P, Kang G. 2002. Some present problems and a proposed experimental phantom for SAR compliant testing of cellular telephones at 835 and 1900MHz. *Phys Med Biol.* 47(5): 1501–18.

George M J, Odgers C L. 2015. Seven fears and the science of how mobile technologies may be influencing adolescents in the digital age. *Perspect Psychol Sci.* Nov; 10(6): 832–51, access mode https://www.ncbi.nlm.nih.gov/pmc/articles/PMC4654691/

Gittleman H, Ostrom Q T, Rouse C D et al. 2015. Trends in central nervous system tumor incidence relative to other common cancers in adults, adolescents, and children in the United States, 2000 to 2010. *Cancer.* 121(1): 102–12.

Grigoriev Y G, Grigoriev O A. 2013. Cellular communication and health. The electromagnetic environment. Radiobiology and hygiene problems. Forecast of danger. M.: Economy, 567 (in Russian).

Grigoriev Y G, Khorseva N I. 2014. Mobile communications and health of children. Risk assessment of the use of mobile communication by children and adolescents. Recommendations to children and parents M.: Economics, 230p (in Russian).

Hardell L, Carlberg M, Hansson Mild K. 2009. Epidemiological evidence for an association between use of wireless phones and tumor diseases. *Pathophysiology.* 16: 113–22.

Hardell L, Carlberg M, Söderqvist F, Mild H. 2013. Pooled analysis of case-control studies on acoustic neuroma diagnosed 1997-2003 and 2007-2009 and use of mobile and cordless phones. *Int J Oncol.* 43:1036–44.

Hardell L, Carlberg M. 2015. Mobile phone and cordless phone use and the risk for glioma—Analysis of pooled case-control studies in Sweden, 1997–2003 and 2007–2009. *Pathophysiology*. Mar; 22(1): 1–13, doi: 10.1016/j.pathophys.2014.10.001. Epub 2014 Oct 29.

Hardell L, Vild H, Carlberg M et al. 2004. Cellular and cordless telephones and the association with brain tumours in different age group. *Arch Environ Health*. 59: 132–7.

Huss A, van Eijsden M, Guxens M, Beekhuizen J et al. 2015. Environmental radiofrequency electromagnetic fields exposure at home, mobile and cordless phone use, and sleep problems in 7-year-old children. *PLoS One*. Oct 28; 10(10): e0139869, access mode https://www.ncbi.nlm.nih.gov/pmc/articles/PMC4625083/

Hysing M, Pallesen S, Stormark KM et al. 2015. Sleep and use of electronic devices in adolescence: Results from a large population-based study. *BMJ Open*. Feb 2; 5(1): e006748, access mode https://www.ncbi.nlm.nih.gov/pmc/articles/PMC4316480/

IARC WHO. 2011. *Classifies Radiofrequency Electromagnetic Fields as Possibly Carcinogenic to Humans*. Press release No 208, 31 May 2011, 3 p.

Inyang I, Benke G, Dimitriadis C et al. 2010a. Predictors of mobile telephone use and exposure analysis in Australian adolescents. *J Pediatr Child Health*. 46(5): 226–33.

Inyang I, Benke G, McKenzie R et al. 2010b. A new method to determine laterality of mobile telephone use in adolescents. *Occup Environ Med*. 67(8): 507–12.

Kabali H K, Irigoyen M M, Nunez-Davis R et al. 2015. Exposure and Use of Mobile Media Devices by Young Children. *Pediatrics*. 136(6): P1044–50, doi: 10.1542/peds.2015-2151

Kazarin I P, Shvaiko I I. 1983. Age-related sensitivity of the animal to electromagnetic fields of ultrahigh frequency. *Hygiene and Sanitation*. 3: 86–9.

Kazarin I P, Shvaiko I I. 1988. Comparative characteristics of the biological action of electromagnetic fields of superhigh and frequency. *Hygiene and Sanitation*. 7: 11–3 (in Russian).

Kheifets L, Repacholi M. 2005. Sensitivity of children to electromagnetic fields. *Pediatrics*. 4: 303–13.

Khorseva N I. 2004. Ecological significance of natural electromagnetic fields in the period of intrauterine development of humans. *Diss PhD- M*, 144p (in Russian).

Khorseva N I, Zakharova I E. 2011a. Psychophysiological indicators as the criterion for evaluating the effectiveness of correctional work of the logopedist. Educational Horizons. *Scientific-Methodical Journal*. 3(33): 87–91 (in Russian).

Khorseva N I, Zakharova I E. 2011b. Psychophysiological indicators as the criterion for evaluating the effectiveness of correctional work of the logopedist Part 2. Monitoring psycho-physiological parameters and efficiency of correctional work of the logopedist. Educational Horizons. *Scientific-Methodical Journal*. 1(33): 60–8 (in Russian).

Khurana V, Teo C, Kundi M et al. 2009. Cell phones and brain tumors: a review including epidemiologic data. *Surg Neurol*. 72(3): 205–15.

Lahkola A, Salminen T, Raitanen O et al. 2008. Meningioma and mobile phone base—A collaborative case-contril stude in five North European countries. *Int J Epidemiol*. 37: 1304–13 (in Russian).

Li Y, Shi C, Lu G et al. 2012. Effects of electromagnetic radiation on spatial memory and synapses in rat hippocampal CA1. *Neural Regen Res*. Jun 5; 7(16): 1248–55, access mode https://www.ncbi.nlm.nih.gov/pmc/articles/PMC4336960/

Lukyanova S N. 2015. *Electromagnetic Field of Super High Frequency Range of Non- Thermal Intensity as a Stimulus to the Central Nervous System*. Moscow, 200 p (in Russian).

Maganioti A, Papageorgiou C, Hountala C et al. 2010. Wi-Fi electromagnetic fields exert gender related alterations on EEG. *VIth International Workshop on Biological Effects of Electromagnetic Fields*. access mode http://www.istanbul.edu.tr/6internatwshopbioeffemf/cd/pdf/poster/WI-FI%20ELECTROMAGNETIC%20FIELDS%20EXERT%20GENDER.pdf

Microwave News, May 2016, access mode http://bit.ly/WSJsaferemr

Mohammed B, Jin J, Abbosh A et al. 2017. Evaluation of children exposure to electromagnetic fields of mobile phones using age-specific head models with age-dependent dielectric properties. *IEEE Access*. 99(5): 27345–27353. http://ieeexplore.ieee.org/stamp/stamp.jsp?reload=true&arnumber=8086149.

Narayanan S N, Kumar R S, Potu B K et al. 2010. Effect of radio-frequency electromagnetic radiations (RF-EMR) on passive avoidance behaviour and hippocampal morphology in Wistar rats. *Ups J Med Sci*. May; 115(2): 91–6, access mode https://www.ncbi.nlm.nih.gov/pmc/articles/PMC2853785/

Navakatikyan M A. 1988. Changes in the activity of conditioned reflex dejatelnostnyj rats during chronic microwave irradiation and after it. *Radiobiology*. 28(1): 121–5 (in Russian).

Navakatikyan M A. 1992. Methodology of the study of defensive conditioned reflexes of active avoidance. *J High Nerv Act*. 42(4): 812–8 (in Russian).

O'Connor R P, Madison S D et al. 2010. Exposure to GSM RF fields does not affect calcium homeostasis in human endothelial cells, rat pheocromocytoma cells or rat hippocampal neurons. *PLoS One*. 5(7): e11828, access mode https://www.ncbi.nlm.nih.gov/pmc/articles/PMC2910734/

Ostrom Q, Gittleman H, Fulop J et al. 2015. CBTRUS statistical report: Primary brain and central nervous system tumors diagnosed in the United States in 2008-2012. *Neuro Oncol*. (Suppl 4): 62p.

Panda N K, Jain R, Bakshi J. 2007. Audiological disturbances in long-term mobile phone users. *J Otolaryngol Head Neck Surg*. 137(2)(Suppl.): 131–2.

Panda N K, Jain R, Bakshi J, Munjal S. 2010. Audiologic disturbances in long-term mobile phone users. *J Otolaryngol Head Neck Surg*. 39(1): 5–11.

Panda N K, Modi R, Munjal S, Virk R S. 2011. Auditory changes in mobile users: is evidence forthcoming? *J Otolaryngol Head Neck Surg*. 144(4): 581–5.

Papageorgiou C, Hountala C, Maganioti A et al. 2011. Effects of Wi-Fi signals on the p300 component of event-related potentials during an auditory haling task. *J Integr Neurosci*. 10(2): 189–202.

Pol'ka N S. 1989. The functional state of the developing organism, as a criterion of hygienic regulation of electromagnetic field 2750 MHz. *Hygiene and Sanitation*. 10: 36–9 (in Russian).

Pryakhin E A, Tryapitsyna G A, Andreev S S et al. 2007. Evaluation of the effect of modulated electromagnetic radiation of radio frequency on cognitive function in rats of different ages. Radiation biology. *Radioecology*. 47(3): 339–44 (in Russian).

Reykjavik. 2017. *Appeal on Wireless Technology in Schools*. 3p.

Salford L, Brun A, Eberhardt J et al. 2003a. Microwaves emitted by mobile phones damage neurons in the rat brain. *Proceedings 3rd International EMF Seminar in China EMF and Biological Effects*. Guilin (China). Oct. 2003; 33–4.

Salford L, Brun A, Eberhart J et al. 2003b. Nerve cell damage in mammalian brain after exposure to microwaves from GSM mobile phones. *Environ Health Perspect*. 111(7): 881–3.

Schoeni A, Roser K, Röösli M. 2015a. Memory performance, wireless communication and exposure to radiofrequency electromagnetic fields: A prospective cohort study in adolescents. *Environ Int*. Oct 13; 85: 343–51, doi: 10.1016/j.envint.2015.09.025.

Schoeni A, Roser K, Röösli M. 2015b. Symptoms and Cognitive Functions in Adolescents in Relation to Mobile Phone Use during Night. *PLoS One*. Jul 29; 10(7): e0133528, doi: 10.1371/journal.pone.0133528. eCollection 2015 access mode https://www.ncbi.nlm.nih.gov/pmc/articles/PMC4519186/

Sillanpaa M, Anttila P. 1996. Increasing prevalence of headache in 7-year-old schoolchildren. *Headache*. 36: 466–70.

Sudan M, Kheifets L, Arah O A et al. 2012. Prenatal and postnatal cell phone exposures and headaches in children. *Open Pediatr Med J.* 6: 46–52.

Sudan M, Kheifets L, Arah O A, Olsen J. 2013. Cell phone exposures and hearing loss in children in the Danish National Birth Cohort. *Paediatr Perinat Epidemiol.* 27(3): 247–57.

Thomas S, Heinrich S, von Kries R, Radon K. 2010. Exposure to radio-frequency electromagnetic fields and behavioural problems in Bavarian children and adolescents. *Eur J Epidemiol.* 25(2): 135–41.

US NPCR—United States National program of Cancer Registries (NPCR). 2015. access mode http://www.liquisearch.com/cancer_registry/national_program_of_cancer_registries_npcr

Van den Bulck J. 2007. Adolescent use of mobile phones for calling and for sending text messages after lights out: results from a prospective cohort study with a one-year follow-up. *Sleep.* 30(9): 1220–3.

WHO. 2003. Backgrounder N 3. 5p.

Zheng F, Gao P, He M et al. 2015. Association between mobile phone use and self-reported well-being in children: A questionnaire-based cross-sectional study in Chongqing, China. *BMJ Open.* May 11; 5(5): e007302, access mode https://www.ncbi.nlm.nih.gov/pmc/articles/PMC4431134/

Index

D

E

I

L

M

P

Q

R